FORREST GENERAL MEDICAL CENTER

ADVANCED MEDICAL TRANSCRIPTION COURSE

third edition

Donna L. Conerly-Stewart, Ed.D.
Professor Emeritus
Business Technology Education
The University of Southern Mississippi
Hattiesburg, MS

Wanda L. Lott, A.R.T.
Retired Director
Medical Records Department
Forrest County General Hospital
Hattiesburg, MS

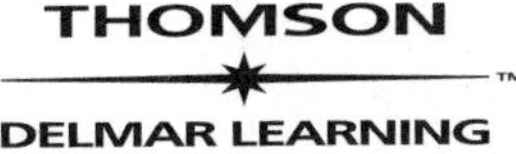

Australia Canada Mexico Singapore Spain United Kingdom United States

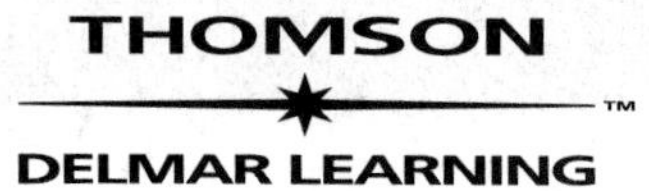

Forrest General Medical Center
Advanced Medical Transcription Course
THIRD EDITION
by
Donna L. Conerly-Stewart and Wanda L. Lott

Executive Director, Health Care Business Unit:
William Brottmiller

Editorial Director:
Cathy L. Esperti

Acquisitions Editor:
Maureen Rosener

Developmental Editor:
Maria D'Angelico

Marketing Director:
Jennifer McAvey

Editorial Assistant:
Matthew Thouin

Project Editor:
Shelley Esposito

Production Coordinator:
Jessica Peterson

Art/Design Coordinator:
Robert Plante

Printed in the United States of America
3 4 5 XXX 07 06 05 04

For more information, contact Delmar Learning, 5 Maxwell Drive, Clifton Park, NY 12065
Or find us on the World Wide Web at http://www.delmarlearning.com

Library of Congress Cataloging-in-Publication Data

Conerly-Stewart, Donna L., 1943–
Forrest General Medical Center advanced medical transcription course / Donna L. Conerly-Stewart, Wanda L. Lott.—3rd ed.
p. ; cm.
title: Advanced medical transcription course.
Includes bibliographical references and index.
ISBN 1-4018-3348-9
1. Medical transcription—Handbooks, manuals, etc. 2. Medicine—Terminology—Handbooks, manuals, etc.
[DNLM: 1. Medical Records. 2. Medical Secretaries. 3. Terminology. WX 173 C747f 2004] I. Title: Advanced medical transcription course. II. Lott, Wanda L. III. Title.
R728.S745 2004
651.7'4—dc21

2003011012

Notice to the Reader

Publisher does not warrant or guarantee any of the products described herein or perform any independent analysis in connection with any of the product information contained herein. Publisher does not assume, and expressly disclaims, any obligation to obtain and include information other than that provided to it by the manufacturer.

The reader is expressly warned to consider and adopt all safety precautions that might be indicated by the activities described herein and to avoid all potential hazards. By following the instructions contained herein, the reader willingly assumes all risks in connection with such instructions.

The publisher makes no representations or warranties of any kind, including but not limited to, the warranties of fitness for particular purpose or merchantability, nor are any such representations implied with respect to the material set forth herein, and the publisher takes no responsibility with respect to such material. The publisher shall not be liable for any special, consequential, or exemplary damages resulting, in whole or part, from the reader's use of, or reliance upon, this material.

TABLE OF CONTENTS

PREFACE TO THE THIRD EDITION

Forrest General Medical Center, third edition, has been completely revised and updated. This comprehensive text is designed primarily for advanced medical transcription students. One should possess a good foundation in medical terminology and transcription before beginning study of these materials.

The text may be used in a traditional classroom setting or as a self-paced resource for practitioners who wish to upgrade their medical transcription and terminology skills. Written for persons in allied health or court-reporting fields, a medical office, or a business office, this educational package presents learning activities that will develop and/or refine transcription skills to a competitive level.

Organization and Design

This third edition contains 20 chapters organized into an introductory chapter, 18 medical specialty chapters, and one chapter of critical thinking/decision-making activities. Chapter 1 presents a thorough review of transcription rules; selected confusing medical terms; AAMT formatting guidelines; discussion of the "big four" reports—history & physical, consultation, operative report, and discharge summary; sample model reports; and pertinent information on professionalism.

Information presented in Chapters 2–19 includes an introduction to a specialty, a list of related abbreviations typically used in dictation, and anatomical illustrations (in most chapters) that will help the student more readily assimilate the anatomical parts associated with the particular specialty. Presented next are terminology words with phonetic pronunciations (some of which occur in the dictation) and transcription tips to aid in transcription of the realistic dictation material provided on accompanying audio for each chapter. New to the "Transcription Tips" section of each chapter is a list of helpful Web sites one can go to for additional help.

Chapter 20 includes challenging exercises arranged in three sections. In Section I the student will hear dictation of a white paper (journal article), continuation notes, letters, and an emergency room record. Section II presents 20 realistic on-the-job dilemmas, and Section III contains documents to be edited.

New and Updated Features

Using this third edition, students have the opportunity to transcribe 62 new dictation exercises, among which are a heart/lung transplant, Gamma knife stereotactic radiosurgery, cochlear implant, bone marrow harvest, stem cell transplant, abdominoplasty, and ankle replacement. The dictation is offered on CDs, audio cassettes, and as a download from the online companion web site to suit the needs of the individual.

The pronunciations that appear with the terminology lists are repeated on the CDs and tapes. The printed versions will be a useful quick reference, as they use the familiar "long vowel" marks (e.g., ā, ē, ī, ō) and primary and secondary accent marks (e.g., ', ") to guide the reader in understanding generally accepted pronunciations.

Another new feature is the addition of helpful Web sites in each specialty chapter. With these resources, one can find more specific information on particular disease processes, new equipment, and new drugs related to the specialty.

Some new continuation notes have been added in Section I of Chapter 20. Also, new critical thinking exercises appear in the specialty chapters.

Other Key Features

The basic features of *Forrest General Medical Center* have remained the same. They are:

- Realistic dictation in 18 specialties by professionals from various ethnic groups
- Comprehensive terminology lists in each chapter
- Realistic anatomical visuals
- Comprehensive appendices, including types of incisions, sutures, suture materials, dressings, instruments, anesthesia, operative positions, common lab tests, common drugs, prefixes, combining forms, and suffixes
- Index of all the medical terms in the terminology sections of each chapter
- Selected recommended resources

Ancillary Materials for the Instructor

The following materials are provided to assist the instructor:

- *Instructor's Manual*
- Online companion

Instructional Aids for the Student

- Terminology words presented at the beginning of each chapter included on audio before transcription exercises
- Transcription tips, including a list of helpful Web sites, in each chapter
- Index of dictated reports included on each CD or tape
- Extensive review of transcription rules, including grammar, punctuation, numbers, etc.
- Comprehensive lists in the Appendix of helpful information

Acknowledgments

Many people have assisted in the production of this third edition. We are particularly indebted to the following professionals:

Linda Haywood, RN, MS, Director, Health Information Management, Forrest General Hospital
Paula Long, Transcription Team Manager, Forrest General Hospital
Ladoris Nicholson, Systems Administrator for Health Information Management, Forrest General Hospital
Mary Reeves, RHIA, Director, Medical Information Services, Vanderbilt University Medical Center, Nashville, Tennessee
Liz Colwart, RHIA, Manager, Health Information Management, Terrebonne General Medical Center, Houma, Louisiana

Our sincerest appreciation is extended to the following reviewers who provided significant feedback to this edition:

Terrie Ortego, RN, CCM
Louisiana Technical College
T. H. Harris Campus
Opelousas, LA

Esther Storvold
Selkirk College
Trail, BC, Canada

Connie Regener, MA
Formerly with Saddleback College
Mission Viejo, CA

A special note of thanks goes to these physicians for lending their expertise to this product:
Nagan Bellare, MD
A. Dean Cromartie, MD
Larry Day, MD
Joel R. Flynt, MD
H. Creed Fox, MD
John M. Guice, MD
E. Randy Henderson, MD
Jason D. Hutto, DDS
D. G. Kobs, MD
Lynn McMahan, MD
M. B. Moore, Jr., MD
Charles J. Parkman, MD
Richard Pecunia, MD
Doug Rouse, MD
Clay Thames, DDS
Donald Townsend, MD

The following healthcare professionals were also instrumental in this revision:

Sandy Arnold, RN
Serina Carpenter, RN, MSN, CNRN
Sandy Cooley, RN
Linda Hanly
Brenda Holloway
Helena Lasseter, LSW, MPH
Woody Mathis, RT
Alice McCann, CRNP
Charlotte McDonnell, RN, BS, OCN
Shelia Morse, RN, BSN
Jan Odom, RN, MSN
Mary Ann Purvis, RN, MSN
Barnard Shows, RTT
Sandi Thames, MT (ASCP) (CLS) (NCA)
Janice Tisdale, BSN, MBA
Steve Zary, BS

Very special thanks go to Sara Jane Jones, RHIA, Instructor, Office Administration/Medical Option at Nashville State Tech, Nashville, Tennessee, for her many helpful suggestions, valuable critique of materials, and constant encouragement.

We could never have completed this edition without the encouragement and support of our families: Vic, Brett, Keith, Vivian, Brittney, Michelle, Smitty and Hayward, Kim, Larry, and Ryan.

Above all, we are thankful to our Lord and Savior, Jesus Christ, without whom none of this would have been possible.

Donna Conerly-Stewart
Wanda Lott

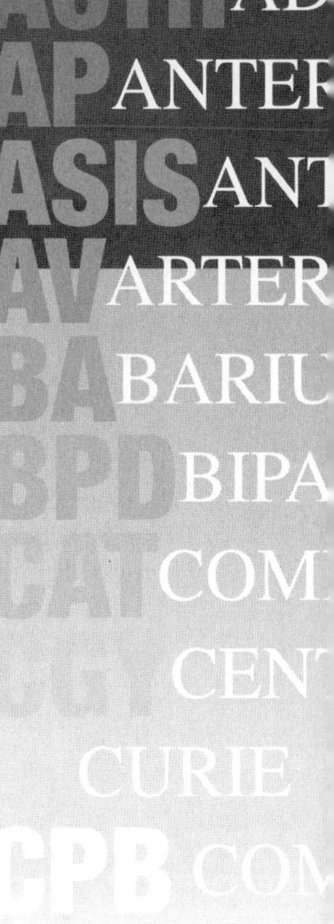

NOTES TO THE STUDENT

You are about to enter the exciting world of "realistic" medical transcription. The task will be much easier if you have had exposure to medical terminology and basic transcription skills; if you have not, these materials will really offer a challenge. With a lot of hard work, though, you can be successful in your study of these advanced transcription activities.

This third edition of *Forrest General Medical Center Advanced Medical Transcription Course* presents learning activities that will equip you with very competitive skills. Because the exercises you will transcribe were dictated in realistic settings, you will become accustomed to transcribing dictation that is very similar to that encountered on the job. This exposure should enable you to be productive from your first day as a medical transcriptionist. If you presently work in a medical setting, your skills should be sharpened and your production rate increased.

Structure of the Learning Materials

Chapter 1 presents valuable information on the following aspects of and/or resources for medical transcription:

- Suggested medical transcription guides
- Typical grammar and punctuation reference books
- Comprehensive transcription rules
- Detailed information on professionalism opportunities

In Chapters 2–19, the materials are organized as follows:

- An introduction to the specialty
- Critical thinking exercises
- A list of abbreviations typically used in dictation
- Visuals (in most chapters)
- Terminology specific to the specialty
- Transcription tips
- Supportive Web sites

A new feature of this edition is the inclusion of supportive Web sites for each chapter. Accessing and studying the information available on these sites will assist in your transcription activities.

The "Transcription Tips" section of each chapter includes other valuable information as well—knowledge that will make your transcription task easier. You will see confusing terms that you might encounter in the dictation, combining words and/or forms, and specialized treatment methods employed in patient care in each particular specialty.

When you have become familiar with the introductory materials for each chapter and have listened to the terminology words, you should be ready to begin transcribing the medical reports given on the audio component correlated with each chapter. For most chapters, you will be transcribing types of medical reports frequently encountered in a hospital setting, such as operative reports, discharge summaries, x-ray reports, consultations, and the like.

The transcription exercises you will hear at the beginning of most chapters are new in this edition. These exercises represent some of the newer, most innovative medical procedures being performed in hospitals and/or outpatient facilities, such as a heart/lung transplant, Gamma knife stereotactic radiosurgery, cochlear implant, bone marrow harvest, stem cell transplant, abdominoplasty, and ankle replacement. Because each chapter is independent of the others, your instructor may have you begin transcribing documents from Chapter 5 rather than from Chapter 2.

Chapter 20 includes challenging exercises arranged in three sections. Section I presents opportunities to transcribe different types of medical reports from those presented in Chapters

2–19. The realistic on-the-job dilemmas contained in Section II will test your knowledge of ethical decision making as it applies to the medical transcriptionist job. Section III contains documents to be edited. This task requires you to apply knowledge of grammar, punctuation, spelling, and similar rules, and also research skills.

Successful completion of the exercises presented in Chapter 20 should give you confidence that you are ready to assume a productive role as a medical transcriptionist.

Be sure to become completely familiar with the lists provided in the Appendix. These lists include types of incisions, sutures, suture materials, dressings, instruments, anesthesia, operative positions, common lab tests, common drugs, prefixes, combining forms, and suffixes. There are also more references and helpful Web sites. As you transcribe, you will find these reference materials invaluable.

An index of all the medical terms from each chapter is provided in the back of the text. This list will serve as a quick spelling reference as you transcribe.

Good luck as you begin this exciting study of advanced medical transcription!

CHAPTER 1

INTRODUCTION

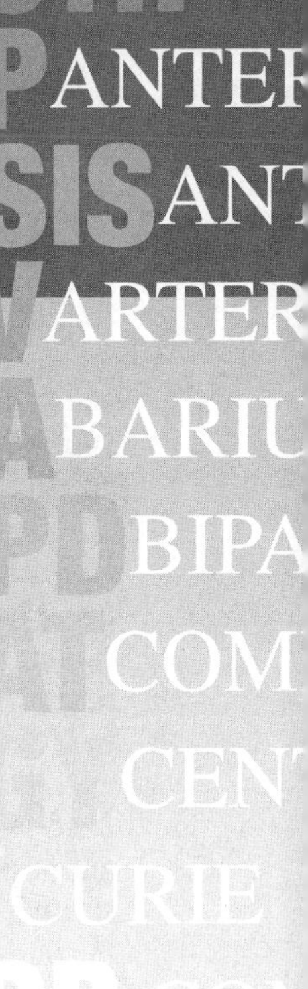

This chapter reviews the information you will need to successfully complete the transcription activities presented in the remaining chapters. In order to produce quality work with efficiency, carefully study the information presented here before beginning the transcription activities.

The following pages contain information on

- Selected medical transcription guides
- Selected office reference manuals
- Transcription rules recommended by the American Association for Medical Transcriptionists (AAMT)
- Opportunities to demonstrate and enhance your professionalism
- Selected confusing medical terms
- AAMT report-formatting guidelines
- The "big four" reports
- Model reports

The information in this chapter will be indispensable as you complete the transcription exercises in Chapters 2 through 20.

References

To work efficiently and accurately, you need to have references at hand to support your transcription activities. Several guides for medical transcription are available. You should select one and follow it consistently. Your employer may have a preference; if so, adopt that one as your guide.

The following publications are examples of selected medical transcription guides:

Blake RS. *The Medical Transcriptionist's Handbook.* 2nd ed. Clifton Park, NY: Delmar Publishers; 1998.

Hughes P, ed. *The AAMT Book of Style for Medical Transcription.* 2nd ed. Modesto, CA: American Association for Medical Transcription; 2002.

Pfeiffer M, ed. *Medical Transcription Do's and Don'ts.* Philadelphia: WB Saunders Company; 1999.

Pugh, MB, ed. *American Medical Association Manual of Style.* 9th ed. Philadelphia: Lippincott Williams & Wilkins; 1998.

Selected references to assist you with grammar and punctuation rules and other transcription trouble spots are:

Clark JL, Clark LR. *How 9: A Handbook for Office Workers.* 9th ed. Cincinnati: South-Western College Publishing; 2001.

Jaderstrom S, Kruk L, Miller J. *Complete Office Handbook.* 3rd ed. New York, NY: Random House; 2002.

Sabin W. *Gregg Reference Manual.* 9th ed. Blacklick, OH: Glencoe McGraw-Hill; 2001.

For a more extensive list of suggested references, see the Appendix, page 255.

Important Tips for Transcriptionists

The transcriptionist is a very important member of the patient-care team. As a transcriptionist, you are charged with the responsibility of assuring that the physician's words are recorded promptly and accurately. You must be a good proofreader and exhibit excellent editing skills.

Technology developed over the last few years has entered the medical field in many ways. Voice recognition systems, electronic patient records, and electronic signatures directly affect the transcriptionist's job.

Today many medical facilities are using *voice recognition systems* as the primary means of obtaining physician dictation. This process makes the transcriptionist's job easier in some respects: production rate accelerates and keying errors are reduced. If the facility where you work changes to a voice recognition system, your job becomes primarily one of editing.

Additionally, more and more facilities are turning to *electronic (computer-based) patient records* rather than paper-based patient records, to make the clinical decision-making process more efficient. The electronic patient record stores comprehensive information on the patient from a variety of sources, such as clinic, laboratory, and pharmacy. Clinical examination results can be entered by clinicians at or near the point of care with the aid of portable computers. Automatic date- and time-stamping of entries facilitates documentation and tracking of patient care and outcomes over time.

An electronic record also makes it easier for the physician and other clinicians to quickly locate accurate and readily usable information about the patient at the point of care. If necessary, the physician and other personnel can view a document as soon as it is transcribed, even before it is edited or signed. However, the record must still be authenticated by the physician's signature to be considered legal.

Today many physicians use *electronic signatures* rather than taking the time to personally sign each document. The typist should key in the words "electronically signed by [physician's name]" underneath the signature.

At the end of this chapter, you will find model reports, which are examples of how you can arrange the information you hear on the tapes. These reports have been formatted in the style recommended by the AAMT in *The AAMT Book of Style for Medical Transcription.* AAMT guidelines represent a "standard" organizational pattern for medical reports. Formatting guidelines begin on page 10.

On the model reports, notice the name of the physician at the end of each report. The name of the physician has been typed, followed by his/her title and reference initials. Sometimes the reference initials are typed in lowercase letters. Always be sure to include your initials after the physician's. After typing the reference initials, you should type the date the report was dictated and the date it was transcribed. These dates can be critical; be sure to type in the correct date. Although you will not hear dates on the tapes, you should supply the information so as to produce a complete transcript. Today, the computer program used by the transcriptionist automatically inserts the time the report was transcribed. You will see this indicated on some new reports included in this edition.

Model Report #4 illustrates the way to indicate that the report has been electronically signed. Note that the time and date when the signature was affixed are included. In the reference lines, the physician's complete name is typed, followed by the transcriptionist's initials. The time the document was dictated and transcribed, together with the document number, are also included. Some facilities follow this practice to improve the audit trail.

Although we have made an attempt to be consistent in all the reports, several correct ways exist to transcribe many things you will hear in medical transcription. For example, if the physician dictates "one 0 nylon suture," you may type it either "1–0 nylon suture" or "0 nylon suture." However, "2–0" should be keyed as "2–0," not "00," and "4–0" as "4–0," not "0000." You should be guided by the preference of the physician or medical facility for which you work. You must learn to be flexible.

Before "beginning work" at Forrest General Medical Center, you should review the following aspects of medical transcription:

1. Prefixes, suffixes, word roots, and/or combining forms (see Appendix and tips within each chapter)
2. Types of medical reports (see page 10 and model report forms, beginning on page 12)
3. Transcription and/or grammar rules, beginning on page 2
4. Confusing words (pages 8 and "Tips" section of each chapter)
5. Types of sutures, anesthesia, dressings, incisions, operative positions, frequently used drugs, instruments, and laboratory tests (see Appendix)
6. Components of the "big four" reports (page 10)
7. Spellings of difficult words you may have had trouble with in past transcription situations

Although a medical transcriptionist should be more concerned with transcribing the correct words than with placing each punctuation mark properly, strive to apply grammar and punctuation rules correctly as you would in any other setting.

The following section is a review of grammar, punctuation, and formatting guidelines.

Transcription Rules

The following selected rules adhere to *The AAMT Book of Style for Medical Transcription.* You should consult that book when you encounter situations that are not addressed in the information that follows.

Capitalization

General Rules

1. Capitalize the trade names of drugs and brand names of manufactured products and equipment. **Do not** capitalize the generic names of drugs.

Advil	ibuprofen
Pepcid AC	famotidine
Lanoxin	digoxin
amoxicillin	
penicillamine	

2. Capitalize eponyms but not the word(s) that accompany them. You will see an apostrophe in some eponyms. The *AAMT Book of Style for Medical Transcription* recommends that the apostrophe be dropped; other references retain the apostrophe. Words derived from eponyms (such as adjective forms) are not capitalized.

Parkinson disease	parkinsonism
Banks graft	
Down syndrome	
Deaver skin incision	

NOTE: In Forrest General Medical Center, 3rd ed., solutions to the transcription exercises DO retain the apostrophe if indicated in *Dorland's Medical Dictionary*.

3. Capitalize the name of a genus used in the singular form and its abbreviation, but do not capitalize the plural form or the adjective form. Species names should not be capitalized.

Streptococcus	streptococcal
S. pneumoniae	
Pseudomonas	pseudomonas
P. aeruginosa	
Escherichia	
E. coli	

NOTE: Some reference books suggest capitalizing and underlining the singular form of the name of a genus.

4. Do not capitalize general references to departments or rooms in a medical facility. For example, *emergency room* and *recovery room* should not be capitalized. You can think of these as generic terms. Specially designated rooms, however, should be capitalized; for example, the Crystal Room.

5. When indicating positive allergy information, use some format that will highlight the data. Acceptable formats are:

ALLERGIES: CODEINE AND PENICILLIN
ALLERGIES: codeine and penicillin
ALLERGIES: codeine and penicillin
ALLERGIES: codeine and penicillin

6. Capitalize acronyms but not the words from which the acronym is obtained. Avoid using acronyms unless they will be recognized readily. When using an acronym that is not widely recognized, use the complete term first and place the acronym in parentheses. You may then use the acronym throughout the rest of the report.

AIDS	acquired immunodeficiency syndrome
CABG	coronary artery bypass graft
CT	computed tomography
AICD	automatic implantable cardioverter-defibrillator

7. Do not capitalize *stage* and *grade* when used in connection with cancer stages and grades. Do not capitalize *grade* when describing neurological classifications and diastolic and systolic murmurs.

stage I	grade 1
stage IV	grade 2
stage II	grade 3

8. Do not capitalize disease names except for eponyms that form part of the name.

endometriosis	osteosclerosis
Lyme disease	Alzheimer's disease
Crohn disease	arthritis

9. Capitalize all major section headings in medical reports (i.e., PREOPERATIVE DIAGNOSIS, FAMILY HISTORY, HEENT, LUNGS, RECOMMENDATIONS, PHYSICAL EXAMINATION, HEART, etc.). For subsection headings, capitalize only the first letter of the word (i.e., under REVIEW OF SYSTEMS, Cardiac: Pulmonary:, etc.)

10. Do not capitalize the names of medical specialties such as "orthopedics"; these are common nouns. Likewise, reference to one practicing orthopedics, an "orthopedist," should not be capitalized.

11. Capitalize brand names for items such as dressings, sutures, instruments, and the like. Do not capitalize generic names or the adjectives and common nouns that accompany the brand names.

Heyer-Schulte clamp	Adaptic gauze dressing
milk of magnesia	catgut sutures
Babcock forceps	Prolene sutures

Numbers

In general, follow rules of accepted convention in the expression of numbers. Because figures (arabic numerals) are more distinguishable from surrounding text than are spelled-out numbers, AAMT recommends the use of figures except in certain instances. Refer to the following rules for specific situations.

General Rules

1. Use arabic numerals when typing units of measure, ages and other vital statistics, and lab values. In other instances when communication has to be quick and clear, use arabic numerals as well.

3-year-old male
4 inches
hemoglobin 14.5
4 eosinophils

2. Use ordinal numbers (1st, 2nd, 3rd, . . .) to express position in a series or order. When referring to part of a series, use arabic numerals with *st, nd, rd, th,* etc.

   Ms. Davis is in her 5th month of pregnancy.
   The 5th lumbar vertebra . . .
   The 7th entry on the . . .
   Andy is to return on the 11th and 24th of . . .

3. Follow the standard rules concerning the expression of dates. If the day precedes the month, use ordinal numbers; if it follows the month, use figures. Note the correct use of the comma when the year appears with the day and month and the correct format when only the year appears with the month.

   On the 13th of January . . .
   The report is due on October 23.
   On April 4, 2002, Mary is to return to my office.
   In December 2002 Ann's surgery is scheduled. *OR*
   In December, 2002, Ann's surgery is scheduled.

   In textual material, spell out the month and format as one of the previous examples. Use numbers with virgules (forward slashes) in the "date dictated/date transcribed" section.

   D: 6/17/03
   T: 6/18/03

4. Spell out a number that begins a sentence or rewrite the sentence to place the number elsewhere. Keep numbers that relate to specific terms with the term. Keep numbers with their associated units of measurement or an associated abbreviation.

   NOT . . . . 2 and 10 o'clock *BUT* . . . . 2 and 10 o'clock

   NOT . . . . 4-0 Prolene suture *BUT* . . . . 4-0 Prolene suture

   NOT . . . . The uterus measured 5 cm in diameter. *BUT* . . . The uterus measured 5 cm in diameter.

5. Use a comma for numbers of more than four digits, except in a number that includes a decimal. In four-digit numbers the commas may be omitted.

   Platelet count was 304,000.
   White count was 6600.
   76098.67

6. When a value less than one is dictated, place a "0" before the decimal.

   0.4 mg *BUT* 4.5 cm

7. Roman numerals are generally used in the following situations. Sometimes, however, arabic numerals may be used. Follow the preference of your institution and/or reference manual.

   a. For expression of "types"
      type II tympanoplasty
      type IV imperforate anus
      type I mastoidectomy
      BUT type 2 diabetes mellitus
   b. For designation of cranial nerves
      cranial nerve II *OR* cranial nerve 2
      cranial nerve XI *OR* cranial nerve 11
   c. For some operation and instrument names
      Orthocor II pacemaker
      Frickman II operation
   d. With eponyms*
      LeFort II fracture
   e. With clotting "factor"
      factor V thromboplastin
      factor VII antihemophilic factor

For expression of stages, the trend is away from use of Roman numerals, although cancer stages are still expressed in Roman numerals. Cancer *grades* are expressed in arabic numerals.

PUNCTUATION

Commas

General Rules

1. In most cases, follow the standard rules concerning the use of commas, but avoid overuse. Use a comma to improve clarity, enhance readability, or avoid confusion or misunderstanding.

2. Use a comma between coordinate adjectives—adjectives that modify the same noun.

   Physical examination revealed a tall, emaciated, sick man.
   (*NOTE:* No comma is placed between the last adjective and the noun.)

3. If an adjective or adjective phrase follows the noun it modifies, set it off in commas.

   She has tendinitis, right shoulder, with much discomfort.

---

*Eponyms are names for anything (operations, tests, diseases, structures) derived from the name of a person or place.

4. Use commas between independent clauses that do not contain internal commas. If either (or both) contains internal commas, use a semicolon to separate the clauses. Remember, a *phrase* is a group of words that does not have a subject and verb, and a *clause* is a group of words that does contain a subject and verb.

   The patient was begun on Ativan, and her symptoms subsided.
   (Independent clauses that do not contain internal commas and are joined by conjunction.)

   The patient, who was brought in by his mother, was begun on Ativan; and after about two hours, his symptoms subsided. (Independent clauses that contain internal commas and are joined by conjunction.)

5. Use commas to set off dependent nonrestrictive (or nonessential) clauses. Remember, a dependent clause is a group of words that "depends" on the rest of the sentence to make sense. It cannot stand alone as a sentence.

   The patient, who was brought in by his mother, was. . . .
   "Who was brought in by his mother" is a dependent clause.

6. Do not set off dependent restrictive (essential) clauses with commas.

   The cut that was from the shoulder to the elbow was bleeding profusely. ("that was from the shoulder to the elbow" is restrictive; it tells which cut and is therefore necessary for the sense of the sentence.)

7. When typing information concerning weights, spell out *pounds* and *ounces* and do not separate with a comma.

   The infant weighed 6 pounds 10 ounces.

Periods

1. Do not use periods after or within most abbreviations. Most English units of measurement should be written out. Do use periods in drug-related abbreviations that are in lower case. If a sentence ends with an abbreviation that requires periods, do not use another period to end the sentence.

RBC	p.r.n.
rbc	t.i.d.
AMA	inch

2. For plural forms of capitalized abbreviations, use a lowercase *s*.

   EOMs PVCs RBCs

3. To form the plural of abbreviations written in lower case, use '*s*.

   wbc's cbc's

4. For the correct format of unusual abbreviations, consult a reference guide.

Semicolons

1. Use a semicolon to separate two independent clauses not joined by a conjunction.

   Mrs. Davis has emphysema; her quality of life is very poor.

   The patient was taken to a private room; his wife was taken to surgery.

2. Use a semicolon to join independent clauses, one or both of which contain internal commas.

   Jesse, who is Jane's brother, was injured seriously in the accident; Jane was not injured.

   There was some spasm in the sigmoid colon; but otherwise, there were no mucosal lesions, mass lesions, friability, or ulceration seen throughout the colon.

3. Use a semicolon to separate two independent clauses joined by an adverbial connective (conjunctive adverb).

   The patient was considered to be terminally ill; therefore, no further parenteral measures were to be taken.

Colons

1. Use a colon to introduce a list, series, or enumeration; an example; and sometimes a quotation. Only one space should follow the colon; capitalize the word immediately following the colon.

   Andrew was given the following medications: Platinol, kitasamycin, and Trental.

   HEART: Regular rate and rhythm.

2. Use a colon to express a ratio but not a range.

   1:100,000
   70–150 *NOT* 70:150

Hyphens

1. Use a hyphen to join compound modifiers occurring before a noun.

   The well-developed, well-nourished young man was admitted to the hospital for observation.

When compound modifiers occur after the noun, the hyphens are omitted except when listed in the dictionary with hyphens. Compound adjectives shown in the dictionary with hyphens are considered permanently hyphenated. Regardless of whether the compound appears before or after a noun, it retains the hyphens. Examples of some of these permanently hyphenated compounds are:

first-class	short-term
up-to-date	well-known
old-fashioned	well-rounded

When the parts of compound adjectives are separated (or suspended), hyphenate each part.

The six-, seven-, and eight-year-old patients are to be moved from the pediatric floor to the surgery floor until the windows are repaired.

Adjective/adverb combinations should not be hyphenated.

The terminally ill young man is in desperate need of financial help.

2. When hyphenated compound words become well established, many times the hyphen is dropped and the words are joined to form one word. When such words can be used as either nouns, verbs, or adjectives, the noun/adjective forms are joined without a hyphen. When the compound word is used as a verb and one of the words is a preposition, the compound remains as two separate words.

VERB	NOUN, ADJECTIVE
follow up	followup
follow through	followthrough
check up	checkup
work up	workup

Abbreviations and Symbols

1. Abbreviate units of measurement as *cm* for centimeters and *g* for gram but spell out other abbreviations. Do not use a period after the abbreviation.

2. Write out terminology that is dictated in full except for units of measurement. A sentence may begin with a dictated abbreviation, acronym, or brief form.

3. If an abbreviation is used in the admission, discharge, preoperative, or postoperative diagnosis, spell it in full. Also, a conclusion in a consultation and information in the title of an operation should be written out, not abbreviated.

4. Selected symbols that you might see used in medical reports are:

Ⓛ	left	Ⓜ	murmur
♂	male	♀	female
*	birth	†	death
p̄	after	ā	before
c̄	with	s̄	without
>	greater than	<	less than
≥	greater than or equal to	~	approximate
±	not definite, plus/minus	(+)	significant
(±)	possibly significant	↓	decreased
↑	increased	→	causes, no change
←	is due to	O	normal
V	systolic blood pressure	Λ	diastolic blood pressure
#	number, weight	°	degree
′	foot	″	inch
:	ratio	+	positive, present
–	absent, negative	≠	does not equal
⌢	combined with	/	per one, two, or three (as in number of grams, etc.)

Miscellaneous Rules

1. For words that require accent marks, the trend is to omit them in transcription because of equipment limitations and/or the possibility of making errors in placement. Never place them in handwritten form.

2. When an acronym is dictated, you may either type it in the abbreviated form or type the words in full. Do not, however, use the abbreviated form in sections of reports that give names of diagnoses or operations.

3. Use of the ampersand (&) should be limited to certain single-letter abbreviations (i.e., D&C). No space should precede or follow the ampersand. Do not use between operative titles or diagnoses.

4. Limit use of the degree sign to information in tables except when giving temperature. Write out *degrees* in text when expressing angles.

   The knee was bent to 30 degrees flexion.

   Temperature was 48 degrees. *OR* 48° if degree symbol is available.

5. Do not abbreviate *beats per minute;* spell out.

   Her pulse rate was 40 beats per minute.
   NOT 40 bpm.

6. When transcribing dimensions, use a lowercase *x* or the multiplication symbol and space before and after it.

   The cut measured 4 × 6 inches.

Use of Dates within Medical Reports

1. Spell out the month within the context of a report. Use numerals to represent the month within the "date dictated, date transcribed" section of the report.

   The patient was brought to the hospital via ambulance on September 12, 2003.

   On May 29, 2003, Mrs. Jones was involved in a tragic car accident and expired on June 26. (Note the use of commas to set off the year in the first date.)

   Mr. Jonathan Andrews was named director of the hospital in October 2003. (A comma between the month and year is not necessary here but could be used.)

2. "date dictated, date transcribed"

   D: 5/20/97
   T: 5/21/97

3. When typing dates, always keep the month with the day; the year can be typed on the next line if necessary.

   NOT . . . . October 24, 1997 *BUT* . . . . October 24, 1997.

Decimals

When metric measures are dictated, always use the decimal form of the number, not a fraction.

The incision was 4.5 cm long. *NOT* 4 1/2 cm long.

Percent

When "percent" is dictated, use % or *percent* within the report. Do not abbreviate pct. except in tables. Use % after a number but use *percent* when the number is written in full.

. . . 40% or 40 percent *NOT* 40 pct.
Twenty percent . . . .

Punctuation with Quotation Marks

1. Periods and commas always go inside the final quotation marks. Colons and semicolons always go outside. Placement of the question mark and exclamation mark depends on the wording of the sentence.

   The physician said, "Mrs. Anderson should be taken to an extended-care facility."

2. If the quotation is asking the question, place the question mark inside the quotation marks. If, however, the sentence is stated in the form of a question but the quotation is not, place the mark outside the quotation marks.

   The social worker asked, "Is he to be admitted to the drug treatment facility?"

   Did the social worker say, "We cannot accept his admission"?

Drug Information

1. When typing information relating to drug dosage, use lowercased abbreviations with periods. If the physician dictates "penicillin four milligrams three times a day," you should type

   . . . penicillin 4 mg t.i.d.

   If he/she dictates "Keflex two hundred fifty milligrams every four hours," you should type

   . . . Keflex 250 mg q.4h.
   NOT Keflex 250 mg
   q. 4 hours

2. Do not separate drug names from instructions and doses with commas.

   The patient was instructed to take erythromycin 250 mg q.i.d., Keflex 500 mg q.6h., and Reglan 10 mg at bedtime.
   NOT . . . Keflex, 500 mg, q.6h.

Formatting of Reports

See sample reports on pages 12–32 for formatting procedures recommended by AAMT.

Professionalism

Your professionalism can be demonstrated in several ways. It is imperative that medical transcriptionists keep everything they hear and/or transcribe about a patient confidential. Another way to exhibit professionalism is by joining appropriate professional organizations and striving to become a Certified Medical Transcriptionist (CMT).

The American Association for Medical Transcriptionists (AAMT) is the largest national professional association for medical transcriptionists. Members receive the *Journal of the American Association for Medical Transcription (JAAMT),* gain opportunities to network with other practitioners, and reap other benefits.

The CMT designation is awarded by AAMT to those who successfully complete the certification examination. The exam is administered for AAMT by the Medical Transcription Certification Commission (MTCC). One who has completed three years of experience as a medical transcriptionist can apply to sit for the exam.

The certification exam consists of two parts. Part I is written and includes 120 multiple-choice questions from the following six major content areas: medical terminology, English language and usage, anatomy and physiology, disease processes, healthcare record, and professional development. Part II consists of about 15 minutes of dictation from a variety of report types and specialties that must be transcribed, proofread, and printed within two hours. For more specific information about the exam and registration procedures, visit AAMT's web site at www.aamt.org/. There you can read more about the organization and find answers to questions about the benefits of AAMT membership, resources, certification, and other relevant topics.

Confusing Terms

abduction – the act of drawing away from the axis of the body

adduction – the act of drawing toward a center

aberration – deviation from the usual course or condition

abrasion – the wearing away of a substance or structure through some unusual or abnormal mechanical process

absorption – the soaking up of a substance by skin or other surface

adsorption – the adherence of a substance to a surface

afferent – designates nerves or neurons that convey impulses from sense organs and other receptors to the brain or spinal cord

efferent – designates nerves or neurons that convey impulses from the brain or spinal cord to muscles, glands, and other effectors

aphagia – inability to swallow

aphasia – a disorder of language affecting the generation of speech and its understanding and not simply a disorder of articulation

areola – a circular area of a different color surrounding a central point

areolae – plural of areola

areolar – pertaining to or containing areolae

arteriosclerosis – a group of diseases characterized by thickening and the loss of elasticity of arterial walls

arteriostenosis – ossification of an artery

atherosclerosis – hardening of the arteries caused by the deposition of calcium and cholesterol in the arterial walls

aural – pertaining to the ear

oral – pertaining to the mouth

calculous – pertaining to, of the nature of, or affected with calculus

calculus – a hard, pebble-like mass formed within the body, particularly in the gallbladder

callous (adj) – unfeeling; the adjective form of callus

callus (n) – a callosity

cancellous – of a reticular, spongy, or lattice-like structure; said mainly of bony tissue

cancellus – any structure arranged like a lattice

canker – an ulceration, primarily of the mouth and lips

chancre – the primary lesion of syphilis

cerebellum – that part of the brain behind the cerebrum

cerebrum – the main portion of the brain

cite – to quote

site – a location

sight – the function of seeing, a view, or to take aim

cystoscopy – direct visual examination of the urinary tract with a cystoscope

cystostomy – the formation of an opening into the bladder

cystotomy – surgical incision of the urinary bladder

dysphagia – difficulty in swallowing

dysphasia – impairment of speech

dysplasia – abnormality of development

enervation – lack of nervous energy

innervation – the supply of nervous energy or of nerve stimulus sent to a part

enterocleisis – closure of a wound in the intestine

enteroclysis – the injection of a nutrient or medicinal liquid into the bowel

facial – pertaining to the face

fascial – pertaining to the fascia

fossa – a trench or channel; a general term for a hollow or depressed area

fossae – plural of fossa

ileum – part of the small intestine

ilium – part of the pelvis

malleolus – a bone of the ankle

malleus – a bone of the ear

mucosa – a mucous membrane

mucosal – pertaining to the mucous membrane

mucous (adj) – pertaining to or resembling mucus

mucus (n) – secretion of the mucous membrane

myelitis – inflammation of the spinal cord

myositis – inflammation of a voluntary muscle

palpation – the act of feeling with the hand

palpitation – unduly rapid action of the heart

para – combining form meaning beside, near, past, beyond, the opposite, abnormal

peri – prefix meaning around or about

pericardium – the membrane surrounding the heart

precordium – the region of the thorax immediately over the heart

perineal – pertaining to the perineum, or genital region

peritoneal – pertaining to the peritoneum, or membrane lining the abdominal wall

peroneal – pertaining to the fibula

pleural – referring to the pleura

plural – more than one

psittacosis – an infectious disease of parrots and other birds that may be transmitted to humans

psychosis – a general term for any major mental disorder of organic and/or emotional origin

sycosis – a disease marked by inflammation of the hair follicles

radical – directed to the cause; directed to the root or source of a morbid process

radicle – any one of the smallest branches of a vessel or nerve

scirrhous – pertaining to a cancer that is stony hard to the touch

scirrhus – scirrhous carcinoma

supination – the act of rotating the arm so that the palm of the hand is forward or upward

suppuration – the formation or discharge of pus

ureter – the tube through which urine travels to the bladder

urethra – a membranous canal through which urine travels from the bladder to the surface

ureteral – pertaining to the ureters

urethral – pertaining to the urethra

vesical – pertaining to the bladder

vesicle – a small bladder or sac containing liquid

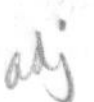

villous – shaggy with soft hairs; covered with villi

villus – a small vascular process or protrusion

viral – pertaining to a virus

virile – possessing masculine traits

AAMT Report Formatting Guidelines

Adhering to the following guidelines and studying the model reports will assist you in formatting your reports correctly. Although the AAMT guidelines are the "standard," your facility may prefer and/or require you to use a different style guide for formatting reports.

1. Use block format for all reports with left justification.
2. Leave 1/2- to 1-inch top, bottom, left, and right margins.
3. Hyphenate words at the end of lines only when typing words with preexisting hyphens.
4. Paragraph where the dictator indicates except when paragraph use is excessive. If no paragraphs are dictated, paragraph when appropriate.
5. Type major headings in all capitals as dictated. Type vertically admitting diagnoses, preoperative diagnoses, postoperative diagnoses, impressions, discharge diagnoses, names of operations, and similar entries.
6. If the dictator uses "same" for the postoperative diagnosis (meaning it is the same as the preoperative diagnosis), rekey the diagnosis; do not type "same."
7. For enumerated items, number them if the dictator does. If he/she numbers some and not all, you should be consistent. Either number all or none.
8. Double space between major sections of reports but single space between subheadings that are listed vertically.
9. Even if dictated, do not abbreviate headings except for widely used and readily recognizable abbreviations such as HEENT.
10. If information concerning a heading follows on the same line as the capitalized heading, use a colon after the heading, followed by one space.
11. If the information is to begin on the next line at the margin, omit the colon after the heading.
12. The signature block should begin at the left margin four spaces after the last line of type. Type the dictator's full name followed by "MD" (or other appropriate title). A title accompanying the name should be typed on the left margin one single space beneath the name.
13. At a double space below the dictator's name and/or title, type the reference initials of the dictator followed by your initials. Acceptable styles are

    RT:al *OR* rt:al *OR* RT:AL
    RT/al *OR* rt/al *OR* RT/AL

14. When a report continues onto a second and/or succeeding page, type "continued" at the bottom of each page and insert a heading at the top of each succeeding page. See page 12 of the model reports for a correct example.
15. Use the "widow/orphan" feature of your word processor to avoid having a single line of a paragraph appear as the last line on the page or the first line of a new page.

Major Types of Medical Reports

The "big four" include the *history and physical, operative report, consultation,* and *discharge summary.* The radiology report and pathology report are two more frequently encountered reports. Other types of reports are dictated when specialized procedures are done, such as the report of a catheterization procedure, electrophysiology study, phacoemulsification, refractive procedure, death summary, and so on.

Becoming familiar with the following information about the "big four" reports and radiology and pathology reports will help you understand the components of each of these reports.

1. History and physical—This report is usually dictated by the admitting physician or resident when a patient is admitted to a hospital. The "history" includes the chief complaint, history of present illness, and historical information about the patient's past, social, and family history that contributed to the present illness. In addition, a review of systems and physical findings present upon examination by the physician are part of this report. The "physical" is not historical but includes information from the physician's physical evaluation of the patient at the time of admission. Vital signs and information about systems and organs are dictated in this section. (See Model Report #1, p. 12)

2. Consultation report—When an attending physician desires a second opinion about a patient's condition or diagnosis, he/she requests a consulting physician to evaluate the patient and dictate findings. This report is dictated by the consultant, addressed to the attending physician, and generally includes the date of and reason for the consultation, the physical and laboratory evaluation of the patient, and the consultant's impression and recommendations. A note of appreciation for the consultation may also be dictated by the consulting physician. (See Model Report #3, p. 15)

3. Operative report or operative note—This report is dictated by the operating physician or assistant and includes specific information about an operative procedure. Preoperative and postoperative diagnoses, surgeons' names, anesthesiologist(s) name(s), anesthesia, findings, and a detailed description of the procedure are typical parts of this report. Information about sponge and/or instrument counts and estimated blood loss is also generally dictated. (See Model Report #2, p. 14)

4. Discharge summary—This report is dictated by the physician when the patient is dismissed from the hospital. It includes a review of why the patient was admitted and a history of the hospital stay. It can also include information on laboratory data, followup instructions, discharge medications, condition of the patient on discharge, and prognosis. The primary focus of the discharge summary is a summary of events that occurred while the patient was in the hospital and the discharge diagnoses. (See Model Report #4, p. 16)

5. Radiology report—This report is dictated by a radiologist upon completion of a diagnostic procedure and includes the radiologist's impression of the findings. Example procedures are CAT scans, MRI scans, basic x-rays, nuclear medicine procedures, and fluoroscopic examinations. (See Model Reports #6 and #7, pp. 20 & 21)

6. Pathology report—A pathologist dictates this report, which describes findings relating to disease and/or pathology of a tissue sample. Samples can be taken during surgery, special procedures, or biopsies. The focus of the report is on the gross and microscopic findings and the pathological diagnosis. Information in this report is generally limited to tissue, whereas laboratory data usually includes information about body fluids. A separate report is not prepared to report lab data, but the information appears within the history and physical and/or discharge summary reports. (See Model Reports #8 and #9, pp. 22 & 23)

Some practitioners dictate the *problem-oriented record (POR)* so that specific problems are defined, numbered, and referred to by number throughout the record. Components of the POR may vary according to the particular setting in which the system is used. However, every system includes the following:

1. The *initial data base,* which consists of the patient's comprehensive health history, a complete physical exam, and available laboratory data.

2. The *problem list.*

3. The *progress notes,* which may be organized in different formats, yet the basic format remains the same. The note begins with the problem and its number and then continues as follows:

S	=	subjective data (history, consultation)
O	=	objective data (physical exam, lab reports)
A	=	assessment of the S and O
P	=	plan—a statement specifying what is to be done regarding the problem. (See Model Report #5, p. 18)

MODEL REPORTS

History and Physical — Model Report No.1

HISTORY AND PHYSICAL

Aultman, Johnny
3798670
Sachi Dazai, MD
March 14, 20 - -

CHIEF COMPLAINT
Black, tarry stools.

PRESENT ILLNESS
This is a 76-year-old white male who presented to the ER because of black, tarry stools. He had been having these for just a short period of time and has had only two stools. He has not been having any indigestion or heartburn. He has a past history of peptic ulcer disease twice in the past with bleeding. Each of those two times he had no pain or indigestion. He has not had any nausea or vomiting.

PAST HISTORY
He has been in relatively good health. He has had hypertension for about 6 years. No history of thyroid disease or history of asthma, TB, or pneumonia. He has been a borderline diabetic about 6 years. He has had no previous surgery.

FAMILY HISTORY
Father had a CVA. He has a brother with prostate CA and a sister with CA of the spleen.

SOCIAL HISTORY
He smoked about 2 packs a day for about 25 years but stopped about 16 years ago. He does not drink.

ALLERGIES
He has no known allergies.

CURRENT MEDICATIONS
Dyazide one daily; a 1500-calorie ADA diet.

REVIEW OF SYSTEMS

HEENT: Has a cataract on the right eye. He has decreased vision in that eye.
PULMONARY: He has some chronic productive cough and does have
some shortness of breath with exertion. There is no hemoptysis. He has no PND or orthopnea.
CARDIOVASCULAR: No chest pains, palpitations, or fluttering.
GASTROINTESTINAL: See PRESENT ILLNESS.
GENITOURINARY: No dysuria, hematuria, frequency, or urgency. He does have some decrease in size and force of his stream at times. He also has some terminal dribbling. He has nocturia one to two times per night.
NEUROMUSCULAR: He has stiffness in his left shoulder. He has some pain at times in the right shoulder.

PHYSICAL

GENERAL: Well-developed white male in no acute distress.
VITAL SIGNS: Blood pressure 142/70. Respirations 18.
Pulse 100. Temperature 97.5°.

(continued)

HISTORY AND PHYSICAL
Patient Name: Aultman, Johnny
Hospital No.: 3798670
March 14, 20 - -
Page 2

HEENT: Pupils are equal, round, and reactive to light and accommodation. He has a right cataract. Fundi are normal. He has dentures.
NECK: There are no carotid bruits. There is some fullness over the thyroid but no palpable gland.
HEART: Regular without a murmur, rub, or gallop.
LUNGS: Clear to auscultation and percussion.
ABDOMEN: Soft and nontender. No masses are palpable. He has no bruits. There is no palpable organomegaly. No masses palpable.
RECTAL: He has some black, tarry stool in the rectal vault that is hemoccult positive. His prostate is 1 to 2+ enlarged but there are no hard nodules.
NEUROLOGICAL: He moves all extremities well. Sensory and motor function is normal. DTRs are symmetrical.
EXTREMITIES: No clubbing, cyanosis, or edema.

IMPRESSION
Melena; rule out bleeding peptic ulcer disease.

Sachi Dazai, MD

SD:BJ

D: 3/14/ - -
T: 3/14/ - -

Operative Report

Model Report No.2

OPERATIVE REPORT

Toups, Wallis
5439207
Susan Woods, MD
March 15, 20 - -

SURGEON: Susan Woods, MD

PREOPERATIVE DIAGNOSIS
Intermittent atrial flutter/fibrillation with severe ventricular bradycardia.

POSTOPERATIVE DIAGNOSIS
Intermittent atrial flutter/fibrillation with severe ventricular bradycardia.

PROCEDURE
Implantation of permanent transvenous cardiac pacemaker (Medtronic model 5985).

ANESTHESIA
Local, 1% Xylocaine.

FINDINGS (including the condition of all organs examined)
The patient was admitted with episodes of atrial flutter/fibrillation with very slow ventricular response in low 40s. The patient was entirely uncooperative and combative during the course of operation. It took five people to hold him on the cath table. Also, his heart rate was between 140 and 180. He had very small veins in the region of the deltopectoral groove. All these problems led to great difficulty putting this pacemaker in. However, the electrode was finally positioned in the apex of the right ventricle, and I assumed that his threshold was satisfactory; but we could not be entirely sure of this because of his very fast ventricular rate of 140 to 160. It appeared that the threshold was an MA of 0.8, voltage 0.5, with resistance of 610 ohms. R-wave sensitivity was 7.3.

PROCEDURE IN DETAIL
With the patient in the supine position, the right pectoral region was prepped and draped in the usual fashion. As mentioned above, the patient was entirely combative and uncooperative so that five people had to hold him down. After satisfactory local anesthesia and regional anesthesia were induced, a transverse incision was made and the deltopectoral groove was dissected. One vein appeared to be slightly larger than the rest of the very small venules in this area; and it was cannulated with a cardiac electrode, which with some difficulty was gotten into the apex of the right ventricle under fluoroscopic control. As mentioned above, the patient's threshold appeared to be satisfactory, though this was not entirely certain. Electrode was ligated in place with heavy silk, after which it was attached to the Medtronic pacemaker model 5985. The unit was implanted into the subcutaneous pocket. It should be noted that the patient had practically no subcutaneous fat, so that only a very, very thin layer of subcutaneous tissue and skin overlies the pacemaker. The wound was closed in two layers. Dressings were applied, and the patient was taken back to his room.

Susan Woods, MD

SW:BJ

D: 3/15/ - -
T: 3/15/ - -

Consultation

Model Report No.3

CONSULTATION

Levi, Moses T.
3059486
George M. Presley, MD
March 11, 20 - -

CONSULTANT
Michael S. Terry, MD

The patient is a 25-year-old right-handed black male who around 6 a.m. on March 10 was going to work. He states he lost control of his car and was involved in a motor vehicle accident. He was brought to Wallis Emergency Room where he was seen and evaluated by Dr. Presley. He had a fracture involving his mandible and also a fracture involving his left clavicle. He complained of pain in the same region plus pain in the thoracic region of his back.

Examination of his left shoulder reveals he has a large area of ecchymosis over the clavicle. The area is tender. The skin is intact. He has full passive range of motion involving the left shoulder. All muscle tendon units in the left upper extremity were tested and found to be intact.

Examination of his neck revealed that he had some tenderness in the region of the left sternocleidomastoid muscle and left pericervical muscles. He could put his chin on his chest without any difficulty. He had full rotation of his cervical spine.

Examination of his back revealed tenderness over the region of the dorsal spinous process to T6. No swelling or increased heat and no tenderness elsewhere.

X-rays taken of the thoracic spine revealed no fractures or dislocations. X-ray performed of the left clavicle reveals undisplaced fracture involving the left clavicle.

IMPRESSION
1. Undisplaced fracture involving the left clavicle.
2. Multiple abrasions and contusions.
3. Fracture involving the mandible.

I discussed the care of the fractured clavicle with the patient and his wife in detail. He is currently in figure-of-eight clavicular strap. This may be removed for hygiene following his discharge. We need to follow him up in the office regarding this particular fracture. Potential complications of this fracture were discussed with the patient and his family in detail.

Thank you for this consultation.

Michael S. Terry, MD

MST:BJ

D: 3/11/ - -
T: 3/11/ - -

Discharge Summary — Model Report No.4

DISCHARGE SUMMARY

Donaldson, Gayle
4903982
David Hammett, MD
June 14, 20 - -

ADMITTED
June 10, 20 - -

DISCHARGED
June 14, 20 - -

DIAGNOSIS
1. Atrophic gastritis.
2. Irritable bowel syndrome.

OPERATION
Esophagogastroduodenoscopy 6/11/ - -

This 78-year-old white female was admitted for evaluation of abdominal pain, nausea, and vomiting and reports of coffee-ground emesis. Several weeks ago she was evaluated at the Danielson Hospital for similar symptoms and was told she had several ulcers in her distal esophagus and that she would require surgery. She was subsequently started on medications; however, she was told that she might have to have surgery. She did fairly well after the initiation of medication; but over the three days prior to admission, she had increasing left upper quadrant discomfort along with nausea, vomiting, and hematemesis. She also gives history of 35-pound weight loss over the last 18 months. In October 1990 she underwent evaluation at Speed Hospital and was found to have erosive gastritis with duodenitis as well as reflux esophagitis. She also had some left upper quadrant pain at that time which was attributed to some postherpes zoster neuritis. The patient has previously had cholecystectomy and appendectomy.

Physical exam on admission showed multiple well-healed abdominal scars. No masses were palpable. There was some mild discomfort in the left upper quadrant on palpation and bowel sounds were normal.

LABORATORY DATA ON ADMISSION
Hemoglobin 13.8. WBC 8000. Urinalysis showed 3+ protein with 1 to 3 RBCs/HPF. SMAC was normal except for slight elevation of BUN at 38.

HOSPITAL COURSE
The patient underwent EGD by Dr. Andrew Friend on June 11 with findings of some mild erythema in the prepyloric area, but otherwise was unremarkable. CT scan of the abdomen was normal. Serum Gastrin was slightly elevated at 256 and gastric analysis was done which showed basal of 0.3 mEq/hr which was quite low, maximal acid output 7.1 which is also low, and peak acid output of 10 mEq/hr. The Zantac had been discontinued about 24 hours prior to gastric analysis. Lactose tolerance test was done and this showed normal curve. Barium enema was done which was grossly normal.

(continued)

DISCHARGE SUMMARY
Patient Name: Donaldson, Gayle
Hospital No.: 4903982
June 14, 20 - -
Page 2

My impression is that the patient has elements of atrophic gastritis. She was started on Reglan while in the hospital and has shown marked improvement with regard to her nausea and abdominal discomfort. I suspect that she has some element of irritable bowel syndrome, and we are instituting high-fiber diet and continuing Reglan and Zantac. She has been instructed to continue bland diet and to add additional foods one at a time. She is to return to my office in three weeks for followup.

MEDICATIONS AT TIME OF DISCHARGE
1. Zantac 150 mg p.o. b.i.d.
2. Reglan 10 mg p.o. a.c. and h.s.
3. Restoril 30 mg h.s. p.r.n. sleep.
4. Darvocet-N 100 1 q.4h. p.r.n. pain.

Electronically signed by
David Hammett, MD 6/16/ - - 6:20 p.m.

David Hammett, MD /ds
DD: 6/14/ - - 2:45 p.m. DT: 6/14/ - - 5:15 p.m. DOC#: 1284954

Discharge Summary — Model Report No.5

DISCHARGE SUMMARY

Winters, Janet
9068591
George Sullivan, MD
March 9, 20 - -

ADMITTED
February 25, 20 - -

DISCHARGED
February 28, 20 - -

PROBLEM #1
Hemorrhagic vaginitis.

SUBJECTIVE
As per history.

OBJECTIVE
Hemorrhagic vaginitis, negative culture for Neisseria gonorrhea, see GYN note; hematocrit 15%. The patient transfused four units to bring hematocrit up to 25%.

ASSESSMENT
Severe anemia related to vaginal bleeding. Treated with transfusion and topical therapy with good results. The patient was discharged in stable condition for outpatient followup. Coomb negative, creatinine level 352, free plasma hemoglobins have been elevated at 6.5, but was not consistent with hemolytic anemia.

PROBLEM #2
End-stage renal disease (ESRD).

OBJECTIVE
BUN 35, potassium 4, CO_2 20, creatinine 10.9, albumin 3.3.

ASSESSMENT
ESRD requiring dialytic therapy.

PROBLEM #3
Decrease of serum protein.

ASSESSMENT
Albumin decreased as above, probably related to stress, bleeding, and decreased intake. Will follow nutrition on an outpatient basis, as is our routine.

PROBLEM #4
Diastolic heart disease.

SUBJECTIVE
Weakness associated with anemia.

(continued)

DISCHARGE SUMMARY
Patient Name: Winters, Janet
Hospital No.: 9068591
March 9, 20 - -
Page 2

OBJECTIVE
Echocardiogram showed E:A ratio of 0.83.

ASSESSMENT
Diastolic heart disease.

PLAN
Calan. Will use Calan to slow the heart rate to increase diastolic filling time and will follow on an outpatient basis.

PROBLEM #5
Anemia.

ASSESSMENT
See above, also related to ESRD. Will use Epogen as necessary.

George Sullivan, MD

GS:BJ

D: 2/28/ - -
T: 3/09/ - -

X-Ray Report

Model Report No.6

X-RAY REPORT

Welch, Leona
4693802
Thomas P. Ghetti, MD
March 14, 20 - -

HISTORY
Left ureteral stone.

IVP
The scout film shows a large calcification measuring about 4.0 × 6.0 mm in the left pelvis. There is also a calcification overlying the right kidney region. There is good excretion of contrast material bilaterally. The size and shape of both kidneys are normal. There is a dromedary hump on the left side. There is minimal dilatation of the collecting system on the left, and there is moderate dilatation of the left ureter. The calyceal system on the right shows partial duplication but is otherwise normal. The right ureter is normal.

The bladder is also within normal limits. The distal left ureter does point right towards the stone seen on the scout film.

IMPRESSION
Large left ureteral stone in the distal left ureter which is causing only minimal obstructive symptoms.

Thomas P. Ghetti, MD

TPG:BJ

D: 3/14/ - -
T: 3/14/ - -

X-Ray Report

Model Report No.7

X-RAY REPORT

Presley, Andrea
4096082
Salem Poole, MD
March 15, 20 - -

RENAL DYNAMIC AND STATIC SCINTIGRAPHY

HISTORY
Long history of recurrent urinary tract infections, small atrophic right kidney.

NUCLIDE
Technetium glucoheptonate complex 10 mCi - IV

SERIAL POSTERIOR PHOTOSCINTISCANS
There is prompt progression of photon activity down the abdominal aorta with good visualization of the bifurcation and prompt appearance of activity in both renal vascular beds simultaneously.

BLOOD POOL AND DELAYED POSTERIOR AND OBLIQUE PHOTOSCINTISCANS
The renal functioning parenchyma vary in size. Diameters are on the right 7.5 × 5.5 cm and on the left 11.0 × 6.5 cm. Distribution of photon activity is homogeneous and there is collecting system activity in both collecting systems on delayed scan.

SCAN
Hippuran-tagged iodine 131-200 uCi - IV

SERIAL POSTERIOR TWO-MINUTE PHOTOSCINTISCANS
There is activity in both parenchyma at two minutes and collecting system activity bilaterally at four minutes and bladder activity at six minutes. Parenchymal washout is identified bilaterally at eight minutes. No obstruction is present.

HISTOGRAMS
Activity curves are generated over both kidneys and on the right, Phase I curve is initially sharp with a decreasing rate in the last part of the curve peaking at 250 seconds at a 500-count intensity followed by an efficient-appearing washout curve.

On the left, Phase I curve is sharp and peaking occurs at about 270 or 280 seconds at 600-count intensity followed by a sharp washout curve.

Michi Iwasaki, MD
Pathologist

MI:BJ

D: 3/15/ - -
T: 3/15/ - -

Pathology Report

Model Report No.8

PATHOLOGY REPORT

Andrews, Jane
Case Number 40-S-397
Michi Iwasaki, MD
May 18, 20 - -

SPECIMEN
Gallbladder.

GROSS EXAMINATION
There is a single calculus that is yellow to brown, 0.7 cm, mulberry in type. The previously opened gallbladder consists of two portions, one showing abundant fat and multiple staples. The other portion is the portion of the fundus that was previously opened, presently measuring 6.0 × 3.5 × 1.2 cm, the remaining portion measuring 6.0 × 3.0 × 1.5 cm. Representative portion of soft tissue embedded.

MICROSCOPIC DIAGNOSES
1. Chronic cholecystitis—no evidence of malignancy on these sections.
2. Cholelithiasis.

Michi Iwasake, MD
Pathologist

MI:BJ

D: 5/18/ - -
T: 5/18/ - -

Pathology Report

Model Report No.9

PATHOLOGY REPORT

Jordan, Shannon
Case Number 40-S-102
Joel Sundeen, MD
April 8, 20 - -

SPECIMENS
A. Right spermatic cord lipoma.
B. Right inguinal node.

CLINICAL
Not given.

GROSS EXAMINATION
A. Received is a fragment of fibromembranous and fatty tissue which measures 4.4 × 3.0 × 2.0 cm. On cut section most of the tissue appears to be fat which is circumscribed and appears to be partially encapsulated. One representative section is submitted.

B. Received is a fragment of yellow fatty tissue measuring 1.5 × 1.4 × 0.8 cm. On cut section all of the tissue appears to be fat, and it appears to be partially encapsulated. No evident lymph node structure is identified grossly. Representative section is submitted.

MICROSCOPIC DIAGNOSES
A. Hernia sac and lipoma.
B. Lymph node showing extensive fatty replacement.

Joel Sundeen, MD
Pathologist

JS:BJ

D: 4/08/ - -
T: 4/09/ - -

Autopsy Report

Model Report No.10

AUTOPSY REPORT

Delhi, Sanders
Hospital No.: 3869287
Anderson Yates, MD

EXPIRED: May 20, 20 - -

GROSS DESCRIPTION

Autopsy was performed on Saturday, October 13, 20 - -, at Toledo General Medical Center Morgue. Authority for examination of the head only was signed by the son of the deceased.

EXTERNAL DESCRIPTION
The body is that of a well-developed, slightly obese, elderly white female identified by hospital wristband. The head was normal in shape covered with long blond hair. The facial features were normal. The neck was symmetrical. The chest is normal in shape, the breasts slightly atrophic. The abdomen was slightly protuberant. The external genitalia were normal adult female. The extremities were bilaterally symmetrical and grossly not remarkable.

CALVARIUM
The scalp was reflected in the usual manner, and the calvarium removed with a Stryker saw. There is a moderate amount of blood-tinged fluid in the subdural space. The brain is removed and examined externally and found to be grossly symmetrical. There is a massive subarachnoid hemorrhage localized largely around the base of the brain and extending over the cerebral hemisphere on both sides, more prominent on the right side. The vessels at the base of the brain were largely encased and obscured by blood clot. The brain is placed in formalin; further dissection is deferred pending adequate fixation.

GROSS BRAIN DISSECTION
On dissecting away clot from the base of the fixed brain, the vessels of the circle of Willis were found to be intact, showing mild to moderate amounts of atherosclerosis with patent lumens. The clot is more severely impacted around the right middle cerebral artery. On further dissection, the middle cerebral artery seems to disappear in a solid, firm, dark red clot. Further dissection is carried out by multiple coronal sections through the temporal lobe and the remainder of the brain. There is found to be a massive hemorrhage into the cerebral tissue, primarily involving the anterior horn of the temporal lobe. The total area of the destructive hemorrhage is 4.0 cm at greatest diameter. Surrounding cerebral tissue is soft and partially liquefied with a reddish-gray appearance. Hemorrhage extends into and fills the right lateral ventricle. The ventricle is slightly to moderately expanded in size, and the lining has a reddish, yellow-tinged discoloration. Examination of the terminating portion of the middle cerebral artery reveals no gross dilatation or aneurysm formation.

MICROSCOPIC DESCRIPTION
Sections through the involved area of the brain show massive hemorrhage replacing and disrupting cerebral tissue. Erythrocytes were largely laked, and there were layers of fibrin and platelets in some areas. Surrounding brain tissue shows blood staining and phagocytized pigmented material. Relatively few inflammatory cells were encountered. More remote areas of the brain show foci of verification and dilatation and engorgement of the blood vessels. Sections of the main vessels entering the area show a moderate amount of atherosclerosis with thickening of the wall, but the exact site of rupture cannot be identified, and there is no histological evidence of aneurysm formation.

(continued)

AUTOPSY REPORT
Patient Name: Sanders, Delhi
Hospital No.: 3869287
May 20, 20 - -
Page 2

COMMENT
The patient died as a result of a massive hemorrhage in the area of the right middle cerebral artery trifurcation. An aneurysm cannot be definitely demonstrated, though the hemorrhagic nature of the infarct indicated a spontaneous rupture of an arterial vessel. It is not known whether or not the patient had hypertension, which may or may not have been a contributory factor. There is no evidence of a significant herniation of the brain.

DIAGNOSES
1. Spontaneous intracerebral hemorrhagic infarction, predominantly right temporal lobe, area of the trifurcation of the right middle cerebral artery.
2. Cerebral atherosclerosis, mild to moderate.

Ken Ainsworth, MD
Pathologist

KA:NY

D: 5/20/ - -
T: 5/21/ - -

Colonoscopy

Model Report No.11

COLONOSCOPY

Carpenter, Rosa
8968450
Vincent Prell, MD
November 21, 20 - -

INSTRUMENT
Olympus CF1TL flexible colonoscope.

PROCEDURE
The patient was premedicated with Demerol 50 mg and Valium 20 mg, and an additional 10 mg of Valium IV was given during the procedure. The colonoscope was passed to the cecum with mild difficulty.

FINDINGS
The patient was poorly prepped and there was some spasm in the sigmoid colon; but, otherwise, there were no mucosal lesions, mass lesions, friability, or ulceration seen throughout the colon.

IMPRESSION
Normal examination except for some spasm in the sigmoid colon.

RECOMMENDATIONS
1. Antispasmodics.
2. High-fiber diet.

Vincent Prell, MD

VP:BJ

D: 11/21/ - -
T: 11/22/ - -

cc: Milton Toups, MD

Esophageal Motility Study and Bernstein Test

Model Report No.12

ESOPHAGEAL MOTILITY STUDY AND BERNSEIN TEST

Salters, Vivian
3986048
Jim Dews, MD
March 7, 20 - -

The esophageal motility study was done in the usual manner using the Beckman manometer. Using the slow pull-through technique, the lower esophageal sphincter pressure was measured. The mean was 15 mmHg, location at 40 cm, and there was normal relaxation. Using both wet and dry swallows, the peristaltic waves were measured. In the midesophagus, the mean pressure was 41 mmHg, duration 5 seconds; and in the distal esophagus, 38 mmHg, duration of 6 seconds. The upper esophageal sphincter pressure was measured and was 55 mmHg in the anterior and posterior lead and 34 mmHg in the lateral lead. These were all within normal limits. The motility appeared normal even during the episode of chest pain that the patient experienced in the Bernstein test. There was one episode noted on the tracing of some simultaneous waves. However, there were no repetitive waves noted.

IMPRESSION
Positive Bernstein test with a normal esophageal motility study except for a few simultaneous waves.

Jim Dews, MD

JD:BJ

D: 3/07/ - -
T: 3/07/ - -

cc: Endoscopy Lab

Psychological Assessment **Model Report No.13**

JOHNSTON RECOVERY CENTER CHILD/ADOLESCENT UNIT

Clark, Treveria
2679103-6
Rosemary Lowenthal, MD
July 13, 20 - -

ASSESSMENT PROCEDURES
Wechsler Intelligence Scale for Children, III
Woodcock-Johnson Individual Achievement Test - Revised
(administered by hospital personnel)
Bender Gestalt Test of Visual Motor Integration
House-Tree-Person Drawing
Thematic Apperception Test
Rorschach Inkblot Technique
Millon Clinical Adolescent Inventory

REASON FOR REFERRAL
Treveria was referred for assessment by Dr. Elaine Bethell, child psychiatrist, Johnston Recovery Center. Specific information was requested regarding her intellectual potential, achievement, and personality features.

REASON FOR ADMISSION
Treveria is a 13-year-old white female who was admitted to the adolescent treatment unit at Johnston Recovery Center because of problems with oppositional defiant behavior toward her mother and failure to follow directions. She has a history of suicidal and homicidal threats, and her parents reported that she was involved in possible sexual play, acting out with a pimp involved. Treveria denied sexual activity and denied being involved with a pimp. Treveria has a history of school problems but has been recently transferred to an alternative school and her grades are reportedly improving. Treveria's mother and father separated when she was younger. She is the second of five children with the oldest 19 and the youngest 11. She is the only female in the family. When she was younger, she moved frequently to live with both her mother and father and they lived in different states. Her mother was arrested and spent approximately five years in prison for selling drugs. Her mother is reportedly now on probation and doing well.

Treveria has engaged in increased fighting and threats at school and at home. She has threatened to kill her brother on occasion, and she has become increasingly isolated from members of the family. She has been spending increasing amounts of time with older peers, engaging in activities which are not approved of by the family. She has been in outpatient treatment with Johnston Recovery Center but has been uncooperative with treatment. Her mother separated from her husband of three months in June 20 - -. It's stated that Treveria becomes rageful when she does not get her way. She has been involved with Youth Court for disorderly conduct. There's also significant concern on the part of family members regarding Treveria's use of alcohol and substances. She was held back in the third grade and failed the seventh grade. Treveria sleeps 10 to 12 hours a night and occasionally longer. She has admitted to occasional experimentation with alcohol and drugs but denies continuous use. Her mother reportedly used cocaine approximately five years ago during the time she was reportedly selling the substance. It was reported that Treveria's behavior has deteriorated dramatically since her mother divorced in August 20 - -. Treveria's father reports that his relationship with Treveria is conflictual because of his strict rules. Treveria's perinatal period was uneventful and she was born in normal fashion without unusual features. Her developmental milestones occurred at appropriate ages; however, she spoke at eighteen months of age. It was said that Treveria cursed, yelled, and threatened when she had temper tantrums as a young child.

(continued)

PSYCHOLOGICAL ASSESSMENT
Patient Name: Clark, Treveria
Hospital No.: 2679103-6
July 13, 20 - -
Page 2

OBSERVATION OF BEHAVIOR

Treveria presented as a 13-year-old white female of short and chunky build with long blond hair and green eyes. Treveria said she had not worn glasses in the past. She demonstrated no unusual gross or fine motor behaviors. She related verbally in a "slouchy" verbal style. She chewed on a plastic pen top throughout the assessment and spoke in garbled tones while chewing on this object. Her fingernails were noted to be bitten to the quick. She was also noted to have upside-down crosses on the outside end of each middle finger. This may raise questions regarding the possibility she has been involved with satanic activities. Treveria frequently asked questions about the reasons for the assessment and made self-deprecatory comments about her abilities and skills. She occasionally asked whether or not she was doing well and on a couple of occasions she became frustrated and quit trying on difficult items. The test results obtained during this assessment appear to be valid estimates overall; however, the measure of intellectual potential may be an underestimate based on her lack of task persistence and depression.

TEST RESULTS

WECHSLER INTELLIGENCE SCALE FOR CHILDREN III

VERBAL TESTS		**PERFORMANCE TESTS**	
Information	7	Picture Completion	8
Similarities	7	Coding	9
Arithmetic	9	Picture Arrangement	10
Vocabulary	8	Block Design	2
Digit Span	5	Object Assembly	5
		Comprehension	8
VERBAL I.Q.	88	Factor Scores:	
PERFORMANCE I.Q.	80	Verbal Comprehension	80
FULL SCALE I.Q.	83	Perceptual Organization	79
		Freedom from Distractibility	84

Based on the scores obtained by Treveria on this instrument, she is apparently functioning overall with the low-average range of potential. A non-significant 8 point difference between verbal and performance scores was noted. Treveria scored highest on the subtest measuring her ability to put together pictures in the correct sequence so that they match common social interaction patterns. She scored lowest on the subtest measuring visual perceptual ability for abstract designs, short-term auditory memory, and visual perceptual ability for puzzles of familiar objects.

(continued)

PSYCHOLOGICAL ASSESSMENT
Patient Name: Clark, Treveria
Hospital No.: 2679103-6
July 13, 20 - -
Page 3

WOODCOCK-JOHNSON ACHIEVEMENT TEST - REVISED

	Raw Scale	Grade Equiv.	SS	%ile
Letter Word Identification:	43	5.8	87	20
Passage Comprehension:	30	10.0	102	54
Math Calculation:	27	6.4	85	16
Applied Calculation:	39	8.0	95	38
Dictation:	41	7.4	93	32
Writing:	20	11.1	106	65

Based on the scores obtained by Treveria on this instrument, she is functioning within the average range in passage comprehension, applied problems, dictation, spelling, and writing. She is scoring within the low-average range in math calculation.

BENDER GESTALT TEST OF VISUAL MOTOR INTEGRATION

Treveria completed the Bender designs in much less time than is typical. Her manner of responding was impulsive and without due consideration for the task given her. Her errors were considered to be impulsive in nature rather than a reflection of her visual motor skills.

HOUSE-TREE-PERSON DRAWING

Treveria completed a drawing with the required picture elements. A large house dominated the page with prominent windows and curtains. The tree was also large with multiple curly lines used for foliage. The person was drawn in profile with excessive hair. Her drawing suggests that she's resistant to revealing herself and that she may be somewhat flamboyant in behavior. Sexuality may be an issue. The story told by Treveria to accompany her picture suggests that she's resistant and at least mildly oppositional.

THEMATIC APPERCEPTION TEST

Story themes generated by Treveria in response to the TAT materials suggest the following clinical hypotheses. Treveria appears to have feelings of discomfort regarding the aging of older relatives and their approaching death. She is quite capable of being verbally oppositional and impulsive. She seems to be angry regarding discipline and punishment which has been meted out toward her for no appropriate reason (in her perception). Her response to card number 16 clearly demonstrates her anger and opposition to the task at hand. She told a very brief story about a monkey who ate bananas, choked, and died.

RORSCHACH INKBLOT TECHNIQUE

The responses provided by Treveria to the Rorschach suggest the following clinical hypotheses. Treveria appears to miss essential details in her environment. She seems to look and either quickly decide what she is going to do or act impulsively without thinking. Her reality testing and perceptual accuracy appear to be adequate and no evidence of a thought disorder was noted. She seems to have a tendency to be somewhat depressed and to exhibit poorly controlled emotions. She seems to have capacity to understand the world in consensual ways.

(continued)

PSYCHOLOGICAL ASSESSMENT
Patient Name: Clark, Treveria
Hospital No.: 2679103-6
July 13, 20 - -
Page 4

MILLON ADOLESCENT CLINICAL INVENTORY (MACI)

Responses provided by Treveria to the MACI resulted in a protocol which is questionable in terms of its validity. She did not respond in a particularly open manner to the items given her. The scores obtained from her responses suggest that she has a significant delinquent predisposition. Persons who score high on this scale demonstrate behavior that is likely to violate the rights of others. She appears likely to engage in a variety of behaviors which violate societal norms and rules. These behaviors may include threatening others, using weapons, being deceptive, lying persistently, stealing, or engaging in other anti-social behaviors.

Her expressed concerns were all below clinical levels. Two scales, however, were notably higher than the others and near clinical levels. Those scales were social insensitivity and family discord. Persons who score high on these scales tend to be cool and indifferent to the welfare of others and have little empathy for others. In addition, persons who score high on these scales have considerable estrangement from their parents and feel that their families are tense and full of conflict. Personality patterns identified on the basis of her scores included submissive and unruly. These scales suggest that Treveria may be soft-hearted, sentimental and kindly. She may be reluctant to assert herself and she may avoid taking leadership roles. She may be inclined to be dependent and exhibit clinging behavior and fear separation. She may be likely to play down her own achievements and underestimate her abilities. In addition, she appears likely to act out in an anti-social manner and may resist the efforts of others who are trying to get her to follow socially acceptable standards of behavior. She may display a pervasively rebellious attitude that can bring her into conflict with parents and school or legal authorities.

SUGGESTED DIAGNOSIS

AXIS I Oppositional defiant disorder, dysthymia, rule out conduct disorder.
AXIS II Developmental arithmetic calculation disorder and prominent dependent/anti-social personality features.

SUMMARY & RECOMMENDATIONS

Treveria is a 13-year-old white female who was admitted to the adolescent treatment unit at Johnston Recovery Center because of escalating behavior problems including difficulties at school, sexual acting out, threats to harm others, and increased isolation from her family. She has failed several grades and was recently placed in an alternative school where she is doing better. She has been in outpatient treatment but has been uncooperative. Her behavior has reportedly deteriorated since her mother divorced a husband after three months. She has been involved with Family Court for disorderly conduct and has admitted experimentation with alcohol and substances. She currently lives with her biological mother and four siblings. She is the only girl in a family of five and she is second of five children. Treveria's mother was reportedly incarcerated for approximately five years for selling drugs when Treveria was younger. Treveria's relationship with her father is said to be conflictual because of his strict rules.

Based on the information gathered during this assessment, Treveria appears to function intellectually overall within the low average range of potential. Her measure of intellectual potential may be an underestimate of her actual abilities, however. Treveria's achievement was measured within the average range in all areas other than math calculation, which was within the low-average range. A specific learning disability in math calculation was suggested by her score pattern. No significant visual motor integration delays were noted. Personality features identified during the assessment include prominent oppositional and unruly personality traits coupled with a tendency to be dependent, clinging, and deny her independence of leadership. She appears quite resistant to revealing herself and she may be flamboyant and involved

(continued)

PSYCHOLOGICAL ASSESSMENT
Patient Name: Clark, Treveria
Hospital No.: 2679103-6
July 13, 20 - -
Page 5

in sexually provocative behaviors. Her reality testing and perceptual accuracy were found to be adequate and she appears to have a tendency to miss essential details when she tries to understand her environment. This pattern is prominent in children with ADHD.

Based on the information gathered during this assessment, the following recommendations appear to be appropriate:

1. Treveria appears to need continued hospitalization in the adolescent treatment unit at Johnston Recovery Center in order to take full advantage of the treatment milieu provided there.

2. Treveria appears to meet current SDE criteria for a specific learning disability in math calculation. The current test results may be submitted to the special education program developer in the school district where she currently attends school so that eligibility determination can be pursued.

3. Treveria appears to be quite oppositional and non-compliant. She will likely engage in open complaints about tasks which she finds difficult or onerous. She appears to be capable intellectually in sight-oriented therapy; however, her approach to the surrounding environment will make such treatment approaches unfruitful. She appears more likely to benefit from activity-oriented, practical approaches which emphasize behavior management and clear contingencies for inappropriate behaviors.

4. Further investigation of Treveria's possible participation in prostitution should be undertaken. Her scores on the MACI raise interesting questions regarding the personality traits necessary for such behavior. She scored in a manner which suggests an unusual combination of anti-social and dependent personality patterns. It also appears reasonable to investigate whether or not she has been involved in satanic activities as may be indicated by the upside-down crosses placed on the middle fingers of both hands.

Elaine Bethell, MD

EB:WP

D: 6/16/ - -
T: 6/17/ - -

CHAPTER 2

SURGERY

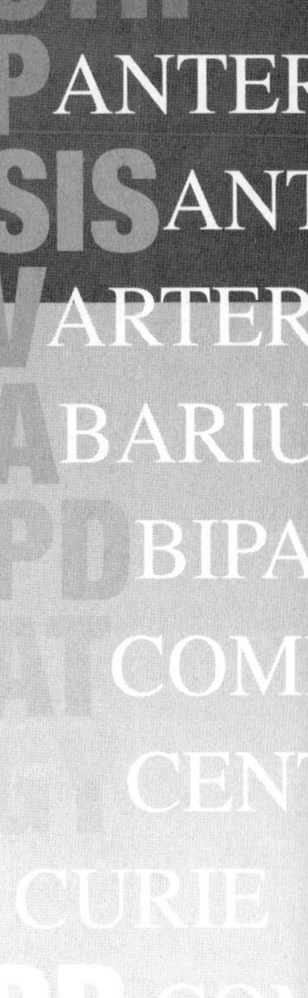

Introduction

Surgery is a specialized field of medicine that requires further educational training—usually four years beyond internship—of one who wishes to become a surgeon. After training in general surgery, one may further specialize into areas such as vascular, orthopedic, urologic, thoracic, or plastic surgery.

Surgeons receive referrals when another physician thinks that a diseased organ or tissue should be removed or when surgical reconstruction is required to make a patient well.

A surgical procedure called a *laparotomy* is frequently performed, because it yields information needed for the diagnosis or treatment of various disease processes. During a laparotomy, a surgical opening is made in the abdomen; examples are procedures performed on the stomach such as *gastrectomy* or *resection* of a portion of the bowel due to disease or obstruction.

When performing a laparotomy, the physician selects the type of incision that will allow the greatest exposure of the involved structures, cause minimal trauma and postoperative discomfort, and provide for primary wound healing with maximal wound strength. The main types of *abdominal incisions* are the *vertical midline* incision, the *McBurney muscle-splitting* incision, the *subcostal* incision, the *Pfannenstiel* incision, the *midabdominal transverse* incision, the *thoracoabdominal* incision, and the *upper inverted-U abdominal* incision.

Another common approach to the abdomen is via the *laparoscopy,* a procedure in which the interior of the abdomen is examined by use of a laparoscope. A laparoscopy necessitates only small incisions. A trocar is placed, CO_2 is insufflated, then the scope is inserted. Multiple procedures can be done with this method, the most common of which is gallbladder removal or laparoscopic cholecystectomy. Marked advantages are the short hospital stay required and the rapid return to normal activities.

Critical Thinking Exercise

Your neighbor, Mr. Palmer, comes to the transcription department and tells you, "I need a copy of my history and physical to carry to the surgeon on Monday. Please make a copy for me."

Would you give him a copy? If not, why not? What would be your advice to him as to how to obtain a copy?

Surgery Abbreviations

abdom	abdomen/abdominal
ABG	arterial blood gas
a.c.	before meals
AD	right ear
a.d.	alternating days
adm	admission
AFB	acid-fast bacilli
AJ	ankle jerk
AK	above the knee
AKA	above-the-knee amputation
alk phos	alkaline phosphatase
ANA	antinuclear antibodies
anes	anesthesia
ant	anterior

A&P	auscultation and percussion
AS	left ear
ASA	acetylsalicylic acid (aspirin)
ASAP	as soon as possible
ASD	atrial septal defect
AU	both ears
AVR	aortic valve replacement
ax	axillary
BE	barium enema
BCC	basal cell carcinoma
bilat	bilateral
BK	below the knee
BPH	benign prostatic hypertrophy
BSO	bilateral salpingo-oophorectomy
BUN	blood urea nitrogen
Bx	biopsy
c̄	with
CA	carcinoma
CABG	coronary artery bypass graft
cath	catheter
CBC	complete blood count
CBD	common bile duct
CEA	carcino-embryonic antigen
CGS	catgut sutures
CNS	central nervous system
C/O	complaining of
coag	coagulation
Con, CON, Cons	consultation
COPD	chronic obstructive pulmonary disease
CPAP	continuous positive airway pressure
CPK	creatine phosphokinase
CR	cardiorespiratory
CRNA	Certified Registered Nurse Anesthetist
CXR	chest x-ray
dc	discontinue
diag	diagnosis
diff	differential
dil	dilute
disch	discharge
DM	diabetes mellitus
DOA	dead on arrival
DOE	dyspnea on exertion
DTR	deep tendon reflexes
Dx	diagnosis
EBL	estimated blood loss
E. coli	Escherichia coli
EDC	estimated day of confinement
EGD	esophagogastroduodenoscopy
EOM	extraocular movement
ESWL	extracorporeal shock wave lithotripsy
EXP LAP	exploratory laparotomy
ext	extremity
FB	foreign body
FBS	fasting blood sugar
FS	frozen section
FUO	fever of unknown origin
Fx	fracture
GB, gb	gallbladder
GI	gastrointestinal
glob	globulin
Glu	glucose
GSW	gunshot wound
GTT	glucose tolerance test
HALS	hand-assisted laparoscopic surgery
HEENT	head, ears, eyes, nose, throat
HNP	herniated nucleus pulposus
Hx	history
IABP	intra-aortic balloon pump
ICU	Intensive Care Unit
I&D	incision and drainage
IM	intramuscular
I&O	intake and output
IJ	internal jugular
IPPB	intermittent positive pressure breathing
IV	intravenous
IVP	intravenous pyelogram; intravenous push
IVPB	intravenous piggyback
jt	joint
KJ	knee joint
KUB	kidneys, ureters, bladder
L	left
L&A, l/a	light and accommodation
lac	laceration
lat	lateral
L.I.F.T.	laser-assisted internal fabrication technique

LKS	liver, kidneys, and spleen
LL	lumbar laminectomy
LLE	left lower extremity
LLL	left lower lobe
LLQ	left lower quadrant
LP	lumbar puncture
LUE	left upper extremity
LUL	left upper lobe
LUQ	left upper quadrant
lymphs	lymphocytes
mEq	milliequivalent
MVR	mitral valve replacement
neg	negative
NG	nasogastric
NKA	no known allergies
noct, noc	night
NPO	nothing by mouth
NSR	nasal septal reconstruction
OR	operating room
PA	posteroanterior
path	pathology
PERLA	pupils equal and react to light and accommodation
PO	by mouth
pos	positive
postop	postoperative
prn	as often as needed
PTA	prior to admission
R	right
RAD	radium
RBC	red blood cell
RLE	right lower extremity
RLL	right lower lobe
RLQ	right lower quadrant
RML	right middle lobe
RO, R/O	rule out
ROM	range of motion
ROS	review of systems
RR	recovery room
RUE	right upper extremity
RUL	right upper lobe
RUQ	right upper quadrant
Rx	prescription/take
SGOT	serum glutamic oxaloacetic transaminase
SGPT	serum glutamic pyruvic transaminase
SMAC	simultaneous multiple automatic chemistries
SOB	short of breath
spec	specimen
Sp. Gr.	specific gravity
S&S	signs and symptoms
staph	staphylococcus
stat	at once
strep	streptococcus
STSG	split thickness skin graft
sub ling	sublingual
subcu, subq	subcutaneous
surg	surgery
sut	sutures
sym	symmetrical
symp, Sx	symptom
TAH	total abdominal hysterectomy
TBA	to be admitted
T&C	type and crossmatch
temp	temperature
TNTC	too numerous to count
tol	tolerate
tr, tinct	tincture
TUR	transurethral resection
TURB	transurethral resection bladder
TURP	transurethral resection prostate
TVH	total vaginal hysterectomy
Tx	treatment
UA	urinalysis

Anatomic Illustrations

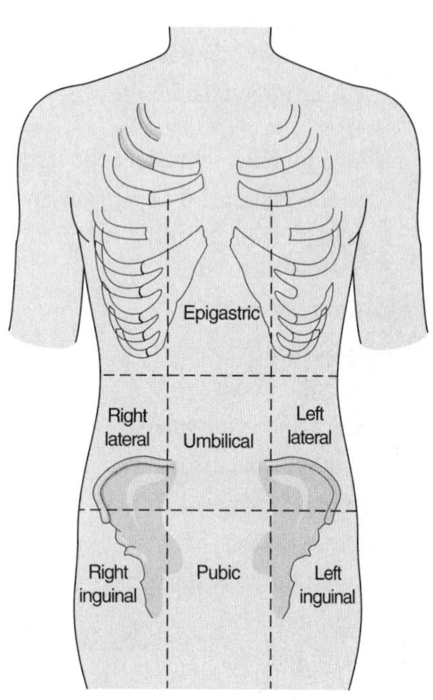

2-1A ABDOMINAL REGIONS

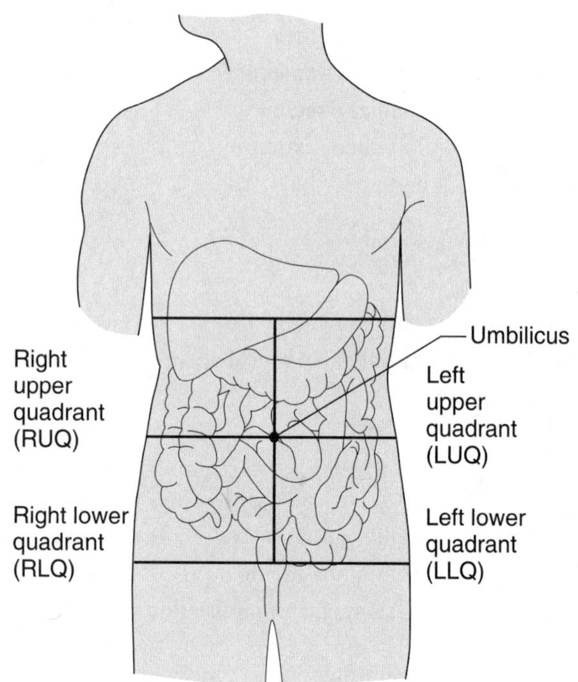

2-1B ABDOMEN DIVIDED INTO QUADRANTS

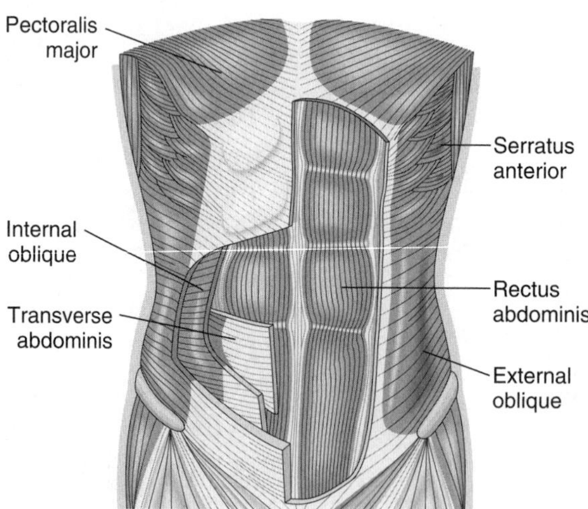

2-2 PECTORALIS MAJOR

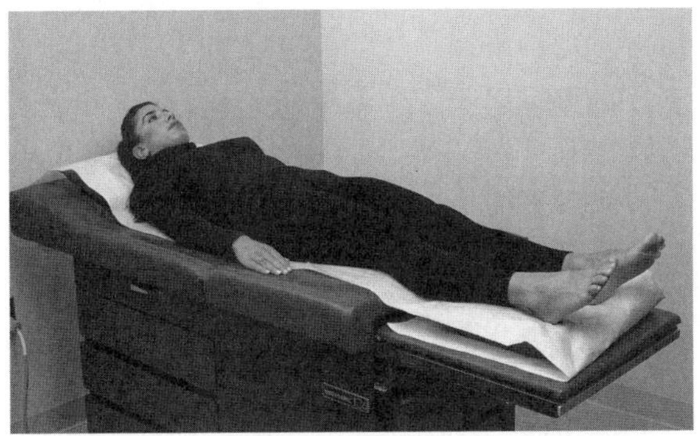
The horizontal recumbent (supine) position.

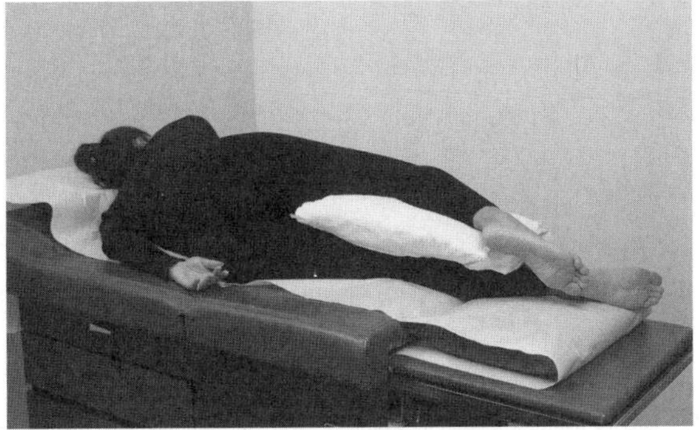
Sims position.

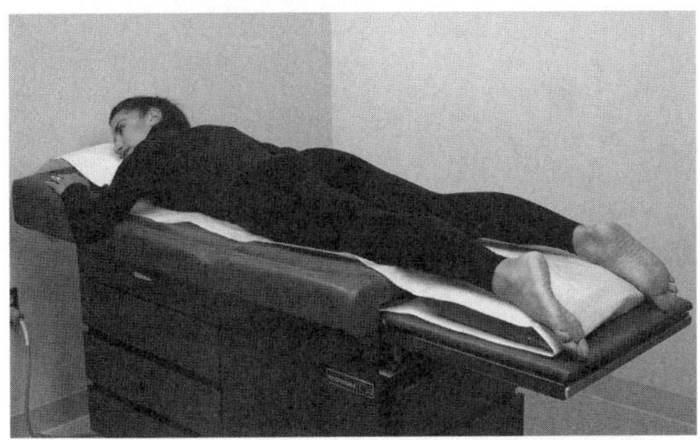
The prone position.

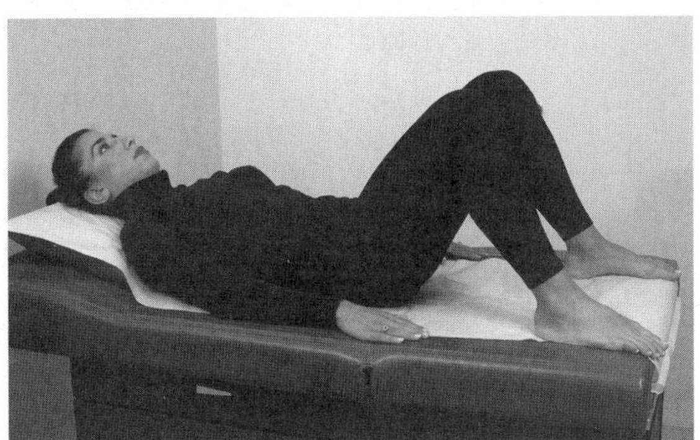
The dorsal recumbent position.

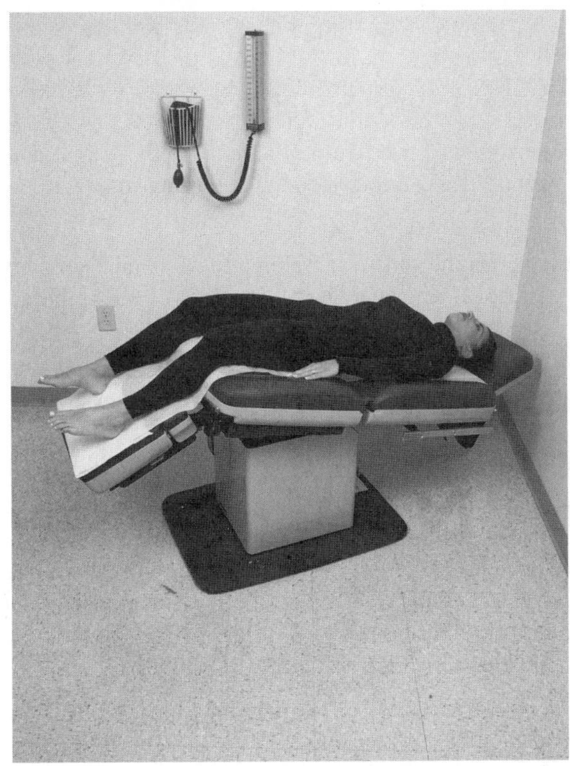
The Trendelenburg position.

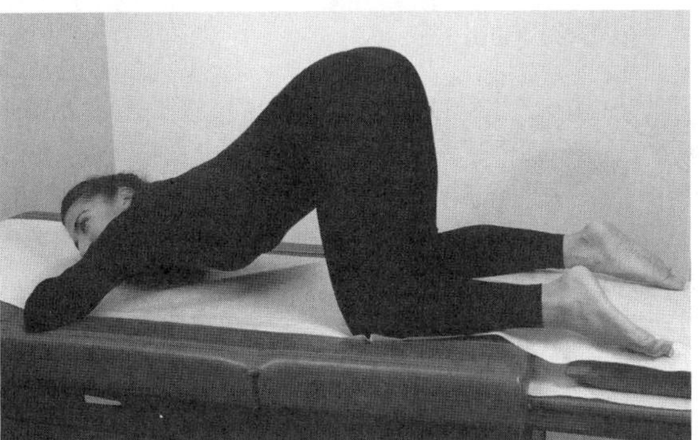
The knee-chest position.

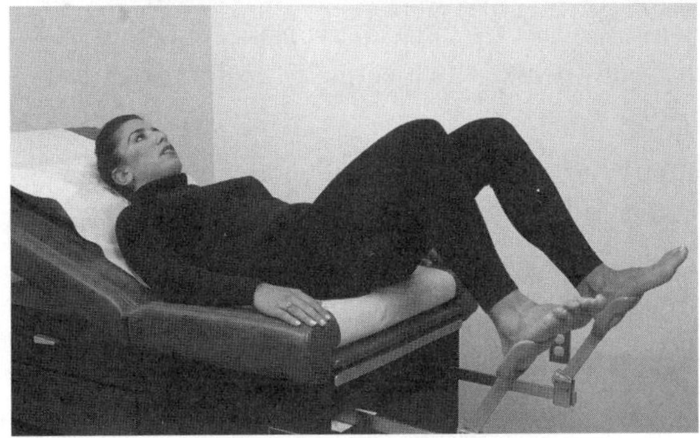
The lithotomy position.

2-3 OPERATION, EXAMINATION, AND TREATMENT POSITIONS

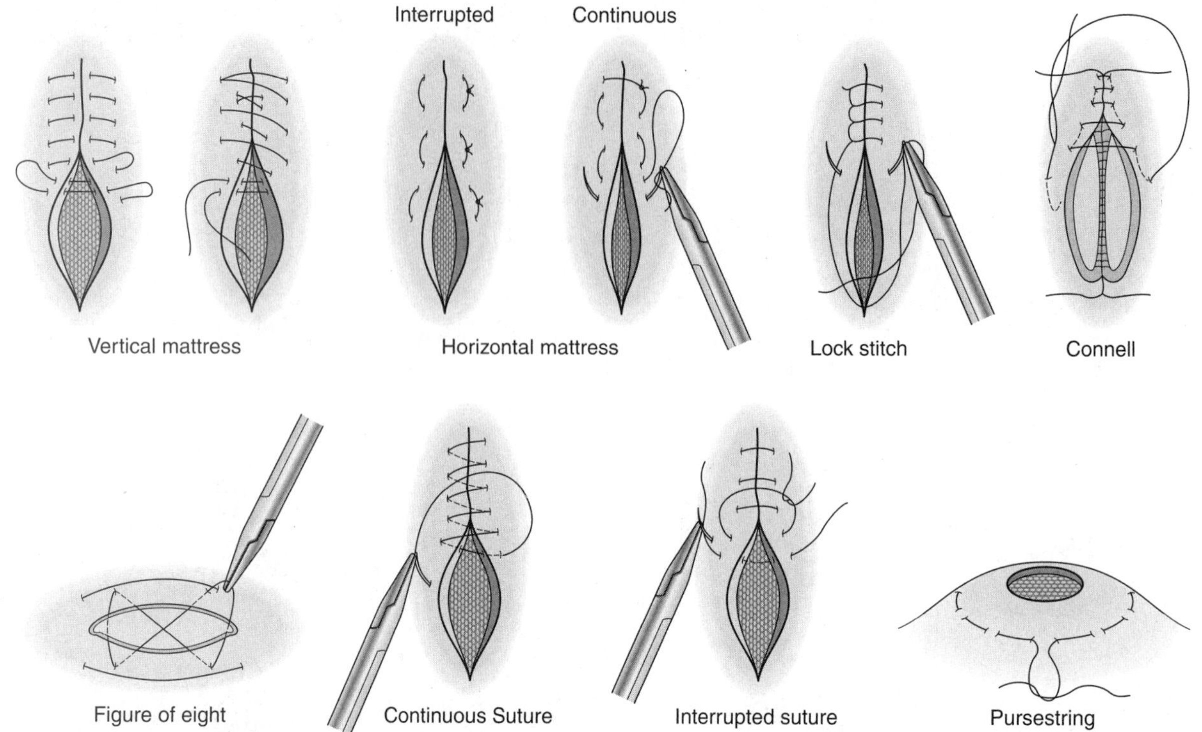

2-4 TYPES OF WOUND CLOSURE

General Surgery Terminology

adenoma (ad"-e-nō'muh) – a benign epithelial tumor in which the cells form recognizable glandular structures or in which the cells are clearly derived from glandular epithelium

adjuvant (ad'-joo-vant) – assisting or aiding; a substance that aids another, such as an auxiliary remedy

anastomosis (ah-nas"-tō-mō'-sis) – a communication between two vessels by collateral channels; an opening created by surgical, traumatic, or pathological means between two normally distinct spaces or organs

antrectomy (an-trek'-tuh-mē) – the procedure of removing the walls of an antrum

aponeurosis (ap"-ō-noo-rō'-sis) – the sheet of connective tissue that attaches muscle to bone or other tissues

areola (ah-rē'-ō-lah) – a circular area in tissue, usually of a color differing from that around it; it may be primary, occurring naturally, such as the areola of the breast, or it may be secondary, caused by some pathological state, such as the red area around a boil or the white area around an allergic reaction

arteriovenous (ar-tē"-rē-ō-vē'-nus) – both arterial and venous; pertaining to or affecting an artery and a vein

asthenic (as-thē'-nik) – pertaining to or characterized by asthenia, which is the lack or loss of strength and energy; weakness

biliary (bil'-ē-air-ē) – of or relating to bile, the bile ducts, or the gallbladder

borborygmus (bor"-buh-rig'-mus) – a rumbling noise caused by the propulsion of gas through the intestines

bougie (boo-zhē') – a slender, flexible, hollow or solid, cylindrical instrument for introduction into the urethra or other tubular organ, usually for the purpose of calibrating or dilating constricted areas

cachectic (kah-kek'-tik) – suffering from cachexia—a general lack of nutrition and wasting occurring over the course of a chronic disease or emotional disturbance

canalization (kan"-uh-lih-zā'-shun) – the formation of canals, natural or morbid

carcinomatosis (kar"-sih-nō-muh-tō'-sis) – the condition of widespread dissemination of cancer through the body; also called carcinosis

carina (kah-rī-'nuh) – a ridge-like structure

cephalad margin (sef'-uh-lad) – toward the head

cholangitis (kō"-lan-jī'-tis) – inflammation of a bile duct

cholecystectomy (kō"-leh-sis-tek'-tuh-mē) – surgical removal of the gallbladder

choledocholithiasis (kō-led"-ō-kō-lih-thī'-uh-sis) – the occurrence of calculi in the common bile duct

choledochoscope (kō-led'-ō-kō-skōp") – an instrument for direct inspection of the interior of the common bile duct by artificial light

choledochotomy (kō-led"-ō-kot'-uh-mē) – incision into the common bile duct for exploration or removal of a calculus

cholelithiasis (kō"-leh-lih-thī'-uh-sis) – the presence or formation of gallstones

cicatrix (sik-a'-triks OR sik'-uh-triks) – a scar; the new tissue formed in the healing of a wound

colostomy (kuh-los'-tuh-mē) – the surgical creation of an opening between the colon and the surface of the body; also used to refer to the opening, or stoma, so created

costophrenic (kos"-tō-frēn'-ik) – pertaining to the ribs and diaphragm

cryosurgery (krī"-ō-sur'-jer-ē) – destruction of tissue by the application of extreme cold; utilized in some forms of intracranial and cutaneous surgery

cul-de-sac (kul'-de-sahk') – a blind pouch or cecum

cystostomy (sis-tos'-tuh-mē) – the formation of an opening into the bladder

d

decortication (dē"-kor-tih-kā'-shun) – removal of portions of the cortical substance of a structure or organ, as of the brain, kidney, lung, etc.

dehiscence (dē-hiss'-enz) – a splitting open

dermatome (der'-muh-tōm) – an instrument for cutting thin skin slices for skin grafts

devascularize (dē-vass"-kyoo-lah-rīz') – to interrupt the circulation of blood to a part causing obstruction or destruction of the blood vessels supplying it

diverticulum (pl. diverticula) (dī"-ver-tik'-yoo-lum) – a circumscribed pouch or sac of variable size occurring normally or created by herniation of the lining mucous membrane through a defect in the muscular coat of a tubular organ

ductus (duk'-tus) – a duct; a general term for a passage with well-defined walls, especially such a channel for the passage of excretions or secretions

duodenum (doo"-uh-dē'-num OR doo-ahd'-eh-num) – the first or proximal portion of the small intestine, extending from the pylorus to the jejunum

e

ecchymosis (ek"-ih-mō'-sis) – a small hemorrhagic spot in the skin or mucous membrane forming a nonelevated, rounded or irregular, blue or purplish patch

empyema (em"-pī-ē'-muh) – accumulation of pus in a cavity of the body

endarterectomy (end"-ar-ter-ek'-tuh-mē) – surgical removal of the lining of an artery

endothelium (en"-dō-thē'-lē-um) – the layer of epithelial cells that lines the cavities of the heart, the blood and lymph vessels, and the serous cavities of the body, originating from the mesoderm

enterocolectomy (en"-ter-ō-kō-lek'-tuh-mē) – resection of the intestines, including the ileum, cecum, and ascending colon

enucleation (ē-noo"-klē-ā'-shun) – the removal of an organ, a tumor, or another body in such a way that it comes out clean and whole, like a nut from its shell

epididymis (ep"-ih-did'-ih-mus) – the elongated, cord-like structure along the posterior border of the testis; spermatozoa are stored in the ducts

epiplocele (ē-pip'-lō-sēl) – a hernia that contains omentum

erythematous (er"-ih-thē'-muh-tus) – characterized by erythemia

eschar (es'-kar) – a slough produced by a thermal burn, by a corrosive application, or by gangrene

esophagogastrectomy (ē-sof"-uh-gō-gas-trek'-tuh-mē) – excision of the esophagus and stomach, usually the distal portion of the esophagus and the entire stomach

esophagogastroduodenoscopy (EGD) (ē-sof"-uh-gō-gas'-trō-doo"-od-eh-nahs'-kuh-pē) – endoscopic examination of the esophagus, stomach, and duodenum

esophagogastroduodenostomy (ē-sof"-uh-gō-gas'-trō-doo"-od-eh-nos'-tuh-mē) – the surgical creation of an opening into the stomach

esophagojejunostomy (ē-sof"-uh-gō-jeh-joo-nos'-tuh-mē) – surgical anastomosis between the esophagus and the jejunum

exacerbation (eg-zas"-er-bā'-shun) – aggravation of symptoms or increase in the severity of a disease

excavation (eks"-kuh-vā'-shun) – the act of hollowing out; a hollowed-out space or pouch-like cavity

extraperitoneal (eks"-truh-pair"-ih-tō-nē'-uhl) – situated or occurring outside the peritoneal cavity

extravasation (eks-trav"-uh-sā'-shun) – a discharge or escape, as of blood, from a vessel into the tissues

extubation (eks"-too-bā'-shun) – the removal of a previously inserted tube

f

fimbriated (fĭm'-brē-ā-ted) – fringed

fingerbreadth (fing'-ger-bredth") – a unit of length based on the breadth of one finger

fistulectomy (fis"-tyoo-lek'-tuh-mē) – excision of a fistulous tract

g

gastroduodenostomy (gas"-trō-doo"-ō-dē-nos'-tuh-mē) – surgical creation of an anastomosis between the stomach and the duodenum

gastroenteroanastomosis (gas"-trō-en"-ter-ō-ah-nas"-tuh-mō'-sis) – anastomosis between the stomach and small intestine in gastroenterostomy

gastroenterostomy (gas"-trō-en-ter-os'-tuh-mē) – surgical creation of an artificial passage between the stomach and intestines

gastroesophagostomy (gas"-trō-ē-sof"-uh-gos'-tuh-mē) – surgical creation of an anastomosis between the stomach and the esophagus

gastrojejunocolic (gas"-trō-jeh-joo"-nō-kol'-ik) – pertaining to or communicating with the stomach, jejunum, and colon

gastrostomy (gas-tros'-tuh-mē) – surgical creation of an artificial opening into the stomach; also, the opening so established

h

Hartmann's pouch of the colon (hart'-manz powch . . . kō'-lun) – an abnormal sacculation of the neck of the gallbladder

hematochezia (hēm"-uh-tō-kē'-zē-uh) – the passage of bloody stools

hemoperitoneum (hē"-mō-pair"-ih-tuh-nē'-um) – an effusion of blood in the peritoneal cavity

hernia (pl. herniae) (her'-nē-uh) – the protrusion of a loop or knuckle of an organ or a tissue through an abnormal opening

hernioplasty (her'-nē-ō-plas"-tē) – operation for the repair of a hernia

Hesselbach's hernia (hes'-ul-boks . . .) – hernia with a diverticulum through the cribriform fascia

Hirschsprung's disease (hirsh'-sproongz . . .) – megacolon due to failure of development of the myenteric plexus of the rectosigmoid area of the large intestine

hydrocele (hī'-druh-sēl) – a circumscribed collection of fluid, especially a collection of fluid in the tunica vaginalis of the testicle or along the spermatic cord

hyperplasia (hī"-per-plā'-zē-uh OR hī"-per-plā'-zhuh) – the abnormal multiplication or increase in the number of normal cells in normal arrangement in a tissue

i

ileostomy (il"-ē-os'-tuh-mē) – surgical creation of an opening into the ileum, usually by establishing an ileal stoma on the abdominal wall

in toto (in tō'-tō) – totally, entirely

insufflation (in"-su-flā'-shun) – the act of blowing a powder, vapor, gas, or air into a body cavity

intraluminal (in"-trah-loo'-mih-nul) – within the lumen of a tube, as of a blood vessel

ischiorectal (is"-kē-ō-rek'-tul) – pertaining to the ischium and rectum

isthmus (is'-thmus) – a narrow connection between two major bodies or parts

j

jejunectomy (jeh"-joo-nek'-tuk-mē) – excision of the jejunum

jejunojejunostomy (jeh"-joo"-nō-jeh"-joo-nos'-tuh-mē) – the operative formation of an anastomosis between two portions of the jejunum; also, the union so established

k

keloid (kē'-loid) – scar formation in the skin following trauma or surgical incision

keratotic (kār"-uh-taht'-ik) – pertaining to or characterized by keratosis

kerotic (ke-rot'-ik) – pertaining to, characterized by, or permitting keratosis, which is any horny growth, such as a wart or callosity

l

laryngectomy (lar"-in-jek'-tuh-mē) – extirpation of the larynx

Levin's tube (le-vinz' toob) – a gastroduodenal catheter of sufficiently small caliber to permit transnasal passage

ligament of Treitz (lig'-uh-ment uv trits) – a small ligamentous extension of the posterior peritoneum reflected upon to the duodenum as it emerges from the retroperitoneal area

liposarcoma (līp"-ō-sar-kō'-muh) – a malignant tumor derived from primitive or embryonal lipoblastic cells that exhibit varying degrees of lipoblastic and/or lipomatous differentiation

lymphadenectomy (lim-fuh"-dē-nek'-tuh-mē) – surgical excision of one or more lymph nodes

marsupialization (mar-soo"-pē-ul-ih-zā'-shun) – the creation of a pouch

Meckel's diverticulum (mek'-ulz dī"-ver-tik'-yoo-lum) – a congenital outpouching of the wall of the ileum 12 to 18 inches from the ileocecal junction

mesentery (mes'-en-ter"-ē) – a membranous fold attaching various organs to the body wall

mesocolon (mes"-ō-kō'-lon) – the process of the peritoneum by which the colon is attached to the posterior abdominal wall

mucocutaneous (myoo"-kō-kyoo-tā'-nē-us) – pertaining to or affecting the mucous membrane and the skin

nasolabial (nā"-zō-lā'-bē-ul) – pertaining to the nose and lip

Nissen fundoplication (nis'-en fun"-doh-pli-kā'-shun) – mobilization of the lower end of the esophagus and plication of the fundus of the stomach up around it, in treatment of reflux esophagitis

omentum (ō-men'-tum) – a fold of peritoneum extending from the stomach to adjacent organs in the abdominal cavity

orchiectomy (or"-kē-ek'-tuh-mē) – removal of one or both testes

paracentesis (pair"-uh-sen-tē'-sis) – surgical puncture of a cavity for the aspiration of fluid

paramedian (pair"-uh-mē'-dē-un) – situated near the midline or midplane

Parietex (pah-rī'-eh-teks) – composite mesh used for hernia surgery

Paritene (pah-rī'-teen) – mesh graft for hernia surgery

phlegmon (fleg'-mun) – acute suppurative inflammation of the subcutaneous connective tissue, often leading to ulceration or abscess; cellulitis

pneumatocele (noo-mat'-uh-sēl) – hernial protrusion of lung tissue, as through a congenital fissure of the chest

Pneumo Sleeve (noo'-mō slēv) – acts as an airlock during hand-assisted laparoscopic surgery (HALS procedure); contains the CO_2 used to fill the abdomen with air and provide working space

porta hepatis (por'-tuh hep'-uh-tis) – the transverse fissure on the visceral surface of the liver where the portal vein and hepatic artery enter the liver and the hepatic ducts leave

Poupart's ligament (poo-partz' lig'-uh-ment) – the inguinal ligament; a fibrous band running from the anterior superior spine of the ileum to the spine of the pubis

pyloromyotomy (pī-lō"-rō-mī-ot'-uh-mē) – incision of the longitudinal and circular muscles of the pylorus; Fredet-Ramstedt's operation

pyloroplasty (pī-lō'-rō-plas"-tē) – surgical repair of the pylorus, especially by stretching the pyloric opening

rectosigmoid (rek"-tō-sig'-moid) – the lower portion of the sigmoid and upper portion of the rectum

retrocolic (ret"-rō-kol'-ik) – behind the colon

salpinx (sahl'-pinks) – a tube

Scarpa's fascia (skar'-puhz fash'-ē-uh) – a sheet of thin, ligament-like tissue passing from the midabdominal line to the dorsal root of the penis and to the symphysis pubis; very low in the pelvis of the male

serosanguineous (sē"-rō-sang-gwin'-ē-us) – pertaining to or containing both serum and blood

sphincteroplasty (sfink'-ter-uh-plas"-tē) – surgical repair of a defective sphincter

splenectomy (spleh-nek'-tuh-mē) – excision or complete removal of the spleen

stent sutures (stent soo'-churz) – stent graft or surgical dressings

stylet/stilet/stilette (stī'-let) – a wire run through a catheter or cannula to render it stiff or to remove debris from its lumen

tomography (tuh-mog'-ruh-fē) – a special technique to show in detail images of structures lying in a predetermined plane of tissue, while blurring or eliminating detail in images of structures in the other planes

tracheostomy (trā"-kē-os'-tuh-mē) – the surgical creation of an opening into the trachea through the neck; also, the opening so created

transversalis fascia (trans"-ver-sal'-is fash'-ē-uh) – part of the inner investing layer of the abdominal wall, continuous with the fascia of the other side behind the rectus abdominis and the rectus sheath

Trendelenburg (tren-del'-en-burg) – surgeon in Leipzig; an examination position

trocar (trō'-car) – a cannula with a sharp-pointed obturator for piercing the wall of a cavity

U

ultrasonography (ul"-truh-sō-nog'-ruh-fē) – the visualization of deep structures of the body by recording the reflection of ultrasonic waves directed into the tissues

Unna's paste boot (oo'-nahz pāst boot) – a dressing for varicose ulcers

V

vagotomy (vā-got'-uh-mē) – surgical division of the vagus nerve

vermilion (ver-mil'-yun) – the exposed red portion of the upper and lower lip

vermilionectomy (ver-mil"-yun-ek'-tuh-mē) – excision of the vermilion border of the lip, the surgically created defect being resurfaced by advancement of the undermined labial mucosa

verruca (veh-roo'-kuh) – an epidermal tumor caused by a papillomavirus

X

xanthelasma (zan"-thel-az'-muh) – the most common form of xanthoma affecting the eyelids; characterized by soft yellowish spots or plaques

Xeroform (zē'-rō-form) – a gauze dressing

xiphoid (zī'-foid) – shaped like a sword; the xiphoid process

Transcription Tips

When transcribing surgery dictation, you will find the process much easier if you are familiar with

- surgical body positions
- names of instruments used
- abdominal regions of the body
- directional terms
- types of catheters used
- types of sutures and suture materials
- names of medications administered
- types of anesthesia administered

Details concerning suture types, confusing words, operative positions, directional terms, and types of anesthesia are presented later in this section. Study the information contained in the figures presented earlier in this chapter and the material presented in the Appendix for details relating to the other topics. Consult one of the Web pages referenced in this chapter or one of the other resources listed in this text for more detailed information concerning the topics.

Tessier's *The Surgical Word Book* and Pyle's *Current Medical Terminology* are valuable resources for locating words used in surgery. To locate a type of suture and/or suture material, for example, look under "suture"; you will find many terms listed. Other entries, such as "forceps," "catheters," "bur," and "prosthesis," for example, also list many types.

The following is a selected listing of suture types. Many others exist; consult a reference for other types.

Bunnell	figure-of-eight	Mersilene	rhabdoid
catgut	fish-mouth	Nurolon	silk
Cloward	Halsted	PDS	Sturmdorf
Dacron	harelip	pledgeted	Teflon-coated
Deknatel	lambdoid	plicating	Tevdek
Dermalon	LeFort	Polydek	Tycron *or* Ti-Cron
Dexon	Lembert	Prolene	Vicryl
Ethibond	limbal	pursestring	Y-sutures

Confusing Terms

colectomy – excision of a portion of the colon

colpectomy – excision of the vagina

epithelial – pertaining to the covering of internal and external surfaces of the body, including the lining of vessels and other small cavities

endothelial – pertaining to or made up of the layer of epithelial cells that link the cavities of the heart

hemithorax – one side of the chest

hemothorax – a collection of blood in the pleural cavity

pneumothorax – accumulation of air or gas in the pleural space

hemostasis – the arrest of bleeding

homeostasis – a tendency to stability in the normal body states of the organism

peritoneum – the serous membrane lining the abdominopelvic walls

perineum – the pelvic floor and the associated structures occupying the pelvic outlet

peroneal – refers to the fibula or to the outer side of the leg

serous – pertains to or resembles serum

serious – said or done in earnest; sincere

Commonly Used Operative Positions

supine – Patient lies flat on back with arms at side, palms down with fingers extended and free to rest on the table; legs are straight with feet slightly separated. This position is commonly used for hernia repair, exploratory laparotomy, cholecystectomy, gastric and bowel resection, and mastectomy.

prone – Patient lies on abdomen with face turned to one side and arms at side with palms pronated and fingers extended. This position is used for surgery on the back, spine, and rectal area.

Trendelenburg – Patient's head and body are lowered into a head-down position; knees are flexed by breaking the table and the patient is held in position by padded shoulder braces. The Trendelenburg position is used for operations on the lower abdomen and the pelvis to obtain good exposure by a displacement of the intestines into the upper abdomen.

Selected Operative Positions for Specialized Surgery

lithotomy – Patient lies on back with buttocks positioned at the break in the operating table; after the patient is anesthetized, the thighs and legs are flexed at right angles and simultaneously placed in stirrups; the lithotomy position is used in perineal, rectal, and vaginal surgery.

lateral – Various versions of the lateral position are used for surgery on the kidney and the chest; the kidney position is used for nephrectomy and pyelolithotomy.

Special positions may be necessary to place the operative site in the best possible position. One example would be the thyroid exposure. The patient lies on his or her back with the head hyperextended and a small sandbag, pillow, or thyroid rest under neck and shoulders to provide exposure of the thyroid gland.

Directional Terms

anterior – used synonymously with "cranial" in quadrupeds and with "ventral" in bipeds

caudal – the tail end (caudad—toward the tail)

cephalic – toward the head

cranial or **cephalic** – the head end (cephalad—toward the head)

distal – used in conjunction with proximal, meaning farther away from the trunk; farthest from point of attachment (distad—away from the trunk)

dorsal – the back side (dorsad—toward the back)

exterior – outside

inferior – the lower portion or that which is below

internal – inside

lateral – refers to a location farther from the midline than another location (laterad—away from the midline)

medial – refers to a location nearer to the midline than another location (mediad—toward the midline)

median – the middle or midline

midline – an imaginary plane that bisects the body into right and left halves

peripheral – at or near the suface of the body

plantar – referring to the sole of the foot

posterior – used synonymously with "caudal" in quadrupeds and with "dorsal" in bipeds

proximal – commonly used with reference to the appendages, meaning that portion which is nearer the trunk or main body mass (nearest to point of attachment to the trunk; proximad—toward the trunk)

superior – the upper portion or that which is above

ventral – the belly side (ventrad—toward the belly)

Types of Anesthesia

The choice of anesthesia is based on many factors: the physical condition and age of the patient; the presence of coexisting diseases; the type, site, and duration of the operation; and the personal preference of the anesthesiologist or anesthetist.

General anesthesia is produced by inhalation of gases or vapors of highly volatile liquids or by injection into the bloodstream of anesthetic drugs in solution. Certain drugs that produce general anesthesia such as *thiopental sodium* (Pentothal sodium) are used to put the patient to sleep and are almost always supplemented with other agents to produce surgical anesthesia.

Inhalation anesthesia is produced by having the patient inhale the vapors of certain liquids or gases.

Regional anesthesia is produced by the injection or application of a local anesthetic agent along the course of a nerve.

Topical anesthesia is accomplished by applying or spraying a local anesthetic drug, such as cocaine or lidocaine, directly onto the part to be anesthetized.

Infiltration anesthesia is accomplished by injection of the anesthetic drug directly into the area to be incised or manipulated.

Spinal anesthesia is accomplished by injection of a local anesthetic drug in solution into the subarachnoid space, which contains spinal fluid.

Epidural block occurs when an anesthetic agent is injected between the vertebral spines and beneath the ligamentum flavum in the extradural space; also called peridural anesthesia.

IV sedation is achieved by introduction of an anesthetic agent intravenously.

Conscious sedation (moderate sedation) is a drug-induced depression of consciousness during which patients respond purposefully to verbal commands and are able to maintain a patent airway and spontaneous ventilation.

Types of Intravenous Anesthesia Agents

Thiopental sodium (Pentothal sodium) is the drug used most frequently for induction of anesthesia.

Ketamine is a nonbarbiturate, parenteral anesthetic agent. It produces an anesthetic state termed *dissociative anesthesia.* It is a substance permitting surgical operations on patients who may appear to be awake since movement may occur and the eyes remain open.

Other Types of Anesthesia Agents

Amidate (etomidate) – quick onset, short-acting IV induction agent

Brevital (methohexital) – ultra-short-acting IV agent for induction

Diprivan (propofol) – sedative hypnotic IV agent used for induction and maintenance of general anesthesia

Fluothane (halothane) – highly potent, nonflammable, colorless liquid with a sweet smell

Forane (isoflurane) – volatile inhalation anesthetic agent with a pungent, ether-like odor

Nitrous oxide – nonirritating, odorless, colorless, nonflammable gas

Suprane (desflurane) – one of the newest inhalation agents; has a strong, pungent odor

Ultane (sevoflurane) – the newest inhalation gas; pleasant odor

Versed, Valium (benzodiazepines) – sedatives that can be used for induction

Supportive Web Sites

www.ccspublishing.com (Click on "Journal of Surgery")

www.findarticles.com (Search for "surgery")

www.mayoclinic.com (Search for "surgery")

www.mindspring.com/~videosur/

www.netsurgery.com

www.onlinesurgery.com

Index of General Surgery Reports

(see table of contents for audio information)

Exercise #	Patient Name	Report/Procedure
TE#1	*Boleware, Rebecca*	*Groshong catheter insertion*
TE#2	*Jenkins, Amanda*	*Insertion of vagal nerve stimulator*
TE#3	*Reynolds, Denita*	*Heart/lung transplant*
TE#4	*Powell, Dennis T.*	*Repair of abdominal aortic aneurysm with Ancure device and angioplasty*
TE#5	*Tucker, Dylan*	*Repair of hiatus paraesophageal-type hernia; partial colectomy*
TE#6	*Murdock, Glenn*	*Antrectomy, anastomosis, and jejunostomy*
TE#7	*Jones, Russell*	*Parathyroid resection*
TE#8	*Andrews, Christy*	*H&P and OR—endoscopic gastrostomy*
TE#9	*Zaleski, Jeff*	*Repair of abdominal aortic aneurysm using an endoluminal Ancure device*

CHAPTER 3
CARDIOLOGY

Introduction

The *cardiovascular system* has numerous functions, two of which are carrying oxygen from the lungs to individual cells and transporting carbon dioxide from the cells back to the lungs. This system is composed of the *heart, blood vessels,* and *blood;* blood consists of *cells* and *plasma.*

The primary duty of the heart, which is the functional center of the system, is to act as a muscular pump propelling blood into and through vessels to and from all parts of the body. The heart beats in two phases. In *diastole,* or relaxation, the ventricle walls relax and blood flows into the heart from the venae cavae and pulmonary veins. When the walls of the right and left ventricles contract *(systole),* blood is pumped into the pulmonary artery and the aorta. This cycle of relaxation and contraction occurs approximately 100,000 times a day, pumping about 2000 gallons of blood through the body. After the heart performs the function of pumping the blood, the network of blood vessels *(vascular system)* carries the blood to all parts of the body.

The blood travels in a circular route beginning and ending at the same place. This course starts at the heart and is composed of the *arteries, arterioles, capillaries, vessels,* and *veins.* An artery is a blood vessel that carries blood away from the heart; a vein is a blood vessel that carries blood back to the heart.

The rhythm of the heart is controlled by the *sinoatrial node,* or pacemaker, of the heart. Normal rhythm is called *sinus rhythm.* The force exerted on arterial walls by blood is called *blood pressure.* Medical personnel use a *sphygmomanometer* to measure blood pressure, which is recorded as a fraction with systolic pressure over the diastolic pressure.

Diagnostic procedures for treating heart problems consist of laboratory tests and clinical procedures. A *lipid profile* is a blood test that measures the amounts of *cholesterol* and *triglycerides* in a blood sample. *Lipoprotein electrophoresis* is a laboratory test that separates lipoproteins (proteins that transport lipids, or fats, in the blood) from a blood sample. A *serum enzyme* test is used to measure enzymes released from the dying heart muscle into the bloodstream during a *myocardial infarction.*

Examples of clinical procedures employed to assess cardiovascular fitness and/or problems are x-ray tests such as angiography and digital subtraction angiography. Other procedures include *echocardiogram, Doppler ultrasound, catheterization, cardiac scan, cardiac MRI, Holter monitoring, stress test,* and *angioplasty.* During angioplasty, physicians may insert either a balloon or a *stent* to open an occluded artery.

The specialty of vascular surgery concerns itself with the diagnosis, repair, and reconstruction of heart and blood vessel defects.

Critical Thinking Exercise

You work for Dr. Brett Liuji, a cardiologist. Your friend Deanna calls you one night and says, "Jennifer told me she was going to see Dr. Liuji today. What did he find wrong with her?"

How do you respond to Deanna?

Cardiology Abbreviations

A2	aortic second sound
AAA	abdominal aortic aneurysm
ABG	arterial blood gas
ACLS	advanced cardiac life support
ACT	activated clotting time

AF, A Fib	atrial fibrillation
A Flt	atrial flutter
AI	aortic insufficiency
AICD	automatic implantable cardioverter defibrillator
AIVR	accelerated idioventricular rhythm
AMI	aortic myocardial infarction
AP	anteroposterior
AR	aortic regurgitation, aortic insufficiency
AS	aortic stenosis
ASD	atrial septal defect
ASH	asymmetrical septal hypertrophy
ASHD	arteriosclerotic heart disease
ASPVD	atherosclerotic peripheral vascular disease
AST	aspartate aminotransferase
ATS	autotransfusion system
AV, A-V	atrioventricular node
AVB	atrioventricular block
AVG	aortic valve gradient
AVR	aortic valve replacement
BBB	bundle branch block
bFGF	basic fibroblast growth factor
BiVAD	bi-ventricular assist device
BP	blood pressure
BVH	biventricular hypertrophy
CAB	coronary artery bypass
CABG	coronary artery bypass graft
CABRI	coronary artery bypass revascularization investigation
CAD	coronary artery disease
cath	catheterization
CAVH	continuous arterio-venous hemofiltration
CC	cardiac catheterization
CCP	Certified Cardiovascular Perfusionist
CCU	coronary care unit
CHD	coronary heart disease
CHF	congestive heart failure
CI	cardiac index
CPB	cardiopulmonary bypass
CPK	creatine phosphokinase (released into bloodstream following injury to heart or skeletal muscles)
CPR	cardiopulmonary resuscitation
CT	cardiothoracic ratio
CTICU	cardiothoracic intensive care unit
CV	cardiovascular
CVA	cerebrovascular accident
cva	costovertebral angle
CVP	central venous pressure
DHCA	deep hypothermic circulatory arrest
DILV	double inlet left ventricle
DOE	dyspnea on exertion
DOLV	double outlet left ventricle
DORV	double outlet right ventricle
DSA	digital subtraction angiography
DVT	deep venous thrombosis; deep vein thrombosis
ECA	external carotid artery
ECC	extracorporeal circulation
ECD	endocardial cushion defect
ECG/EKG	electrocardiogram
ECHO	echocardiography
ECMO	extracorporeal membrane oxygenation
ECT	extracorporeal circulation technology
EECP	enhanced external counter pulsation
EF	ejection fraction
EP	electrophysiology
ERP	effective refractory period
ETT	exercise tolerance test
FHS	fetal heart sound
FRP	functional refractory period
HCVD	hypertensive cardiovascular disease
HDL	high-density lipoproteins
H&L	heart and lungs
HLHS	hyperplastic left heart syndrome
HPCD	hemostatic puncture closure device
HV	hallux valgus
HVD	hypertensive vascular disease
IAPB	intra-aortic balloon pump
IASD	interatrial septal defect
ICA	internal carotid artery
IHSS	idiopathic hypertrophic subaortic stenosis
IMA	inferior mesenteric artery or internal mammary artery
IV	intravenous
IVC	inferior vena cava
IVCD	interventricular conduction defect
IVSD	interventricular septal defect

LA	left atrium
LAD	left anterior descending coronary artery
LBBB	left bundle branch block
LD	lactic dehydrogenase
LDH	lactate dehydrogenase (enzyme released from dying heart muscle)
LDL	low-density lipoproteins
LIMA	left internal mammary artery
LV	left ventricle
LVAD	left ventricular assist device
LVEDP	left ventricular end diastolic pressure
LVF	left ventricular failure
LVH	left ventricular hypertrophy
M2	mitral second sound
MI	mitral insufficiency or myocardial infarction
MIDCAB	minimally invasive direct coronary artery bypass
MR	mitral regurgitation
MS	mitral stenosis
MUGA	multiple-gated acquisition scan (radioactive test of heart function)
MVP	mitral valve prolapse
NSR	normal sinus rhythm
OHS	open heart surgery
OPG	ocular plethysmography
P2	pulmonic second sound
PA	pulmonary artery
PAC	premature atrial contraction
PAT	paroxysmal atrial tachycardia
PCI	percutaneous coronary intervention
PCWP	pulmonary capillary wedge pressure
PDA	patent ductus arteriosus
PICVA	percutaneous in situ coronary venous arterialization
PMI	point of maximum impulse
PND	paroxysmal (sudden) nocturnal dyspnea (often a symptom of congestive heart failure)
PT	prothrombin time
PTCA	percutaneous transluminal coronary angioplasty
PTT	partial thromboplastin time
PV	pulmonary valve
PVC	premature ventricular contraction
PVD	peripheral vascular disease
RA	right atrium
RAH	right atrial hypertrophy
RBBB	right bundle branch block
RCA	right coronary artery
RFA	radio frequency ablation
RHD	rheumatic heart disease
RIMA	right internal mammary artery
RRP	relative refractory period
RSR	regular sinus rhythm
RV	right ventricle
RVH	right ventricular hypertrophy
SA, S-A	sinoatrial
SACT	sinoatrial conduction times
SCD	sudden cardiac death
SGOT	serum glutamic oxaloacetic transaminase or serum glutamic oxalic
SGPT	serum glutamic pyruvic transaminase
SV	stroke volume
SVC	superior vena cava
SVG	saphenous vein graft
SVPT	supraventricular premature contraction
TEE	transesophageal echocardiography
TGA	transposition of the great arteries
TI	tricuspid insufficiency
TIA	transient ischemic attack
TOF	tetralogy of Fallot
tPA	tissue-type plasminogen activator (drug used to prevent thromboses)
TR	tricuspid regurgitation
TS	triscupid stenosis
TV	triscupid valve
VAD	ventricular assist device
VDH	valvular disease of heart
VEGF	vascular endothelial growth factor
VHD	valvular heart disease
VLDL	very low density lipoproteins
VPC	ventricular premature contraction
VSD	ventricular septal defect
VT, V tach	ventricular tachycardia

Anatomic Illustrations

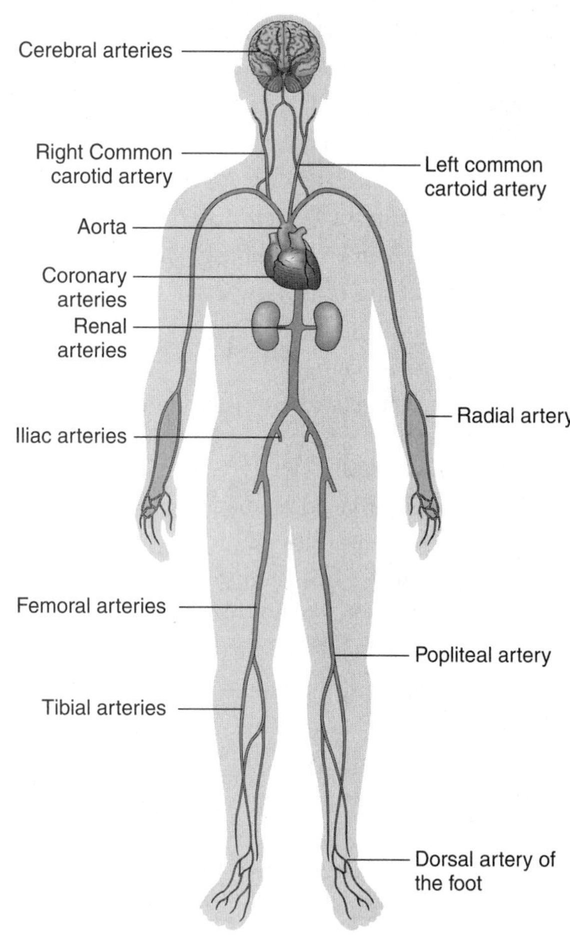

3–1 ARTERIOLE SYSTEM OF THE BODY

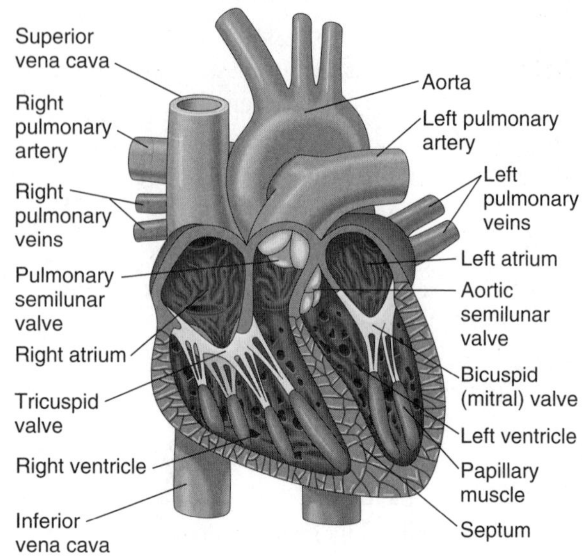

3–2 PULMONARY ARTERIES AND VEINS OF THE HEART

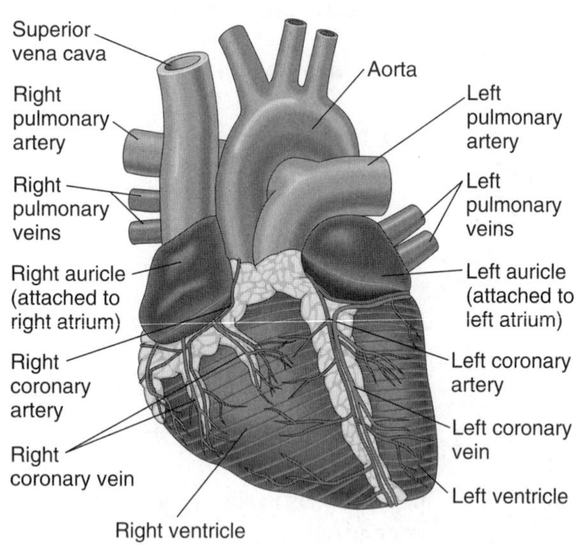

3–3 HEART AND GREAT VESSELS

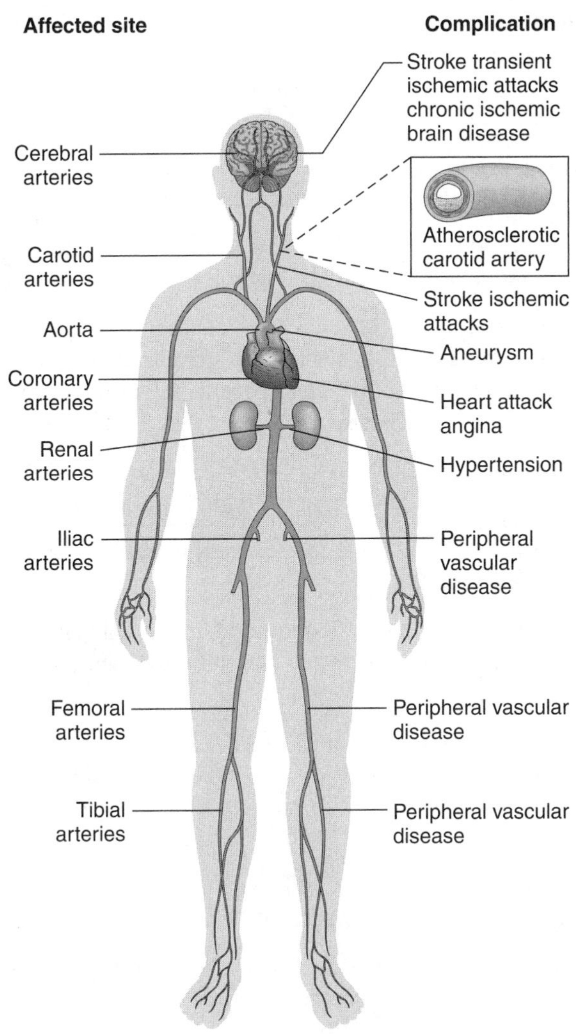

3-4 ARTERIES AFFECTED BY ATHEROSCLEROSIS AND THE RESULTING COMPLICATIONS

Cardiology Terminology

a

ablation (uh-blā'-shun) – to remove or destroy tissue that is suspected of causing irregular heartbeats (arrhythmia)

aneurysm (an'-yoo-rizm) – ballooning out of a portion of a blood vessel (usually an artery) due to a congenital defect or a weakness in the wall of a blood vessel

aneurysmectomy (an"-yoo-riz-mek'-tuh-mē) – the surgical removal of an aneurysm by removing the sac

angina pectoris (an-jī'-nuh OR an'-jih-nah pek-tor'-is) – a paroxysmal thoracic pain with a feeling of suffocation and impending death due most often to anoxia of the myocardium and precipitated by effort or excitement

AngioJet Rheolytic thrombectomy system (an'-jē-ō-jet rē-ō-lih-tik throm-bec'-tuh-mē sis'-tum) – device that employs a minimally invasive catheter system to remove intravascular blood clots from leg and arm arteries and bypass grafts

angioplasty (an'-jē-ō-plas"-tē) – alteration of the structure of a vessel by surgical procedure or by dilating the vessel using a balloon inside the lumen

Angio-Seal (an'-jē-ō-sēl) – a hemostatic puncture closure device used after interventional or diagnostic vascular procedures to seal the arteriotomy

aortic atresia (ā-or'-tik uh-trē'-zē-uh) – small or undeveloped aortic valve

aortocoronary bypass (ā"-or-tō-kōr'-ō-nār-ē bī-pass) – coronary bypass

aortotomy (ā"-or-tah'-tuh-mē) – surgical incision into the aorta

arrhythmia (uh-rith'-mē-uh) – any variation from the normal heartbeat

arteriosclerosis (ar-tē"-rē-ō-skle-rō'-sis) – a group of diseases characterized by thickening and loss of elasticity of arterial walls

arteriotomy (ar"-tē-rē-ot'-uh-mē) – division or opening of an artery by surgery

asynchronous (ā-sing'-kruh-nus) – a fixed-rate type of pacemaker that discharges regular impulses despite the intrinsic rhythm or rate of the heart

atherectomy (ah-ther-ek'-tuh-mē) – procedure done to remove plaque from artery either by blade or rotation (rotablade)

atheromatous (ath"-er-ō'-muh-tus) – affected with a mass or plaque of degenerated, thickened arterial intima occurring in atherosclerosis

atriotomy (ā"-trē-ot'-uh-mē) – surgical incision of an atrium of the heart

automatic implantable cardioverter defibrillator (AICD) (aw-tuh-mat'-ik im-plan'-tuh-bul car-dē-ō-ver'-tur dē-fih'-brih-lā-tur) – a device that is surgically implanted to monitor the heartbeat; if it senses rapid irregular heartbeats, it delivers an electric shock to the patient's heart

b

Beta-Cath System (bā'-tuh-kath sis'-tum) – device designed to prevent an artery from renarrowing following angioplasty or stent placement

bigeminy (bī-jem'-ih-nē) – any arrhythmia that occurs in pairs; sometimes refers to a normal beat followed by a premature beat

brachytherapy (brak"-ē-ther'-uh-pē) – a procedure that employs low-level radiation to reduce recurrence of blockage by scar tissue in previously stented arteries

bradycardia (brā"-dē-kar'-dē-uh) – abnormally slow heart rate (less than 60 beats per minute)

c

cardiac output (CO) (kar'-dē-ak owt'-put) – the amount of blood usually ejected by the left ventricle in one minute

cardiac reserve (kar'-dē-ak rē-zerv) – the ability of the heart to increase its cardiac output during stress, normally 300%–400% above resting values

cardiogenic shock (kar"-dē-ō-jen'-ik shok) – failure to maintain blood supply to tissues because of inadequate cardiac output

cardiomyopathy (kar"-dē-ō-mī-op'-uh-thē) – a general diagnostic term designating primary myocardial disease, often of obscure or unknown etiology

cardioplegia (kar"-dē-ō-plē'-jē-uh) – interruption of contraction of the myocardium as may be induced by the use of chemical compounds or of cold (cryocardioplegia) in the performance of surgery upon the heart

cardiopulmonary bypass (kar"-dē-ō-pul'-muh-nair-ē bī'-pass) – procedure employed during open-heart surgery whereby a heart-lung machine takes over the functions of the heart and lungs

CardioTek (kar'-dē"-ō-tek) – electrophysiologic tracer (a machine that prints out tracings during an EKG)

cardiotomy (kar"-dē-ot'-uh-mē) – surgical incision into the heart to repair cardiac defects

cardioversion (kar"-dē-ō-ver'-zhun) – the restoration of a normal rhythm of the heart by electric shock

cineangiocardiography (sin"-ē-an"-jē-ō-kar"dē-og'-ruh-fē) – study of the chambers of the heart and pulmonary circulation by the use of motion picture techniques (while the structures are in motion) following injection of radiopaque material

congestive heart failure (CHF) (kun-jest'-iv hart fail'-yoor) – inability of the heart to maintain normal circulation, resulting in shortness of breath and abnormal fluid retention

cor pulmonale (kōr pul'-mō-nal) – heart disease due to pulmonary hypertension secondary to diseases of the blood vessels of the lungs

coupling interval (kup'-ling in'-ter-vul) – when utilizing a pacemaker to introduce a premature impulse, the time between the last normal beat and the premature beat

Crafoord clamps, scissors, forceps (krā'-foord . . .) – instruments used in heart and lung operations

d

defibrillation (dē-fib"-rih-lā'-shun) – the termination of ventricular fibrillation by electric shock

depolarization (dē-pō"-lahr-ih-zā'-shun) – when a cardiac muscle cell is electrically stimulated, a change in membrane permeability permits the inside of the cell to become positive with regard to the outside

dextrocardia (deks"-trō-kar'-dē-uh) – location of the heart on the right side of the midline of the chest

dyspneic (disp'-nē'-ik) – characterized by difficult or labored breathing

e

echocardiogram (ek"-ō-kar'-dē-ō-gram") – a diagnostic test used to measure the structure and function of the heart

effective refractory period (ERP) (ē-fek'-tiv rē-frak'-tuh-rē pēr'-ē-ud) – the same as absolute refractory period; that period of time just after depolarization when the cardiac cell cannot be stimulated

electrogram (ē-lek'-trō-gram) – any record produced by changes in electrical potential

embolectomy (em"-bō-lek'-tuh-mē) – surgical removal of an embolus or clot from a blood vessel

endarterectomy (end"-ar-ter-ek'-tuh-mē) – removal of the interior portion of an artery

endocardium (en"-dō-kar'-dē-um) – the innermost lining of the heart

endothelium (en"-dō-thē'-lē-um) – the monocellular lining of blood vessels, heart, and lymphatic system

Ethibond suture (eth'-ih-bond soo'-cher) – a type of suture material

External CounterPulsation therapy (ECP) (eks-ter'-nul kown'-ter-puhl-sā'-shun ther'-uh-pē) – a noninvasive procedure for chronic angina pectoris that stimulates the formation of small branches of blood vessels (collaterals), thereby increasing blood flow around blocked arteries

f

femoropopliteal bypass (fem"-ō-rō-pop-lit'-ē-ul bī-pass) – vascular prosthesis that bypasses an obstruction in the femoral artery

foramen ovale (for-ā'-men ō'-vahl-ē) – in the fetal heart, the oval opening in the septum secundum; the persistent part of the septum primum acts as a valve for this interatrial communication during fetal life and postnatally becomes fused to the septum secundum to close it

fusion beat (fyoo'-zhun bēt) – the result of a normal and abnormal impulse stimulating the ventricles simultaneously

g

Glidewire (glīd'-wīr) – trade (brand) name of a coated, kink-resistant, guided wire used in endourology procedures

h

heparinization (heh'-puh-rin-ih-zā'-shun) – treatment with heparin to increase the clotting time of the blood

hyperperfusion (hī"-per-per-fyoo'-zhun) – increased blood flow to an organ or tissue

hypertrophic cardiomyopathy (hī"-per-trō'-fik kar"-dē-ō-mī-op'-uh-thē) – disease of the myocardium produced by enlargement of the cells of the myocardium

hypoxia (hī-pok'-sē-uh) – oxygen deficiency

i

idioventricular rhythm (ih"-dē-ō-ven-trik'-yoo-lur rih'-thum) – relating to or affecting the cardiac ventricle alone

inotropic agent (in"-ō-trōp'-ik ā'-jent) – that which affects the force of energy of muscular contractions. Negative weakens and positive strengthens; these are usually drugs

interpolated (in"-ter-pō'-lā-ted) – refers to a premature beat that does not interrupt the regularity of the basic rhythm

intramyocardial (in"-truh-mī"-ō-kar'-dē-ul) – within the myocardium, the heart muscle

ischemia (iss-kē'-mē-uh) – deficiency of blood to the heart muscle

isoelectric line (ī"-sō-ē-lek'-trik līn) – on an ECG, the point of departure for the P wave, QRS complex, and T wave; reflects those portions in the cycle when no difference exists in the electrical charges across the myocardial muscle cell wall

j

joule (jool) – a unit of energy equivalent to 1 watt-second

l

LOA cines (el-ō-ā sin'-ēz) – left occipitoanterior position

m

mannitol (man'-ih-tol) – an IV solution used in varying concentrations (5, 10, 15, 20%) as an osmotic diuretic; used to prevent oliguria during surgical procedures

mitral regurgitation (mī'-trul rē-gur"-jih-tā'-shun) – abnormal systolic backflow of blood from the left ventricle into the left atrium, resulting from imperfect closure of the mitral valve

mitral valve (mī'-trul valv) – the valve between the left atrium and left ventricle

morphology (mor-fol'-uh-jē) – the structure and form, often meaning the form of an irregular heart rhythm (arrhythmia)

myocardium (mī"-ō-kar'-dē-um) – the middle and thickest layer of the heart; it lies between the endocardium (the inner lining) and the epicardium (the outer covering) of the heart

n

nodal (nō'-dul) – refers to the atrioventricular (AV) node

NOGA mapping system (nō'-guh map'-ing sis'-tum) – diagnostic procedure that employs magnets to produce a three-dimensional, real-time image of the heart; appreciably reduces x-ray exposure of the patient

o

ostium primum (os'-tē-um prē-mum) – an opening in the lowest aspect of the septum primum of the embryonic heart, posteriorly, in the neighborhood of the atrioventricular valve

ostium secundum (os'-tē-um seh-kun'-dum) – an opening high in the septum primum of the embryonic heart, approximately where the foramen ovale will be later

p

parenchymal (pah"-reng'-kih-mul) – pertaining to or of the nature of parenchyma, which refers to the essential elements of an organ; a general term to designate the functional elements of an organ

Perclose closure device (pur'-klōz klō'-zhur dih-vīs') – a suture device

perfusion scan (per-fyoo'-zhun skan) – a test to determine the status of blood flow to an organ

perfusionist (per-fyoo'-zhun-ist) – uses artificial blood pumps to propel blood through a patient's body tissue, replacing the function of the heart during open-heart surgery

perfusion technologist (per-fyoo'-zhun tek-nol'-uh-jist) – the health professional educated to operate the heart-lung machine and other life support devices

pericarditis (pair"-ih-kar-dī'-tis) – inflammation of the pericardium

peroneal artery (per"-ō-nē'-ul ar'-ter-ē) – artery located on the outer side of the leg; fibular artery

premature ventricular contraction (prē"-muh-choor' ven-trik'-yoo-lur kun-trak'-shun) – an irregular heartbeat that comes before the next regular beat is expected

profunda femoris artery (prō-fun'-duh fem'-uh-ris ar'-ter-ē) – deep femoral artery

pulmonary atresia (puhl'-muh-nair'-ē uh-trē'-zē-uh) – small or undeveloped pulmonary valve

Purkinje fibers (pur-kin'-jē fī-burz) – specialized cardiac muscle fibers that conduct the impulse from the right and left bundle branches to the cells of the ventricle

q

quadrigeminy (kwod"-rih-jem'-ih-nē) – quadrigeminal or four-fold rhythm

r

rami communicans (rā'-mī kuh-myoo'-nih-kanz) – a communicating branch between two nerves; a branch connecting two arteries

reanastomosis (rē-uh-nas"-tuh-mō'-sis) – a reattachment between two vessels by collateral channels

s

saphenous vein (suh-fē'-nus vān) – pertaining to or associated with a saphena, which is either of two larger superficial veins of the leg

supraventricular (soo"-pruh-ven-trik'-yoo-lur) – a heartbeat originating "above" the ventricles

synchronous (sing'-krō-nus) – refers to an on-demand type of pacemaker

syncope (sing'-kuh-pē) – extreme dizziness or fainting due to lack of blood to the brain

systole (sis'-tuh-lē) – portion of the heart cycle in which the heart muscle fibers are contracting

t

tachycardia (tak"-ē-kar'-dē-uh) – a rapid heart rhythm greater than 100 beats per minute

transducer (tranz-doo'-ser) – a device that translates one form of energy to another (e.g., the pressure, temperature, or pulse to an electrical signal)

transmyocardial revascularization (TMR) (tranz"-mī"-ō-kar'-dē-ul rē-vas"-kyoo-lar-ih-zā'-shun) – a state-of-the-art laser used during open-heart surgery to create new pathways in the heart muscle

tricuspid atresia (trī-kus'-pid uh-trē'-zē-uh) – small or undeveloped tricuspid valve

tricuspid valve (trī-kus'-pid) – the valve that lies between the right atrium and right ventricle

u

unifocal (yoo"-nih-fō'-kul) – an irregular heartbeat (arrhythmia) that has one point of origin

v

vagus nerve (vā'-gus nurv) – this nerve slows the heart rate when stimulated; it is the tenth cranial nerve and part of the parasympathetic nervous system

Valsalva's maneuver (val-sal'-vah muh"-noo'-ver) – bearing down, or a forced exhalation effort against a closed throat; this causes stimulation of the vagus nerve and usually slows the heart

valvuloplasty (val'-vyoo-lō-plas"-tē) – plastic operation on a valve

valvulotomy (val"-vyoo-lot'-uh-mē) – an incision into a diseased and stenosed cardiac valve made to increase the valve area

vasodilator (vā"-zō-dī'-lā-tur) – any agent (usually a drug) that causes the blood vessels to dilate, thereby reducing the force against which the heart must pump the blood

vasopressor (vā"-zō-pres'-ur) – stimulating contraction of the muscular tissue of the capillaries and arteries; an agent that stimulates contractions of the muscular tissue of the capillaries and arteries

venotomy (phlebotomy) (vē-not'-uh-mē, fle-bot'-uh-mē) – incision into a vein, as for the letting of blood

ventricular fibrillation (ven-trik'-yoo-lur fih-bri-la'-shun) – rapid random quivering of the ventricles; essentially no blood is pumped during this arrhythmia, which leads to death unless reversed by electric shock (defibrillation)

ventricular tachycardia (ven-trik'-yoo-lur tak"-ē-kar'-dē-uh) – an arrhythmia that originates in the ventricles at a rate of 150–250 beats per minute

visceromegaly (vis"-er-ō-meg'-uh-lē) – enlargement of viscera

Transcription Tips

When transcribing cardiology dictation, you will find the task easier if you are familiar with the structure of the heart and accompanying terms. For example, you should be able to recognize the chambers of the heart, the names of the valves, and the names and locations of arteries.

Familiarity with sound-alike words, combining forms, frequently occurring terms, and common manifestations of heart disease will also make your transcription more accurate.

Heart chambers – right atrium, right ventricle, left atrium, and left ventricle
Valves – tricuspid, bicuspid or mitral, pulmonary semilunar, and aortic semilunar

Names and Locations of Arteries

radial – radial (or thumb side) of the wrist

brachial – in the bend of the elbow

carotid – in the neck

temporal – at the temple

femoral – in the groin

Confusing Terms

arrhythmia – irregular heartbeat

eurhythmia – regular pulse

arteriosclerosis – hardening of the arteries

arteriostenosis – narrowing of the space within an artery

atherosclerosis – a form of arteriosclerosis

arteriotomy – surgical opening of an artery

arteriotony – blood pressure

arteritis – inflammation of an artery

arthritis – inflammation of a joint

atrial – pertaining to the atrium

arterial – pertaining to one or more arteries

arteriole – a small arterial branch

efferent – carrying *away from* a central organ or section (e.g., as efferent arterioles, which carry blood from glomeruli of the kidney)

afferent – carries impulses *toward* a center

cor – muscular organ that maintains the circulation of the blood

core – a central part

crus – term used to designate a leg-like part

crux – a cross

cuspis – a tapering projection applied to one of the triangular segments of a cardiac valve

cuspid – having one point

fundus – the bottom or base

fungus – a vegetable cellular organism that subsists on organic matter

ostial – between two distinct cavities within the body

osteal – bony

palpation – the act of feeling with the hand

palpitation – either regular or irregular rapid action of the heart felt by the patient

perfusion – pouring a fluid over an organ or tissue or forcing it through vessels of an organ

profusion – abundance

pericardial – fibroserous sac that surrounds the heart and roots of the great vessels

precordial – the region over the heart and lower part of the thorax

Confusing Terms

thecal – pertaining to an enclosing case or sheath

fecal – pertaining to excrement discharged from the intestines

vesicle – small sac containing fluid

vesical – shaped like a bladder

fascicle – a small bundle, like muscle or nerve fibers

vesicles – small fluid-containing sacs

vessels – tubes, ducts, or canals that carry body fluids

vesicular – composed of or relating to small, sac-like bodies

fascicular – pertaining to a fascicle (small bundle or cluster)

testicular – pertaining to a testis

vena cava – one of two venae cavae, superior or inferior

venae cavae – the two largest veins in the body

Roots and/or Combining Forms

Root	Meaning	Root	Meaning
angio, angi	vessel	sclero, scler	hard, sclera
arterio	artery	steno	narrowed
atrio	atrium of the heart	tachy	fast
brady	slow	thoraco	chest
cardio, card	heart	thrombo	clot
cyano, cyan	blue	vaso	vessel
hem, hema, hemo, hemat, hemato	blood	veno	vein
		ventriculo	ventricle of heart or brain

Major Cardiovascular Terms

12 lead – refers to the surface electrocardiogram (ECG) electrodes placed on the skin of the patient's extremities and chest. They are called I, II, III, aVR, aVL, aVF, V1, V2, V3, V4, V5, and V6. The last six are often referred to as the *V leads* or the *chest leads.*

anemia – a decrease in the number of red blood cells

aneurysm – a sac formed by dilatation of the wall of a blood vessel or the heart

angina pectoris – acute chest pain

aorta – the body's largest artery, originating from the left ventricle of the heart

apex – the lower, rounded tip of the heart

arteriole – a small arterial branch

artery – a vessel that carries blood from the heart to the tissues

atrium – one of the two smaller upper chambers, or cavities, of the heart

capillary – any one of the tiny blood vessels connecting arterioles and venules

cardiac arrest – stoppage of the heart beat

circulatory system – the system through which the blood is distributed throughout the body, by way of the heart, arteries, capillaries, and veins

coagulation – the formation of a clot

coronary arteries and veins – blood vessels of the heart

diastole – dilatation of the heart cavities during the rest period

embolus – a plug or clot originating in a vessel and carried by the blood to a smaller vessel, causing an obstruction

Major Cardiovascular Terms

endocardium – inner lining of the heart

endothelium – lining of the heart and blood vessels

epicardium – external covering of the heart

heparin – an anticoagulant medication

hypertension – high blood pressure

hypotension – low blood pressure

infarct – an area of necrosis due to lack of blood

ischemia – a decrease in the flow of blood to a part

occlusion – blockage of a blood vessel

pericardium – the membrane surrounding the heart

pulse – the rhythmic expansion and contraction of the wall of an artery

systole – the contraction of the heart

thrombus – a plug or clot in a blood vessel or in one of the cavities of the heart, formed by coagulation of blood; remains at its point of formation

valve – a fold in a passage that prevents backward flow of its contents

ventricle – one of the lower chambers on either side of the heart

Selected Diagnostic Tests

catheterization
cerebral angiogram
coronary angiogram
electrophysiology study
MUGA scan
nuclear stress test
PET scan
radionuclide imaging
SPECT scan
stress test
tilt-table test
transtelephonic monitoring
venogram

Selected Noninvasive or Minimally Invasive Tests/Services

ambulatory blood pressure monitoring
CAT scan
chest x-ray
echocardiogram
Types: one-dimensional (M-mode), two-dimensional (cross-sectional), Doppler ultrasound, stress, chemical stress, transesophageal, intravascular
elective cardioversions
electrocardiogram
exercise treadmill test
Holter monitor (ambulatory EKG)
MRA (magnetic resonance angiography)
MRI (magnetic resonance imaging)
signal-averaged EKG
tilt-table test for syncope
ultrafast computed tomography

Selected Invasive Tests/Services

angiography
atherectomy
cardiac mapping using NOGA
cardiac output
diagnostic and therapeutic electrophysiology procedures
hemodynamic studies
implantation of internal defibrillators
intra-aortic balloon pump insertion
intravascular ultrasound
MUGA scan
myocardial biopsy
oxygen saturation studies
percutaneous transluminal angioplasty
pericardiocentesis
permanent and temporary transvenous pacing
PET test
right and/or left heart catheterization
SPECT test
stent placement
thallium stress test
thrombectomy (using AngioJet)
thrombolytic therapy

Selected Treatment Modalities

implantable cardioverter defibrillator (monitors heart rate and administers shock to heart in life-threatening situations)
pacemaker therapy
radiofrequency ablation (for treatment of specific rhythm disturbances)

Minimally Invasive Bypass Surgery

keyhole surgery (buttonhole surgery or laparoscopic bypass)
MIDCAB (minimally invasive direct coronary artery bypass)
OPCAB (off-pump bypass surgery)
port access bypass surgery

Selected Experimental Techniques

PICVA (percutaneous in situ coronary venous arterialization) – has been used successfully in Germany; procedure redirects blood flow around a blocked artery by rerouting it to an adjacent vein

robotic visualization technique – telerobotic method of heart surgery currently being tested; has not yet been approved by the Food and Drug Administration

Common Manifestations of Heart Disease

dyspnea
chest pain
edema
palpitation
hemoptysis
fatigue
syncope and fainting
cyanosis
abdominal pain or discomfort
distention of neck veins
congestive heart failure
pericardial compression due to effusion

Supportive Web Sites

www.centerwatch. com
Under "Patient and General Resources," select "Drug Directories"; then click on "Drugs Newly Approved by the FDA." Select "Cardiology/Vascular Diseases" for a particular year to see drugs approved for this specialty during that year.

http://www.chorus.rad.mcw.edu
Select "Cardiovascular system" for an extensive list of terminology links.

www.fda.gov
Click on "drugs" for informative links to drug information.

www.heartcenteronline.com
Click on "heart quizzes," then "A to Z topic list" for links to deeper sites.

www.hgcardio.com
Click on the "procedures," "heart disease," "what's new," and "links" buttons for detailed information on heart-related topics.

www.nlm.nih.gov/
Click on "health information," then on "MEDLINEplus," and search on "cardiology."

www.novoste.com
Click on "patient" and "healthcare professional" links for access to other informative links.

Index of Cardiology Reports

(see table of contents for audio information)

Exercise #	***Patient Name***	***Report/Procedure***
TE#1	Saja, Antonio	Transmyocardial revascularization (TMR)
TE#2	Robbins, Tanya	Bypass w/octopus stabilization
TE#3	Strahan, Van	CABG and TMR
TE#4	McDaniel, Joshua	Percutaneous transluminal coronary angioplasty
TE#5	Yuen, Chieko	Left atrial mass excision
TE#6	Hinson, Lawrence	Catheterization
TE#7	Yurich, Vivian	Angioplasty and stent implant
TE#8	Helveston, Scott W.	Resection of atrial myxoma; CABG × two
TE#9	Morrow, Bruce	Electrophysiology study
TE#10	Fowler, August	AICD implantation
TE#11	Burns, Jeremy	Endarterectomy
TE#12	Hagler, Jason	Dual chamber pacemaker

CHAPTER 4

DIAGNOSTIC IMAGING/ INTERVENTIONAL RADIOLOGY

Introduction

The medical discipline of *radiology* originated with the discovery of an unknown ray by German physicist Wilhelm Conrad Roentgen in 1895. He named this unknown ray an x-ray. The specialty of radiology (also called *roentgenology*) employs electromagnetic radiation and ultrasonics for the diagnosis and treatment of injury and disease.

Diagnostic imaging is the medical evaluation of body tissues and functions by means of still or moving radiologic images. Physicians employed in the field of diagnostic imaging are *radiologists, nuclear physicians,* and *radiation oncologists*. Radiologists specialize in the practice of diagnostic, therapeutic, or interventional radiology. Nuclear physicians are radiologists who administer nuclear medicine procedures used in diagnosis. Radiation oncologists are skilled in treating disease using radiation, primarily in the management of malignancies.

Diagnostic techniques employed by personnel in diagnostic imaging are CT (computerized tomography) or CAT (computerized axial tomography) scans, contrast studies, fluoroscopy, interventional radiology, tomography, ultrasound, or magnetic imaging or magnetic resonance imaging (MRI).

Interventional radiology is the nonsurgical treatment of disease using radiologic imaging to guide catheters, balloons, filters, and other tiny instruments through the body's blood vessels and other organs. Fallopian tube catheterization, balloon angioplasty, chemoembolization, and thrombolysis are examples of interventional radiologic procedures.

Nuclear medicine is the branch of radiology that uses small amounts of radioactive substances to image the body, diagnose, or treat disease. The amount of radiation used is quite small and poses little hazard to the patient or to any medical employee. Nuclear medicine personnel consider both the physiology and anatomy of the body in establishing diagnosis and treatment.

Nuclear imaging techniques give physicians a way to look inside the body using computers, detectors, and radioactive substances. These techniques include cardiovascular imaging, bone scanning, positron emission tomography (PET), and single photon emission computer tomography (SPECT). Medical conditions such as tumors, aneurysms, irregular or inadequate blood flow to tissues, blood cell disorders, and inadequate functioning of organs, such as thyroid and pulmonary function deficiencies, can be detected using nuclear imaging techniques.

Various body systems are tested through the administration of intravenous medications found in the nuclear medicine department. Almost all the body systems can be evaluated by this intravenous, or noninvasive, method through the use of one or more different drugs tagged with *technetium,* a *radionuclide.* Because radionuclides emit gamma rays that can be detected and recorded in many ways, thus providing statistical information or images, they are used commonly in all phases of medicine.

Of the techniques mentioned, contrast studies, CT scans, fluoroscopy, and tomography use x-rays. Ultrasonography uses ultrasound waves, and magnetic resonance imaging utilizes magnetic and radio waves.

After these diagnostic studies are made, the reports are interpreted by a radiologist and should be signed by that person, because the definitive report is the radiologist's responsibility.

Critical Thinking Exercise

Your instructor has given you the task of researching production standards for medical transcription. Where would you start?

Complete the assignment and share your findings with other class members through an oral presentation or in a general class discussion.

Diagnostic Imaging/Interventional Radiology Abbreviations

ACTH	adrenocorticotropic hormone
angio	angiography
AP	anteroposterior
ASD	atrial septal defect
ASIS	anterior-superior iliac spine
AV	arteriovenous
Ba	barium
BI-RADS	Breast Imaging and Reporting Data System
BPD	biparietal diameter
CAT	computerized axial tomography
CC	costochondral/cardiac catheterization
cGy	centigray; a rad that is one-hundredth of a gray
Ci	curie
CPB	competitive protein binding
cpm	count per minute
C-spine	cervical spine film
CT	computed tomography
CXR	chest x-ray
Decub	decubitus position (lying down)
DI	diagnostic imaging
DISH	diffuse idiopathic skeletal hyperostosis
DORI	Dynamic Optical Breast Imaging System
DSA	digital subtraction angiography
EGD	esophagogastroduodenoscopy
ERCP	endoscopic retrograde cholangiopancreatography
ESD	esophagus, stomach, and duodenum
FUT	fibrinogen uptake test
Fx	fracture
GM	Geiger-Muller (counter)
Gy	gray; unit of radiation equal to 100 rads
HEG	high energy gamma
HVL	half-value layer
ICA	internal carotid artery
ICS	intercostal space
IHSA	iodinated human serum albumin
IVP	intravenous pyelogram
keV/kev	kilo (thousand) electron volts
kHz	kilohertz
KUB	kidneys, ureters, bladder
LAO	left anterior oblique
LAT	lateral
LD	lethal dose
LS films	lumbosacral spine films
MAA	macroaggregated albumin
mCi	millicurie (measure of radiation)
MDP	methylene diphosphonate
MFB	metallic foreign body
MHz	megahertz
MLD	median lethal dose
MLO	mesiolinguo-occlusal
MPC	maximum permissible concentration
MPD	maximum permissible dose
MPL	maximum permissible level or limit
MRI	magnetic resonance imaging
MUGA	multiple-gated acquisition scan (radioactive test to show heart function)
N	neutron
PA	posteroanterior
PBI	protein-bound iodine
PET	positron emission tomography
PIT	plasma iron turnover
PTA	percutaneous transluminal angioplasty
PTC	percutaneous transhepatic cholangiography

PTEA	pulmonary thromboendarterectomy
R	roentgen
rad	radiation-absorbed dose
RAD	roentgen-administered dose
RAIU	radioactive iodine uptake (test)
RAO	right anterior oblique
RBE	relative biologic effectiveness
REG	radiation exposure guide
RIA	radioimmunoassay
RISA	radioiodinated serum albumin
SFA	superficial femoral artery
SPECT	single-photon emission computer tomography
SVC	superior vena cava
TBI	total body irradiation
Tc	technetium
Tc99m or ^{99m}Tc	radioactive technetium used in brain, skull, thyroid, liver, spleen, bone, and lung scans
TD	total dose
TIPS	transjugular intrahepatic portosystemic shunt
TSD	target-skin distance
UGI	upper gastrointestinal series
US, U/S	ultrasound
V/Q	ventilation-perfusion lung scan
XRT	radiation therapy

Anatomic Illustrations

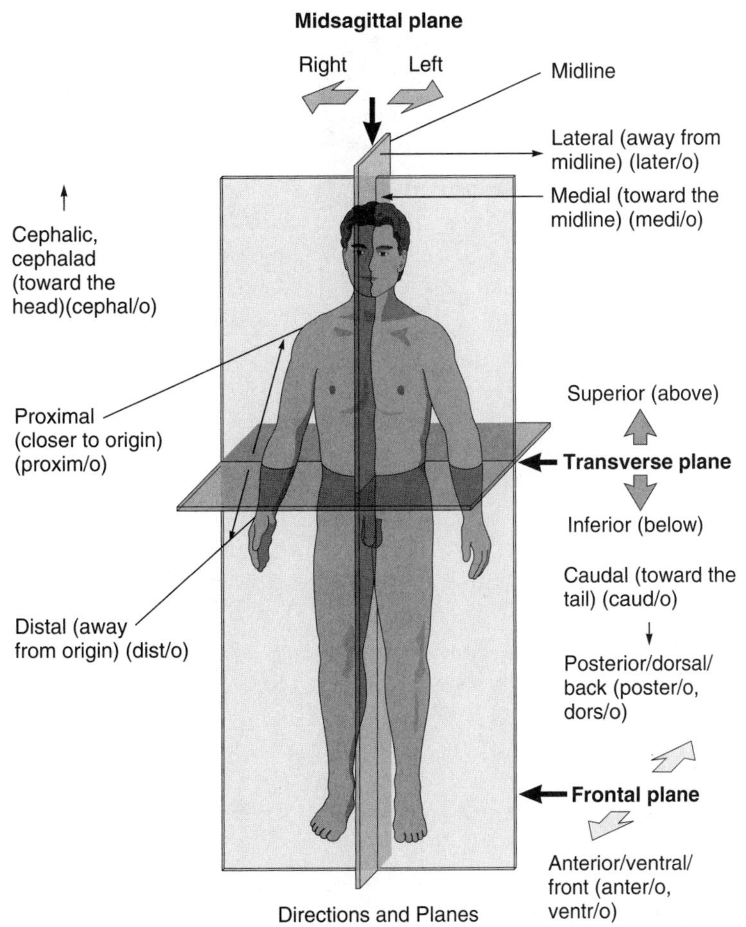

4–1 DIRECTIONS AND PLANES OF THE BODY IN ANATOMIC POSITION

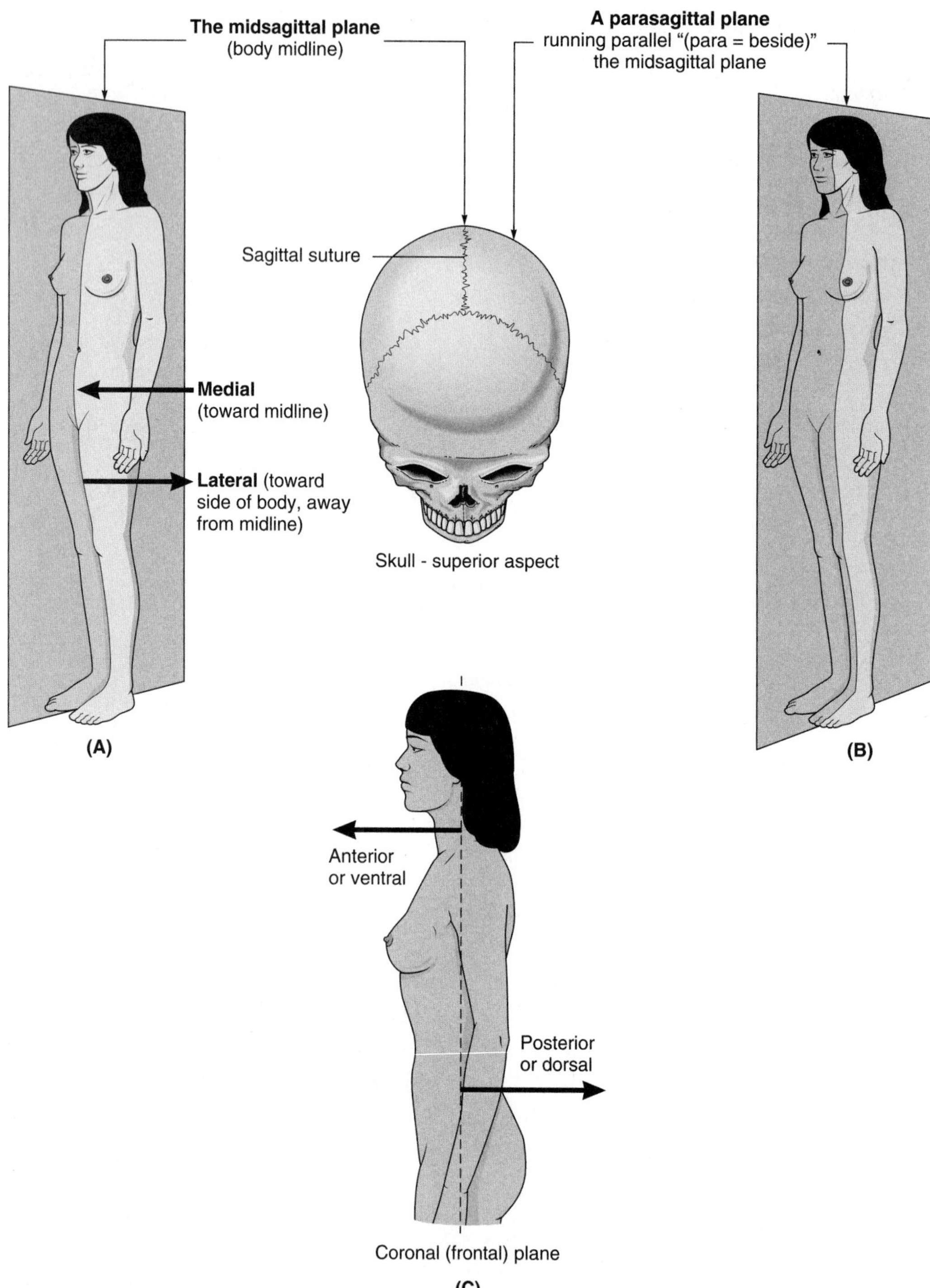
The midsagittal plane
(body midline)
A parasagittal plane
running parallel "(para = beside)"
the midsagittal plane
Sagittal suture
Medial
(toward midline)
Lateral (toward
side of body, away
from midline)
Skull - superior aspect
(A)
(B)
Anterior
or ventral
Posterior
or dorsal
Coronal (frontal) plane
(C)

4–2 *BODY PLANES*

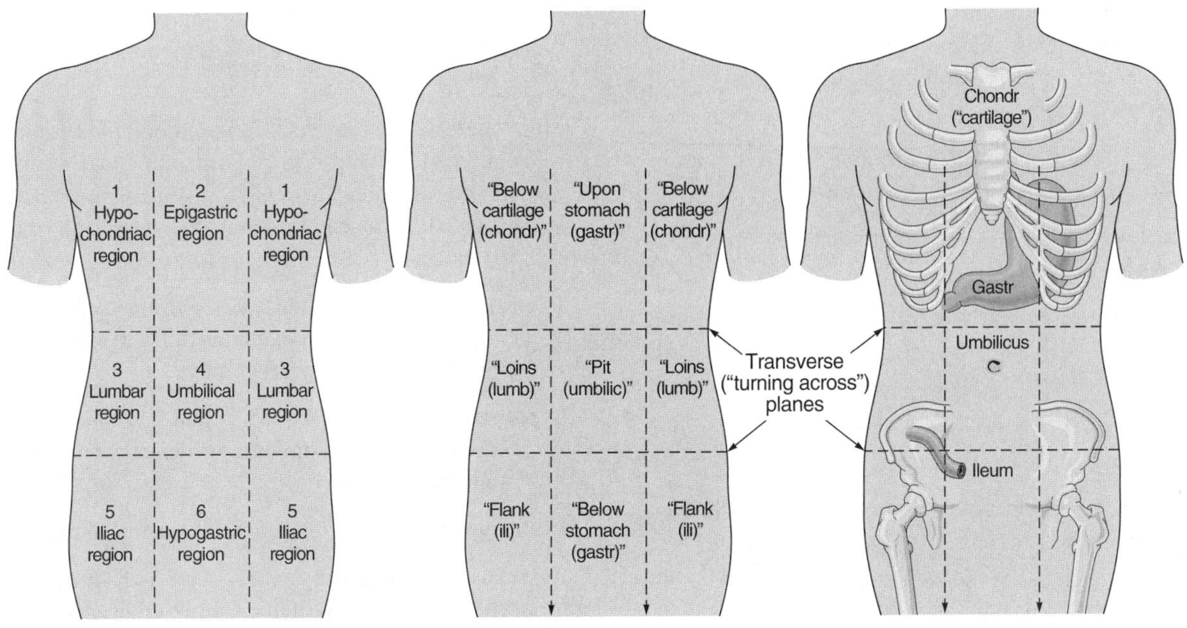

4–3 VERTICAL BODY PLANES

Diagnostic Imaging/Interventional Radiology Terminology

a

air bronchogram (brong'-kō-gram) – radiographic appearance of an air-filled bronchus surrounded by fluid-filled airspaces

angiocardiography (an"-jē-ō-kar'-dē-og'-ruh-fē) – examination of the chambers of the heart and pulmonary circulation after injection of radiopaque material

angiogram (an'-jē-ō-gram") – an x-ray of blood vessels filled with a contrast medium

aortogram (ā-or'-tuh-gram") – an x-ray of the aorta after injection of contrast fluid

appendicolith (uh-pen"-dih-kō'-lith") – a calcified concretion in the appendix visible on an abdominal radiograph

arteriogram (ar-tē'-rē-uh-gram") – an x-ray of an artery

arthropneumoradiograph (ar"-thrō-noo"-mō-rā'-dē-uh-graf") – radiographic examination of a joint after it has been injected with air

attenuation (ah-ten"-yoo-ā'-shun) – the process by which a beam of radiation is reduced in energy when passed through tissue or other material

b

betatron (bā'-tuh-tron) – the machine used in radiotherapy to administer a dose of radiation to a patient

BI-RADS (bī'-radz) – Breast Imaging and Data Reporting System; mammographic findings may be reported by the term BI-RAD followed by an arabic numeral (e.g., BI-RAD 3)

c

cephalometric radiograph (cephalogram) (sef"-uh-lō-meh'-trik rā'-dē-uh-graf) (sef'-uh-lō-gram") – a radiographic view of the jaws and skull permitting measurement

cesium 137 (sē'-zē-um) – radionuclide used for external radiation therapy of cancer

choledochogram (kō-led'-ō-kō-gram") – an x-ray of the common bile duct

cineangiography (sin"-ē-an"-jē-og'-ruh-fē) – the photographic recording of fluoroscopic images of the blood vessels by motion picture techniques

cineradiography (sin"-e-ra"-dē-og'-run-fē) – x-ray motion pictures

cisternography (sis"-ter-nog'-ruh-fē) – the roentgenographic study of the basal cisterns of the brain after the subarachnoid introduction of an opaque or other contrast medium, or a radiopharmaceutical

collimator (kahl'-ih-mā"-tur) – a diaphragm or system of diaphragms made of an absorbing material, designed to identify the dimensions and direction of a beam of radiation

colpostat (kahl'-pō-stat) – an appliance for retaining something, such as radium, in the vagina

Combidex (kahm'-bih-deks) – imaging agent used for lymph nodes

computed tomography (CT) (kum-pyoo'-ted tō-mog'-ruh-fē) – a diagnostic x-ray procedure where a cross-section image of a specific body segment is generated

curie (kyoo'-rē) – the unit for measuring the activity for all radioactive substances

cyclotron (sī'-klo-tron) – a particle accelerator in which charged particles receive repeated synchronized accelerations of "kicks" by electrical fields as the particles spiral outward from their source; a valuable source of radionuclides for medical diagnosis and research

cystogram (sis'-tuh-gram) – an x-ray of the bladder

cystourethrogram (sis"-tō-yoo-rē'-thruh-gram) – an x-ray of the urinary bladder and ureters

d

diathermy (dī'-uh-ther"-mē) – heating of the body tissues due to their resistance to the passage of high-frequency electromagnetic radiation

Digirad 2020tc Imager (dih'-jih-rad ih'-muh-jer) – a digital gamma camera used in nuclear medicine

diskography (dis-kog'-ruh-fē) – radiographic demonstration of an intervertebral disk by injection of contrast media into the nucleus pulposus

dosimeter (dō-sim'-eh-ter) – an instrument for measuring the dose of radiation

e

echogenic (ek-ō-gē'-nik) – containing internal interfaces that reflect high-frequency sound waves

encephalogram (en-sef'-uh-lō-gram") – an x-ray made after the injection of a contrast material, usually air, into the cerebrospinal fluid in order to outline the spinal cord and brain

Explorer X 70 (eks-plor'-eī) – intraoral radiography system

f

fluorescence (floo"-ur-es'-ens) – the characteristic of certain substances to emit light when exposed to certain types of light radiation

fluoroscopy (floo"-ur-os'-kuh-pē) – use of a fluoroscope for medical diagnosis or for testing various materials by roentgen rays

g

GE Senographe 2000D (jē-ē sen'-uh-graf) – the first fully digital system for mammography

Gore 1.5T Torsa Array (gōr' tor'-suh uh-rā') – MRI surface coil for imaging chest, abdominal, and pelvic areas

h

hilar shadow (hī'-lur shad'-ō) – radiographic hilum of the lung; a composite radiographic shadow of the central pulmonary arteries and veins with associated bronchial walls and lymph nodes within the right or left lung

Hypaque (hi-pāk') – used with sodium hydroxide or meglumine as a radiopaque medium in angiocardiography and excretory urography

hyperechoic (hī"-per-ē-kō'-ik) – material that produces echoes of higher amplitude or density than the surrounding medium

hysterogram (hiss'-ter-uh-gram) – an x-ray of the uterus

hysterosalpingography (hiss"-ter-ō-sal"-ping-gahg'-ruh-fē) – an x-ray of the uterus and uterine tubes after injection of a contrast medium

i

in situ (in sē'-too) – in place

interstitial therapy (in"-ter-stih'-shul thair'-uh-pē) – the procedure where radioisotopes are surgically inserted into a tumor

intracavitary therapy (in"-truh-kāv'-ih-tair"-ē thair'-uh-pē) – the process where radioisotopes are placed within a body cavity adjacent to a tumor

iridium (Ir 192) (ih-rid'-ē-um) – a radioisotope used for selected cases of cancer

irradiation (ih-rā"-dē-ā'-shun) – the therapeutic application of roentgen rays, radium rays, ultraviolet rays, or other radiation to a patient

isotope (ī'-suh-tōp) – one of a series of chemical elements that have nearly identical chemical properties but differ in their atomic weights and electric charge; many are radioactive

l

laminagram (lam'-ih-nuh-gram) – an x-ray of a selected layer of the body made by body-section roentgenography

laminagraphy (lam"-ih-nag'-ruh-fē) – the taking of x-rays at varying levels of tissue

lymphangiography (lihm-fan"-jē-og'-ruh-fē) – x-ray study of the lymphatic system after the injection of a contrast medium

m

megavoltage (meg"-uh-vōl'-tij) – high-energy radiation generated by a machine and used in curative x-ray therapy for cancer

meglumine (meg'-loo-mēn) – a chemical used in the preparation of certain radiopaque media

microcurie (mī"-krō-kyoo'-rē) – unit for measuring the energy of a radionuclide in a tracer dose

millicurie (mCi) (mil"-ih-kyoo'-rē) – unit for measuring the energy of a radionuclide in a therapeutic dose

myelogram (mī'-eh-lō-gram) – an x-ray of the spinal cord

myelography (mī"-eh-log'-ruh-fē) – an x-ray of the spinal cord after injection of a radiopaque substance into the subarachnoid space

myelopathic (mī"-eh-lō-path'-ik) – relating to myelopathy (disease of the spinal cord)

Myoview (Cardiolite) (mī'-ō-vyoo, kar'-dē-ō-līt") – radionuclide used in cardiac myocardial scans

n

NeoSpect (nē'-ō-spekt") – imaging agent used for the diagnosis of suspected lung cancer

nephrogram (nef'-ruh-gram) – an x-ray of the kidney

nephrotomography (nef"-rō-tuh-mog'-ruh-fē) – body-section roentgenography as applied to the kidney

neurosonography (nyoo"-rō-suh-nog'-ruh-fē) – a diagnostic technique in which pulses of ultrasonic waves are projected through the head from both sides and echoes from the midline structures of the brain are recorded as graphic tracings

nonopaque (non"-ō-pāk') – not opaque to the roentgen ray

nuclide (noo'-klīd) – a general term denoting all nuclear species of chemical elements, both stable and unstable; used synonymously with isotope

o

opaque (ō-pak') – neither transparent nor translucent

orifice (or'-ih-fiss) – the entrance or outlet of any cavity in the body

oxycephalic (ok"-sē-seh-fal'-ik) – pertaining to or characterized by a condition in which the top of the head is pointed

p

Pantopaque (pan-tō-pāk') – a contrast medium or radiopaque dye used in x-ray studies

photoscan (fō'-tō-skan) – a representation of the concentration of a radioisotope outlining an organ in the body

picogram (pī'-kō-gram) – a unit of weight of the metric system; also called a micromicrogram or one-trillionth of a gram

pneumothorax (noo-mō-thor'-aks) – an accumulation of air or gas in the pleural space, which may occur spontaneously or as a result of trauma or a pathological process, or be introduced deliberately

portogram (por'-tuh-gram) – an x-ray of the portal vein

pyelogram (pī'-el-uh-gram") – an x-ray in which the pelvis of the kidney is shown filled with contrast material, which may be injected directly into the urinary system through a catheter or into a vein to reach the kidneys through the blood

pyeloureterography (pyelography) (pī"-el-ō-yoo-rē"-ter-og'-ruh-fē, pī"-el-og'-ruh-fē) – radiologic study of the kidney and renal collecting system, usually performed with the aid of a contrast agent

r

radiodense (rā'-dē-ō-dens") – the property of a substance that does not allow the passage of x-rays

radioimmunoassay (RIA) (rā"-dē-ō-ih"-myoo-nō-as'-ā) – an in vitro procedure where radioactive chemicals and antibodies are combined to detect hormones and/or drugs in blood; also used to monitor quantity of digitalis in the bloodstream

radioisotope (rā"-dē-ō-ī'-suh-tōp) – an isotope of a chemical element made radioactive by bombardment with neutrons; term has become obsolete – radionuclide is the accepted term

radiolucent (rā-dē-ō-loo'-sent) – allows the passage of most x-rays; radiolucent structures appear black on x-ray film

radionuclide (rā"-dē-ō-noo'-klīd) – a nuclide that displays the property of radioactivity

radiopaque (rā"-dē-ō-pāk') – not permitting radiant energy, such as x-rays, to pass

radiopharmaceutical (rā"-dē-ō-fahr"-muh-syoo'-tih-kul) – a radioactive chemical or pharmaceutical preparation labeled with a radionuclide in tracer or therapeutic concentration used as a diagnostic or therapeutic agent

Reno M-DIP (rē'-nō em'-dihp) – a radiopaque contrast agent

roentgen (rent'-gen) – the international unit of x- or y-radiation

roentgenography (rent"-gen-og'-ruh-fē) – picture of an organ or a region by means of roentgen rays

roentgenology (rent"-gen-ol'-uh-jē) – the study of x-rays; radiology

s

scintigram (sin'-tih-gram) – a two-dimensional representation (map) of the gamma rays emitted by a radioisotope, revealing its varying concentration in a specific tissue of the body, such as the brain, kidney, or thyroid gland

scintillation scan (sin-tih-lā'-shun skan) – image made by a scintillation counter to determine the size of a tumor, goiter, or other involvement and to locate aberrant, metastatic lesions

scintiscan (sin'-tih-skan) – the use of scintiphotography to create a map of scintillations produced when a radioactive substance is introduced into the body

scybalum (sib'-uh-lum) – a dry, hard mass of fecal matter in the intestine

selenium (seh-len'-ē-um) – a metallic element chemically similar to sulfur

sialogram (sī-al'-uh-gram) – radiographic visualization of the salivary glands and ducts after injection of radiopaque material

stereoroentgenography (star"-ē-ō-rent"-gen-og'-ruh-fē) – the making of an x-ray giving an impression of depth as well as width and height

strontium (Sr 89) (stron'-shē-um) – radionuclide used for lesions of the eye and removal of benign small tumors

supratentorial (soo"-pruh-ten-tō'-rē-ul) – above the tentorium of the cerebellum

t

tagging (tag'-ing) – the process of attaching a radionuclide to a chemical and following its course in the body

technetium (Tc 99m) (tek-nē'-shē-um) – a radionuclide used in brain, thyroid, parotid, and heart-blood pool scans

Technetium Sulfur Colloid (tek-nē'-shē-um sul'-fur kahl'-oyd) – radionuclide used in liver, spleen, and bone marrow scans

Telepaque (tel'-eh-pāk) – a contrast media, or radiopaque dye, used in x-ray studies

teleroentgenogram (tel"-eh-rent"-gen'-uh-gram) – the picture or film obtained by teleroentgenography

thallium 201 (thal'-ē-um) – radionuclide used in myocardial scans

tomography (tuh-mog'-ruh-fē) – a special technique to show in detail images of structures lying in a predetermined plane of tissue, while blurring or eliminating detail in images of structures in the other planes

transjugular intrahepatic portosystemic shunt (TIPS) (tranz-jug'-yoo-lur in"-truh-hē-pat'-ik por"-tō-sis"-teh'-mik shunt) – an interventional radiology procedure to relieve portal hypertension

u

UltraSure DTU-one (uhl'-truh-shoor" dē-tē-yoo-wun) – imaging system for assessment of osteoporotic fracture risk

uptake (up-tāk) – refers to the rate of absorption of a radionuclide into an organ or tissue

ureteropyelogram (yoo-rē"-ter-ō-pī'-eh-lō-gram") – an x-ray of the ureter and pelvis of the kidney

v

Valsalva's maneuver (val-sal'-vuhz muh"-noo'-ver) – any forced expiratory effort against a closed airway to increase intrathoracic pressure and impede venous return to the right atrium; used to study cardiovascular effects of raised peripheral venous pressure and decreased cardiac filling and cardiac output

ventilation/perfusion studies (ven"-tih-lā'-shun per-fyoo'-zhun stuh'-dēz) – studies in which a radiopharmaceutical is inhaled (ventilation) and injected (perfusion) and its passage through the respiratory tract is imaged

ventriculography (ven-trik"-yoo-log'-ruh-fē) – an x-ray of the head following removal of cerebrospinal fluid from the cerebral ventricles and its replacement by air or other contrast medium

x

xenon (Xe 133) (zē'-non) – a radionuclide used in studies of lung and blood flow

Xplorer (eks"-plor'-er) – a filmless digital radiography imaging system

y

yttrium (Y 90) (ih'-trē-um) – radionuclide used for ascites and effusions associated with malignant metastatic involvement (i.e., hepatomegaly, splenomegaly, chronic leukemia, and polycythemia)

Transcription Tips

When transcribing diagnostic imaging/interventional radiology reports, basic concepts with which you should be familiar are x-ray views (or positions of the patient), anatomical planes of the body, nuclear medicine tests, confusing terms, and typical formats for x-ray reports.

X-ray Views or Positioning

AP view (anteroposterior) – patient positioned so that the front of the body is to the x-ray machine

PA view (posteroanterior) – patient upright with back to x-ray machine and chest to film

lateral view – x-ray beam passes from one side of the body toward the other to reach the film

oblique view – body part to be imaged is positioned at an angle to x-ray tube

supine – patient lying face up with head turned to one side; x-rays pass through body from front to back

prone – patient lying face down with head turned to one side; x-rays pass from back to front of body

Anatomical Planes

sagittal (lateral) – a lengthwise vertical plane through the longitudinal axis of the trunk dividing the body into two portions

midsagittal or **median** – a vertical plane through the anterior-posterior midaxis that divides the body into right and left halves

frontal (coronal) – a plane dividing the body into front (anterior) and back (posterior) portions

transverse (cross-sectional) – a plane running across the body parallel to the ground that divides the body into upper and lower portions

Nuclear Medicine Tests

Scans – scans of the blood and heart, bone, brain, liver and spleen, thyroid, and PET (positron emission tomography)

Radioactive iodine uptake – reflects the rate of hormone synthesis by the thyroid gland

SPECT (single-photon emission computed tomography) – used to detect liver tumors, cardiac ischemia, and bone disease of the spine

Confusing Terms

arthritis – inflammation of a joint

arthritides – plural of arthritis

bursa – a sac or sac-like cavity filled with viscid fluid

bursae – plural of bursa

draped – describes the procedure where a patient has a cloth placed over him or her in a hospital operating room to keep the site of maximum sterility as small as possible

raped – the situation where one has forced another person to submit to sexual intercourse

ilium – bone

ileum – bowel

medium – means; substance that transmits impulses; substance used in the culture of bacteria; preparation used in creating histologic specimens

media – plural of medium

naris – the nostril; nose

nares – plural of naris

plain x-ray – noncontrast

plane x-ray – tomograms

pleural space – space between the parietal and visceral layers of the pleura

plural space – more than one space

Typical Formats for Reports

The formatting of x-ray reports differs from one facility to another in many cases; therefore, you should be prepared to demonstrate flexibility in transcribing reports. In some facilities, x-ray reports are typed on plain paper (sometimes colored to identify them as x-ray reports); other facilities have a prepared form onto which you will type the dictation. Some prepared forms include a line at the bottom of the page for the signature of the radiologist. When this is the case, you should type the name of the radiologist, his or her title, and your initials on the line. The physician should sign above the typed name.

Currently many medical facilities provide equipment that allows the transcriptionist to download patient information directly from the mainframe for the headings of reports. The transcriptionist selects account information on the patient and copies all relevant information automatically into the document. Then the transcriptionist begins keying the dictation concerning the procedure immediately and does not have to enter any patient information manually.

If results of a particular procedure are found to be normal, most physicians have prerecorded a "normal" template. The physician gives the transcriptionist instructions to retrieve a copy of a "normal 1" or a "normal 2," for example. When a "normal" is to be used, the transcriptionist starts a new document and inserts the "normal" text. This saves time for both the transcriptionist and the physician.

Sample Headings and Meanings of Each Line of Information

Example #1

SALINAS, TOOTIE (patient name)
OP (outpatient)
28398765 (outpatient #)
CT THERAPY LOCALIZATION (type of report; name of procedure)
478067 (x-ray #)
YSIDRO TEW, MD (physician who ordered the exam)
BD: 13 JUNE 75 (birthdate)
10 OCTOBER 03 (date exam was performed)
10 OCTOBER 03 20:36:12 (date and time report was transcribed)

Example #2

6/29/03 (date report was transcribed)
11:10 a.m. (time report was transcribed)

RUTHLESS, YALINDA (patient name)
ER (emergency room)
FLAT & UPRIGHT ABDOMEN (type of report; name of procedure)
X-ray #19683 (x-ray #)
AN 25408564 (account #)
MRN 000678432 (medical record #)
ON 3729867 (order # from physician)
SMITH, ANDREW (physician who ordered the exam)
BD: 12/29/72 (birthdate)
ED: 6/28/03 (date procedure was done)

Supportive Web Sites

www.encarta.msn.com
Search on "radiology"; click on other links as desired.

www.howstuffworks.com
Search on "nuclear medicine"; click on other links as desired.

www.nlm.nih.gov/medlineplus
Search on "diagnostic imaging," "nuclear medicine," or "interventional radiology"; click on other links as desired.

Index of Diagnostic Imaging/Interventional Radiology Reports

(see table of contents for audio information)

Exercise #	Patient Name	Report/Procedure
TE#1	Mann, Teresa	Cardiac imaging
TE#2	Timberton, Justin	Duplex carotid Doppler study
TE#3	Cochran, Trent	Nephrostomy tube change
TE#4	Zinn, Luigi	US liver biopsy
TE#5	Larson, Jill	Persantine/Thallium stress cardiac scan
TE#6	Wren, Sara	Quinton catheter placement
TE#7	Styron, Heather	CT guided-needle biopsy of the lung
TE#8	Zak, Anwar	Carotid arteriogram
TE#9	Thu, Milia	MRI spinal canal C spine
TE#10	Gentry, Marietta	Fistulogram with fistuloplasty
TE#11	Michalski, Matt	Cerebral arteriogram
TE#12	Kobs, Ashley	Bilateral mammogram
TE#13	Jorda, Edgar	MRI brain

CHAPTER 5

PATHOLOGY

Introduction

Pathology is a specialized branch of medicine concerned with the detailed study of any deviation from normal in *anatomy* or *physiology.*

The *pathologist* seeks to determine the cause of disease as well as the changes the disease causes in cells, tissues, organs, and the body as a whole. Additionally, the pathologist studies the form the disease may take, together with the complications that may follow. If the disease leads to the individual's death, the *autopsy* can then be performed by the pathologist, providing additional clues to the process and termination of the disease.

One of the methods by which a pathologist obtains tissue for examination is through the removal of specimens during surgery. Such tissue specimens are examined grossly (for structure) and, if warranted, microscopically (for tissue analysis).

A *biopsy,* a small piece of tissue removed for pathological examination, is widely used for detection of malignant cells. Another aspect of the work of the pathologist is obtaining, through various means, body fluids, blood, and other materials that are either brought or sent to the lab for analysis and study. Pathologic examinations, both *gross* and *microscopic,* at the time of autopsy are the ultimate answer in assessing tissue and organ damage to the body. These examinations establish the cause or contributing cause of death.

Critical Thinking Exercise

Keith Rossier, a neighbor, recently heard a report on television about voice recognition technology. He knows that you are a medical transcriptionist, so he assumes that you can explain to him what the reporter was talking about.

What would you tell him?

Pathology Abbreviations

ABG	arterial blood gas
ACTH	adrenocorticotropic hormone
AFB	acid-fast bacilli
A/G	albumin-globulin ratio
AHT	antihyaluronidase titer
ANF	antinuclear fluorescent antibodies
ASLO	antistreptolysin-O
BMP	basic metabolic panel
Bx	biopsy
CMP	comprehensive metabolic panel
CPK	creatine phosphokinase
DJD	degenerative joint disease
DNA	deoxyribonucleic acid
E. coli	Escherichia coli
ERA	evoked response audiometry
ET	etiology; essential thrombocythemia

FAN	fluorescent antinuclear antibodies
FBS	fasting blood sugar
FS	frozen section
FSH	follicle-stimulating hormone
FTA	fluorescent treponemal antibody
GGTP	gamma-glutamyl transpeptidase
GTM	glucose tolerance meal
GTT	glucose tolerance test
HAA	hepatitis-associated antigen
HBD	hydroxybutyrate dehydrogenase
HCG	human chorionic gonadotropin
Hct	hematocrit
Hgb, Hb	hemoglobin
HIAA	hydroxyindoleacetic acid
HNP	herniated nucleus pulposus
hpf	high power field
IgG	gamma G immunoglobulin
LAP	leucine aminopeptidase; leukocyte adhesion protein
LDH	lactic dehydrogenase
LFT	liver function test
MCH	mean corpuscular hemoglobin
MCHC	mean corpuscular hemoglobin concentration
MCV	mean corpuscular volume
MRSA	methicillin-resistant Staphylococcus aureus
OCP	ova, cysts, parasites
PKU	phenylketonuria
PPD	paraphenylenediamine purified protein derivative
PPLO	pleuropneumonia-like organism
PRA	plasma renin activity
QNS	quantity not sufficient
RIA	radioimmunoassay
RPE	retinal pigment epithelium
SP GR	specific gravity
SSKI	saturated solution of potassium iodide
STS	serologic test for syphilis
TNTC	too numerous to count
TSH	thyroid-stimulating hormone
UCG	urinary chorionic gonadotropin
VDRL	Venereal Disease Research Laboratories
VMA	vanillylmandelic acid
VRE	vancomycin-resistant enteric

Anatomic Illustrations

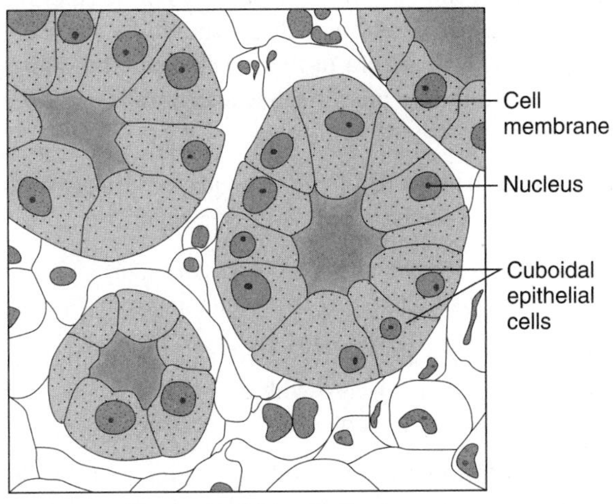

5–1 SIMPLE CUBOIDAL EPITHELIUM

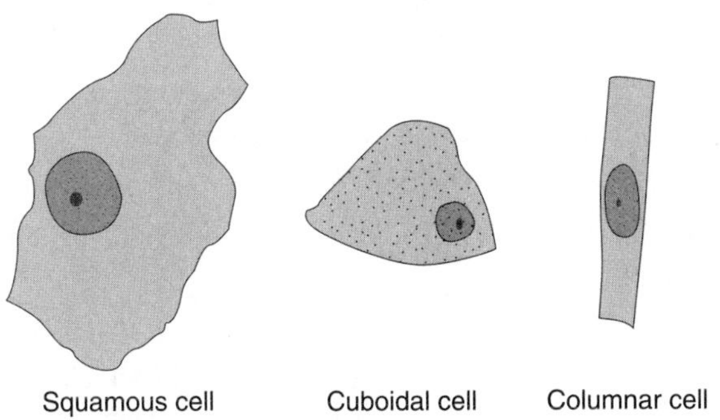

5–2 MAJOR SHAPES OF INDIVIDUAL EPITHELIAL CELLS

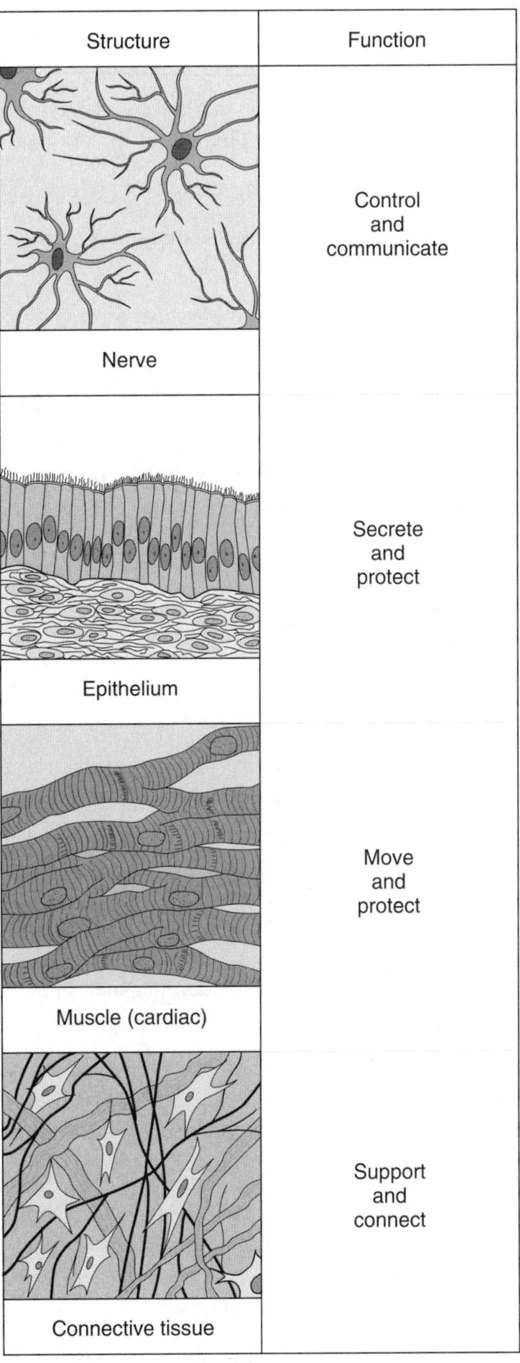

Structure
Function
Nerve
Control and communicate
Epithelium
Secrete and protect
Muscle (cardiac)
Move and protect
Connective tissue
Support and connect

5–3 FOUR TYPES OF TISSUE AND THEIR FUNCTIONS

Pathology Terminology

a

adenomyosis (ad"-ē-nō-mī-ō'-sis) – a benign condition characterized by ingrowth of the endometrium into the uterine musculature

aleukemic (ā"-loo-kē'-mik) – marked by aleukemia, the absence or deficiency of leukocytes in the blood

aleukocytic (ā-loo"-kō-sit'-ik) – showing no leukocytes

amelanotic (ā"-mel-uh-not'-ik) – containing no melanin; unpigmented

amitotic (ā"-mī-tot'-ik) – of the nature of amitosis; not occurring by mitosis

amorphous (uh-mor'-fuss) – without definite shape or form

apocrine (ap'-o-krīn, ap'-uh-krin) – denoting that type of glandular secretion in which the free end or apical portion of the secreting cell is cast off along with the secretory products that have accumulated therein

Armanni-Ebstein changes (ar-mah'-nē-eb-stīn chān-jez) – epithelial tubule containing deposits of glycogen; occurs in diabetes mellitus

arrhenoblastoma (ah-re"-nō-blas-to'-muh) – a neoplasm of the ovary, arising from the ovarian stroma

Askanazy cells (as-kuh-nah'-zē selz) – follicular cells of the thyroid that show increased eosinophilia and nuclear enlargement

astrup (ass'-trup) – an instrument designed to determine the pH, partial carbon dioxide, and bicarbonates of the blood

Auer's bodies (ow'-erz bah-dēz) – elongated bacteria-like inclusions found in the cytoplasm of myeloblasts, myelocytes, monoblasts, and granular histiocytes; thought to be nucleoprotein material

autolysis (aw-tahl'-ih-sis) – the spontaneous disintegration of tissues or of cells by the action of their own autogenous enzymes, such as occurs after death and in some pathological conditions

Autotechnicon (aw-tō-tek'-nih-kahn) – an instrument in which selected tissue sections are successively passed through different solutions by a timed mechanism in preparation for sectioning, staining, and mounting in microscopic slides

azure eosin (azh'-yoor ē'-ō-sin) – a stain for chromaffin

azurophilic (azh"-yoor-ō-fil'-ik) – staining well with blue aniline dyes

b

Bacteroides (bak"-ter-oy'-dēz) – a genus of nonsporulating obligate anaerobic filamentous bacteria occurring as normal flora in the mouth and large bowel; often found in necrotic tissues, probably as secondary invaders

Bartonella (bar"-tō-nel'-luh) – a genus of bacteria; these organisms multiply in fixed tissue cells

Bielschowsky's stain (bē"-el-show'-skēz stān) – a silver stain for demonstrating axons and neurofibrils

Boeck's sarcoid (beks sar'-koyd) – a nonmalignant, granulomatous disease with an unknown cause that affects mainly the lungs, skin, and bone

Bouin's solution (bwahnz' suh-loo'-shun) – a fixation solution for tissue that is especially good for skin and other tissue in which cellular detail is important

c

calcospherite (kal"-kō-sfăr'-īt) – one of the small globular bodies formed during the process of calcification

Call-Exner bodies (kahl"-eks'-ner bah'-dēz) – the accumulations of densely staining material that appear among granulosa cells in maturing ovarian follicles and that may be intracellular precursors of follicular fluid

carbolfuchsin stain (kar"-bahl-fook'-sin stān) – a stain for acid-fast bacteria

celloidin (seh-loy'-din) – a material used for embedding specimens

chondromyxofibroma (kon"-drō-mik"-sō-fī-brō'-muh) – a benign connective tissue tumor in which there are cartilage cells, fibrocytes, and a degenerated granular material spoken of as myxoid tissue

chordoma (kor-dō'-muh) – a malignant tumor arising from the embryonic remains of the notochord

coccidiosis (kok"-sid-ē-ō'-sis) – infection by coccidia

condyloma acuminatum (kon"-dih-lō'-muh ah-kyoo"-mih-nah'-tum) – a papilloma with a central core of connective tissue in a tree-like structure covered with epithelium; caused by a virus, it is infectious and autoinoculable

Coombs' test (koomz tehst) – a test using various antisera, usually employed to detect the presence of proteins on the surface of red cells

corpora amylacea (kor'-pō-ruh am"-ī-lā'-shē-uh) – small hyaline masses of degenerate cells found in the prostate, neuroglia, etc.

corpora arantii (kor'-pō-ruh uh-ran'-tī) – nodules of the aortic valve

cotyledon (kot"-ih-lē'-don) – any one of the subdivisions of the uterine surface of a discoidal placenta

cystosarcoma phyllodes (sis"-tō-sar-kō'-muh fil'-uh-dēz) – a low-grade malignant tumor of the human breast resembling a giant fibroadenoma and often containing cleft-like cystic spaces

d

deciduoma (dē-sid"-yoo-ō'-muh) – an intrauterine mass containing decidual cells

Demodex folliculorum (dem'-ō-deks fahl-ik"-yoo-lō'-rum) – a species of mite found in hair follicles and in secretions of the sebaceous glands, especially of the face and nose

Diff-Quik (dihf'-kwik) – a stain

Diplococcus pneumoniae (dip"-lō-kok'-us noo-mō'-nē-uh) – a species of bacteria that is the commonest cause of lobar pneumonia

Döhle's inclusion bodies (dē'-lēz in-kloo'-zhun bah'-dēz) – small coccus-shaped bodies occurring in the polynuclear leukocytes of the blood in several diseases, especially scarlet fever

dysontogenesis (dis"-ahn-tō-jen'-eh-sis) – defective embryonic development

e

Ehrlichia (ār-lik'-ē-uh) – gram-negative bacteria; transmitted by ticks

Ehrlich's test (ār'-likz tehst) – a test for urobilinogen in the urine

enchondroma (en"-kahn-drō'-muh) – a benign growth of cartilage arising in the metaphysis of a bone

epithelioma of Malherbe (ep"-ih-thē"-lē-ō'-muh uv mal-ārb') – a benign tumor of squamous epithelial cells in which there is some calcification

erythropoiesis (ē-rith"-rō-poy-ē'-sis) – the production of erythrocytes

Escherichia coli (E. coli) (esh"-er-ih'-kē-uh kohl'-ī) – a species of organisms constituting the greater part of the intestinal flora of humans and other animals

f

ferrugination (fuh-roo'-jih-nā-shun) – mineralization (with iron) of the blood vessels of the brain

fetus papyraceous (fē'-tus pap"-ih-rā'-shus) – extreme compression of a dead fetus by its living twin

Fibrindex test (fī'-brin-deks tehst) – a test to determine the adequacy of fibrinogen of the blood

g

gemistocytic (jem-is"-tō-sih'-tik) – composed of large round cells (gemistocytes)

Giemsa's stain (gem'-sahz stān) – a solution used for staining protozoan parasites such as trypanosomes

gitter cell (git'-er sel) – a honeycombed cell packed with a number of lipoid granules

glomangioma (glō-man"-jē-ō'-muh) – a benign, often painful tumor derived from a neuromyoarterial glomus, usually occurring on the distal portions of the fingers and toes, in the skin, or in deeper structures

Gomori methenamine silver stain (guh-mōr'-ē meth"-en-am'-ēn sihl'-vur stān) – stain used specifically for fungus

gynandroblastoma (jī-nan"-drō-blas-tō'-muh) – a rare ovarian tumor containing histological features of both arrhenoblastoma and granulosa cell tumor

h

Hamman-Rich syndrome (ham'-un rich sin'-drōm) – a disease characterized by widespread fibrosis of the lung parenchyma

Hassall's corpuscles (hass'-ulz kor'-puh-suhlz) – small concentrically striated bodies in the thymus

hemangiopericytoma (hē-man"-jē-ō-pār"-ē-sih-tō'-muh) – a tumor composed of spindle cells with a rich vascular network, which apparently arises from pericytes

hematoxylin stain (hēm"-ah-tok'-sih-lin stān) – an intense blue stain used in the preparation of microscopic tissue specimens; stains the nucleus of the cell

hemosiderin (hē"-mō-sid'-er-in) – an insoluble form of storage iron in which the micelles of ferric hydroxide are so arranged as to be visible microscopically, both with and without the use of specific staining methods

Hürthle cells (her'-tul selz) – large eosinophilic cells sometimes found in the thyroid gland

hypereosinophilia (hī"-per-ē"-ō-sin-ō-fil'-ē-uh) – excessive eosinophilia, the formation and accumulation of an abnormally large number of eosinophils in the blood

hypogammaglobulinemia (hī"-pō-gam"-uh-glob"-yoo-lin-ē'-mē-uh) – an immunological deficiency state generally characterized by an abnormally low level of all classes of gamma globulin in the blood

i

iatrogenic (ī"-at-rō-jen'-ik) – resulting from the activity of physicians

j

Jakob-Creutzfeldt disease (yak'-ob-kroytz'-felt dih-zēz') – a progressive dementia involving gray matter and basal ganglia

k

Kaposi's sarcoma (kap'-uh-sēz sar-kō'-muh) – a multifocal, metastasizing, malignant reticulosis with features resembling those of angiosarcoma, principally involving the skin

karyolysis (kār"-ē-ahl'-ih-sis) – destruction or breakdown of the cell's nucleus, at least the loss of affinity of its chromatin for basic dyes

keratoacanthoma (kār"-uh-tō-ak"-an-thō'-muh) – a rapidly growing papular lesion, with a crater filled with a keratin plug, which reaches maximum size and then resolves spontaneously within four to six months from onset

Kerckring's folds (kerk'-ringz foldz) – circular folds of mucous membranes that form elevations in the inner wall of the small intestine

Krukenberg's tumor (kroo'-ken-bergz too'-mur) – a special type of carcinoma of the ovary, usually metastatic from cancer of the gastrointestinal tract, especially of the stomach

Kupffer's cells (koop'-ferz selz) – large star-shaped or pyramidal cells with a large oval nucleus and a small prominent nucleolus

l

Lambl's excrescence (lam'-bulz eks-kress'-ens) – small papillary projections on the cardiac valves seen postmortem on many adult hearts

Langhans' cells (lahng'-hahnz selz) – polyhedral epithelial cells constituting cytotrophoblasts

Letterer-Siwe disease (let'-er-er-sī'-wē dih-zēz') – a serious disease characterized by a proliferation of reticuloendothelial cells in many organs, especially lymph nodes, spleen, and bone

leucine aminopeptidase (loo'-sin am-ē"-nō-pep'-tih-dāz) – an enzyme found in the pancreas

Leydig's cells (lī'-digz selz) – the interstitial cells of the testes that furnish the internal secretion of the testicle

lines of Zahn (līnz uv zahn) – the white lines that are present in thrombosed blood clots and consist of coagulated blood serum that has separated from cellular components

lutein (loo'-tē-in) – a yellow pigment, or lipochrome, from the corpus luteum, from fat cells, and from the yolk of eggs

Lutembacher's syndrome (loo'-tem-bak"-erz sin'-drōm) – atrial septal defect with mitral stenosis

m

macrogametocyte (mak"-rō-gah-mē'-tō-sīt) – the infected red blood cell containing the female form of the malarial parasite which, when transferred from a human to a mosquito, becomes a macrogamete

Malherbe's epithelioma (mahl-ārbz' eh"-pih-thē"-lē-ō'-muh) – a tumor made up of squamous epithelial cells in which heterotopic calcification is present

malpighian corpuscles (mal-pig'-ē-un kor'-puh"-sulz) – ovoid collections of lymphocytes that are present around the small penicilliary blood vessels in the spleen

May-Grunwald stain (mā-groon'-wawld stān) – an alcoholic neutral mixture of methylene blue and eosin

Mayer's mucicarmine stain (mā'-erz myoo"-sih-kar'-mīn stān) – a tissue stain for the substance mucin

megakaryocyte (meg"-uh-kār'-ē-ō-sīt) – the giant cell of bone marrow

mesenchymoma (meh"-zeng-kī-mō'-muh) – a mixed mesenchymal tumor composed of two or more cellular elements not commonly associated, not counting fibrous tissue as one of the elements

molluscum contagiosum (mō-lus'-kum kon-tā'-jē-ō-sum) – a mildly contagious viral disease characterized by lesions in the skin or trunk, face, and genital areas

mosaicism (mō-zā'-ih-sih-zum) – the presence of cells that have different chromosomal constitution

mucicarmine stain (myoo"-sih-kar'-mīn stān) – a reddish stain designed to show selectively the presence of mucinous material

myelophthisis (mī"-eh-lof'-thih-sis) – reduction of the cell-forming functions of the bone marrow

n

necropsy (nek'-rop-sē) – examination of a body after death; autopsy

o

osseocartilaginous (oss"-ē-ō-kar"-tih-laj'-ih-nus) – pertaining to or composed of bone and cartilage

p

pacchionian bodies (pak"-ē-ō'-nē-un bah'-dēz) – smooth, granular structures found in the meninges of the brain

pacinian corpuscles (puh-sin'-ē-un kor'-puh'-sulz) – small, but enlarged, nerve endings concerned with the perception of pressure

Paneth's cells (pah'-natz selz) – narrow, pyramidal, or columnar epithelial cells with a round or an oval nucleus close to the base of the cell

Pel-Ebstein fever (pehl-eb'-stīn fē'-vur) – a fever in which the temperature rises by steps over several days and then goes down in steps the same way; common in Hodgkin's disease

phagocytized (fag'-ō-sit"-īzd) – said of particles engulfed by an active call (a phagocyte), especially a histiocyte

phthisis (tī'-sis) – a wasting away of the body or a part of the body; tuberculosis, especially of the lungs

plicae palmatae (plī'-sē pahl'-mah-tuh) – the grooves in the cervical canal

poikilocyte (poy'-kī-lō-sīt") – a red blood cell showing abnormal variation in shape

proteinaceous (prō"-tē-in-ā'-shus) – compounds to or of the nature of a protein

Proteus vulgaris (prō'-tē-us vul-gār'-is) – the type species of Proteus occurring often as a secondary invader in a variety of localized suppurative pathologic processes; a common cause of cystitis

pseudohypha (syoo"-dō-hī'-fuh) – a chain of easily disrupted fungal cells that is intermediate between a chain of budding cells and a true hypha, marked by constrictions rather than septa at the junctions

Pseudomonas aeruginosa (syoo"-dō-mō'-nus ār-oo-jih-nō'-suh) – the causative agent of a variety of human diseases, including common cases of endocarditis, pneumonia, and meningitis

Purkinje's cells (pur-kin'-jēz selz) – large branching neurons in the middle layer of the cortex cerebelli

pyknosis (pik-nō'-sis) – condensation and increased basophilic staining of a cell's nucleus

q

Queyrat's erythroplasia (kā-rahz' ē-rith"-rō-plā'-zē-uh) – squamous cell carcinoma in situ that manifests as a circumscribed, velvety, erythematous papular lesion on the glans penis, coronal sulcus, or prepuce, leading to scaling and superficial ulceration

r

Recklinghausen's disease (rek'-ling-how"-zenz dih-zēz') – a disease characterized by multiple neurocutaneous fibromas

rete pegs (rē'-tē pegz) – the downward, sawtooth-like projections of the epidermis into the dermis

Rokitansky-Aschoff, crypts of (rō"-kih-tan'-skē-ash'-ahff kriptz) – small folds of the gallbladder mucosa that extend into the muscular wall

Rokitansky's disease, tumor (rō"-kih-tan'-skēz dih-zēz', too'-mur) – acute yellow tumor atrophy of the liver

s

saprophytic actinomycosis (sap"-rō-fit'-ik ak"-tih-nō-mī-kō'-sis) – nonpathogenic form of actinomycosis

Schimmelbusch's disease (shim'-el-boosh"-ez dih-zēz') – a form of productive mastitis marked by the production of many small cysts

scrofuloderma (skrof"-yoo-lō-der'-muh) – suppurating abscesses and fistulous passages opening on the skin, secondary to tuberculosis of lymph nodes, most commonly those of the neck, and sometimes of bones and joints

siderogenous (sid"-er-oj'-eh-nus) – producing or forming iron

squamocolumnar (skwah"-mō-kō-lum'-nahr) – pertaining to the junction between a stratified squamous epithelial surface and one lined by columnar epithelium

sympathicoblastoma (sim-path"-ih-kō-blas-tō'-muh) – a malignant tumor containing sympathicoblasts

syncytium (sin-sish'-ē-um) – a multinucleate mass of protoplasm produced by the merging of cells

syringocystadenoma (sih-ring"-gō-sis"-tad-ē-nō'-muh) – adenoma of the sweat glands

t

telangiectatic (tel-an"-jē-ek-tat'-ik) – pertaining to or characterized by telangiectasia, which is a vascular lesion formed by dilatation of a group of small blood vessels and is the basis for a variety of angiomas

thyroglobulin (thī-rō-glob'-yoo-lin) – an iodine-containing protein secreted by the thyroid gland and stored in its colloid substance

trabeculae carneae (trah-bek'-yoo-lē kar'-nē-ā) – rounded, ridge-like elevations on the interior walls of the ventricles of the heart

v

van Gieson's stain (van-gē'-suhnz stān) – a stain for connective tissue, consisting of acid fuchsin and aqueous solution of trinitrophenol

Vater-Pacini corpuscles (fah'-ter-puh-sē'-nē kor'-puh'-sulz) – sensory nerve structures deep in the hands and feet and around joints serving proprioceptive function

Verhoeff's elastic stain (ver'-hefz ē-lass'-tik stān) – a stain for demonstrating elastic tissue

vernix caseosa (ver'-niks cās-ē-ō'-suh) – the white, clinging, greasy material found on the skin of newborn infants

Verocay bodies (vuhr'-ō-kā bah'-dēz) – small groups of fibrils surrounded by rows of palisaded nuclei; seen in nerve tumors

Virchow-Robin spaces (ver'-kō-rō-bēn' spā'-suhz) – the spaces around the blood vessels where they enter the brain

Z

Zenker's fixation (zeng'-kerz fihks-ā'-shun) – a method of hardening tissue in preparation for section (microscopic slide preparation)

Ziehl-Neelsen's method, stain (zēl-nel'-senz meth'-ud, stān) – a staining procedure for demonstrating acid-fast microorganisms

Transcription Tips

Transcribing dictation from pathology can be one of the most difficult tasks in medical transcription because of the difficult and complex vocabulary in pathology and laboratory medicine. The availability of a reference like *A Word Book in Pathology & Laboratory Medicine* by Sloane and Dusseau will make the task easier.

Pathology reports detail the pathological or disease-related findings from an analysis of tissue. The sample tissue may be taken during a biopsy, surgery, a special procedure, or an autopsy. An autopsy report may be requested by the attending physician or coroner when the cause of death is in question (see Model Report #10).

You will note on Model Reports #8 and #9 that the reports include a section for the "gross" description and another for the "microscopic" description. The gross description is done with the naked eye before the specimen is prepared for microscopic analysis. The microscopic description is given after the tissue has been prepared, mounted on a glass slide, and examined under a microscope.

Many times the gross description is dictated and transcribed some time prior to dictation of the microscopic description. When this is done, you should indicate by typing reference initials and the "date dictated" and "date transcribed" a double space after the information dictated for the gross description. A double space below that, you would continue with information of the microscopic description. When this section is complete, you should space four times and type the pathologist's name and title. End the report with the appropriate reference initials and "date dictated" and "date transcribed" for the microscopic examination.

Knowledge of bacteria, viruses, microorganisms, and eponymic syndromes you might encounter in pathology dictation is helpful. The following are selected lists of such terms.

Selected Bacteria

Achromobacter	facultative anaerobe	pneumococcus
Acinetobacter	Flavobacterium	pneumosintes
aerogenes	fragilis	Proprioni
Aeromonas	fragilis isle	Pseudomonas
aeruginosa	Francisella tularensis	ramosus
Aeruginosum	funduliformis	rickettsia
bacillus (pl. bacilli)	fusiform	sonnei
Chlamydia	melaninogenicus	Spirillum
Choleraesuis	meningococcus	Staphylococcus
Cloacae	Mycobacterium	Streptococcus
Clostridium botulinum	Nocardia	tularemia
corrodens	obligate aerobe	tularense
diplococcus (pl. diplococci)	obligate anaerobe	typhosum
dysenteriae	Pestis bubonica	
enteromycosis	plague	

Selected Viruses

avian leukosis
Colorado tick fever
Coxsackie A, B, C
croup-associated (CA)
cytomegalic inclusion disease (CMID)
cytomegalovirus (CMV)
dengue
eastern equine encephalomyelitis (EEE)
Ebola
encephalomyocarditis (EMC)
enteric cytopathic human orphan (ECHO)
Epstein-Barr (EBV)
granulosis
Hantaan
hepatitis A, B, C, D
herpes simplex
human immunodeficiency virus (HIV)
human papilloma (HPA)
human T-cell leukemia-lymphoma virus (HTLV)
influenza
Japanese encephalitis
lactic dehydrogenase (LDH)
leukemia
lymphocytic choriomeningitis (LCM)
measles
Mengo
mononucleosis
mumps
oncogenic (RNA and DNA viruses)
panleukopenia
papilloma
pneumonitis
poliomyelitis
psittacosis
rabies
respiratory syncytial (RS)
roseola infantum
rubella
serum hepatitis
smallpox
St. Louis encephalitis
teratogenic
tickborne
trachoma
vaccinicum
varicella
varicella-zoster
verruca
vesicular stomatitis
West Nile

Selected Microorganisms

Acinetobacter
aerobic
Alcaligenes
anaerobic
anthrax
Bacteroides (anaerobes)
B. fragilis group
Campylobacter
Capnocytophaga
Cardiobacterium hominis
Citrobacter
Clostridium difficile
Cryptosporidium
Enterobacter
enterococcus
E. (Escherichia) coli
Fusobacterium nucleatum
Haemophilus influenza
Klebsiella
Legionnaires' disease, legionella
Lyme disease (Borrelia burgdorferi)
Morganella
mycobacterium
pathogenic
Pneumococci
pneumococcus
pleuropneumonia-like
Pseudomonas
proteolytic gram-negative
Proteus
Rickett's
salmonella
Serratia
Siderobacter
Staphylococcus aureus
streptothrix
Vincent's
Xanthomonas
Yersinia enterocolitica

Eponymic Syndromes

Aarskog-Scott
Abercrombie
Achard
Adair-Dighton
addisonian
Alezzandrini
Angelucci
Axenfeld
Beckwith-Wiedemann
Berardinelli
Bernard-Horner
Brugsch
Caner-Decker
Capgras
Caplan
Chauffard-Still
Chiari
Chotzen
Clouston
Conradi
Cronkhite
Danlos
de Lange
Del Castillo
Dennie-Marfan
Dighton-Adair
Dresbach
Dressler
Duplay
Eagle
Eddowes
Eisenlohr
Ekbom
Faber
Fanconi
Felty
Fitz
Flynn-Aird
Forney
Foville
Fraser
Fuchs
Gailliard
Gard-Girnoux
Gasser
Gerstmann
Gianotti-Crosti
Goldberg-Maxwell
Goltz-Gorlin
Gopalan
Guillain-Barré
Hakim
Hallervorden
Horner
Houssay
Hunter-Hurler
Hurler-Scheie
Irvine
Ivemark
Jackson
Jaffe-Lichtenstein
Job-Buckley
Kallmann
Kartagener
Kasabach-Merritt
Kiloh-Nevin
Kimmelstiel-Wilson
Klauder
Klemperer
Klippel-Feil
Klumpke-Déjerine
Kocher
Kostmann
Krause
Kuskokwim
Laband
Ladd
Lambert-Eaton
Landry-Guillain Barré
Launois
Lawford
Lennox
Leredde
Lesch-Nyhan
Loffler
Looser-Milkman
Louis-Bar
Lutembacher
Mallory-Weiss
Marchesani
Margolis
Marinesco-Garland
Marshall
Martorell
Mauriac
Meckel
Mengert's shock
Meniere
Meyer-Schwickerath and Weyers
Millard-Gubler
Miranda
Monakow
Moore
Morris
Muckle-Wells
Muir-Torre
Munchausen
Naegeli
Nelson
Noack
Nonne-Milroy-Meige
Nothnagel
Ogilvie
Ostrum-Furst
Pancoast
Parinaud
parkinsonian
Parry-Romberg
Patau
Paterson-Kelly
Pellizzi
Pendred
Perlman
Peutz
Pfaundler-Hurler
pickwickian
Pierre Robin
Polhemus-Schafer-Ivemark
Potter
Prader-Willi
Ramsay Hunt
Renpenning
Rett
Reye
Richards-Rundle
Richter
Rieger
Riley-Day
Robinow
Romano-Ward
Rosenbach
Rosenthal-Kloepfer
Rosewater
Rossbach
Rothmann-Makai
Rotor
Rubinstein
Sabin-Feldman
Sanchez Salorio
Schanz
Schwartz

Eponymic Syndromes

Seabright bantam
Seckel
Selye
Senear-Usher
Sheehan
Shwachman
Shy-Drager
Sicard
Simopoulos
Sipple
Sluder
Sotos
Spens
Speransky-Richen-Siegmund
Sprinz-Dubin
Steiner
Stewart-Morel
Stewart-Treves
Stickler
Still-Chauffard
Stilling-Turk-Duane
Stokvis-Talma
Strachan
Sturge-Kalischer-Weber
Tapia
Taussig-Bing
Thibierge-Weissenbach
Thiele
Tolosa-Hunt
Touraine-Solente-Gole
Troisier
Turcot
Uehlinger
Unna-Thost
Van der Woude
Verner-Morrison
Vinson-Plummer
Vogt-Koyanagi
Waardenburg
Wallenberg
Waterhouse-Friderichsen
Wegener
Wenckebach
Wernicke-Korsakoff
Weyers' oligodactyly
Wildervanck
Willebrand
Wilson-Mikity
Wiskott-Aldrich
Wolff-Parkinson-White
Young
Zellweger
Zieve
Zinsser-Cole-Engman
Zollinger-Ellison

Supportive Web Sites

www.labx.com
Search by name of instrument or other equipment.

www.med.uiuc.edu/
Click on "Urbana Atlas of Pathology"; click on other links of interest as desired.

http://medmark.org/path/
Click on links of interest.

www.mic.ki.se
Click on "Diseases, Disorders, and Related Topics"; click on other links of interest as desired.

www.nlm.nih.gov/medlineplus
Search for pathology, organisms, viruses, and so on.

www.oncli.com/pathology/
Click on links of interest.

www.pathinfo.com/
Click on links of interest.

Index of Pathology reports

(see table of contents for audio information)

Exercise #	***Patient Name***	***Tissue Examined/Reports***
TE#1	Farris, Jon	Antrum biopsy; polyp biopsy, right colon
TE#2	Ruckel, Sue	Spleen
TE#3	Rominger, Amber	Uterus
TE#4	Grayson, Micah	Gallbladder and contents
TE#5	Dagget, Danny	Autopsy
TE#6	Haag, Misty	Placenta
TE#7	Atterberry, Shannon	Right breast mass
TE#8	Florimonte, Danny	Right lung mass

CHAPTER 6

OBSTETRICS/ GYNECOLOGY

Introduction

Obstetrics and gynecology (OB/GYN) is the medical specialty that attends to the care of women during pregnancy, childbirth, contraception, and periods of disease. *Ovaries, fallopian tubes, uterus, vagina, vulva,* and *breasts* comprise the female reproductive system. Activity of the ovaries, the primary sex organs, is regulated by the anterior lobe of the *pituitary gland.*

The ovaries produce *ova* and *hormones.* The fallopian tubes convey the ovum from the ovary to the uterus and sperm from the uterus toward each ovary.

The uterus has an upper portion, a central area (called the *isthmus*) and the *cervix* or lower portion. Within the uterus, the wall is made of three layers—the *peritoneum* or outer layer, the *myometrium* or middle layer, and the *endometrium* or inner layer.

Because the uterus is supported by ligaments that affect its position, it may become malpositioned due to weakness of one or more of the ligaments. Four terms describing such abnormal positions are *anteflexion, retroflexion, anteversion,* and *retroversion.*

The vagina is the organ of copulation and receives the semen from the male penis. It also serves as the passageway for the bloody discharge during *menstruation* and the birth of a fetus.

The *vulva* is composed of the *mons pubis, labia majora, labia minora, vestibule,* and *clitoris,* which make up the external female genitalia. The breasts are the mammary glands that produce milk for newborns.

Physicians who attend to the reproductive problems of women are *gynecologists* and/or *obstetricians.* A gynecologist is a doctor who diagnoses and treats medical problems of the reproductive organs of women and, when necessary, also performs surgery. An obstetrician is the doctor who cares for pregnant women before, during, and after delivery.

All gynecologists are also obstetricians, but not all obstetricians are gynecologists. Some general practitioners also perform obstetrical services and call in an obstetrician only when difficulties arise in the delivery process.

Anyone working as an assistant for a gynecologist or obstetrician should have a basic understanding of the processes of pregnancy, childbirth, and its aftermath.

Critical Thinking Exercise

In your opinion, where do personal ethical beliefs, such as those concerning abortion, come into play in your job as a medical transcriptionist? Would you refuse to transcribe an abortion procedure report? Why or why not?

Respond as a professional and be specific in your response.

Obstetrics/Gynecology Abbreviations

AB	abortion
AFP	alpha-fetoprotein
AH	abdominal hysterectomy
AP	anteroposterior (AP vaginal vault repair)
AROM	artificial rupture of membrane
BBT	basal body temperature
BOW	bag of waters (BOW rupture)
B&S	Bartholin and Skene (glands)

BUS	Bartholin gland, urethra, and Skene (glands)
CIS	carcinoma in-situ
CPD	cephalopelvic disproportion
CS, C-section	cesarean section
CVS	chorionic villus sampling
Cx	cervix
D&C/D & C	dilatation and curettage
DES	diethylstilbestrol (estrogen)
DUB	dysfunctional uterine bleeding
EBL	estimated blood loss
ECC	endocervical curettage
EDC	expected (or estimated) date of confinement
EMB	endometrial biopsy
ERT	estrogen replacement therapy
EUA	examination under anesthesia
FHT	fetal heart tone
FSH	follicle-stimulating hormone
FT	full term
G	gravida (pregnant)
GIFT	gamete intrafallopian transfer
GPA	gravida, para, abortio
Gyn/GYN	gynecology
HCG/hCG	human chorionic gonadotropin
HRT	human replacement therapy
HSG	hysterosalpingography or hysterosalpingogram
IUD	intrauterine device
IUP	intrauterine pregnancy
IVPB	intravenous piggyback
LASH	laparoscopic supracervical hysterectomy
LAVH	laparoscopic-assisted vaginal hysterectomy
LEEP	loop electrosurgical excision procedure
LH	luteinizing hormone
LMP	last menstrual period
LNMP	last normal menstrual period
L/S	lecithin/sphingomyelin ratio (a test on amniotic fluid to determine the maturity of the fetal lungs)
MH	marital history
multip	multipara; multiparous
NB	newborn
OB	obstetrics
OCPs	oral contraceptive pills
Para 3-1-1-3	woman's reproductive history; 3 full-term infants, 1 preterm, 1 abortion, and 3 living children
PAP/ Pap smear	Papanicolaou (smear)
PDS	polydioxanone suture
PG	pregnant
PID	pelvic inflammatory disease
PMP	previous menstrual period
PMS	premenstrual syndrome
POC	products of conception
PSA	polyethylene sulfonic acid
PUD	pregnancy undelivered
Rh neg.	Rhesus factor negative
Rh pos.	Rhesus factor positive
SAB	spontaneous abortion
SROM	spontaneous rupture of membranes
TAH-BSO	total abdominal hysterectomy with bilateral salpingo-oophorectomy
TSS	toxic shock syndrome
UC	uterine contractions
UV	uterovesical
VBAC	vaginal birth after cesarean
VIP	voluntary interruption of pregnancy

Anatomic Illustrations

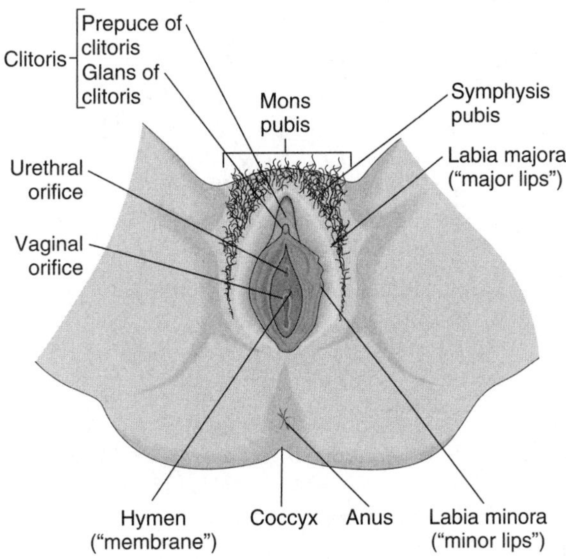

6–1 EXTERNAL FEMALE GENITALIA

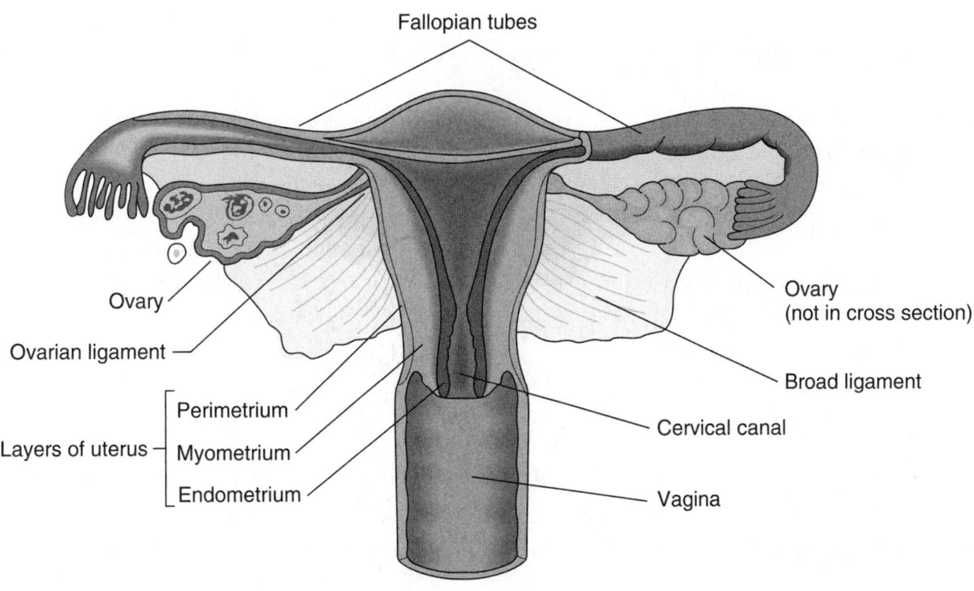

6–2 INTERNAL GENITAL ORGANS OF THE FEMALE

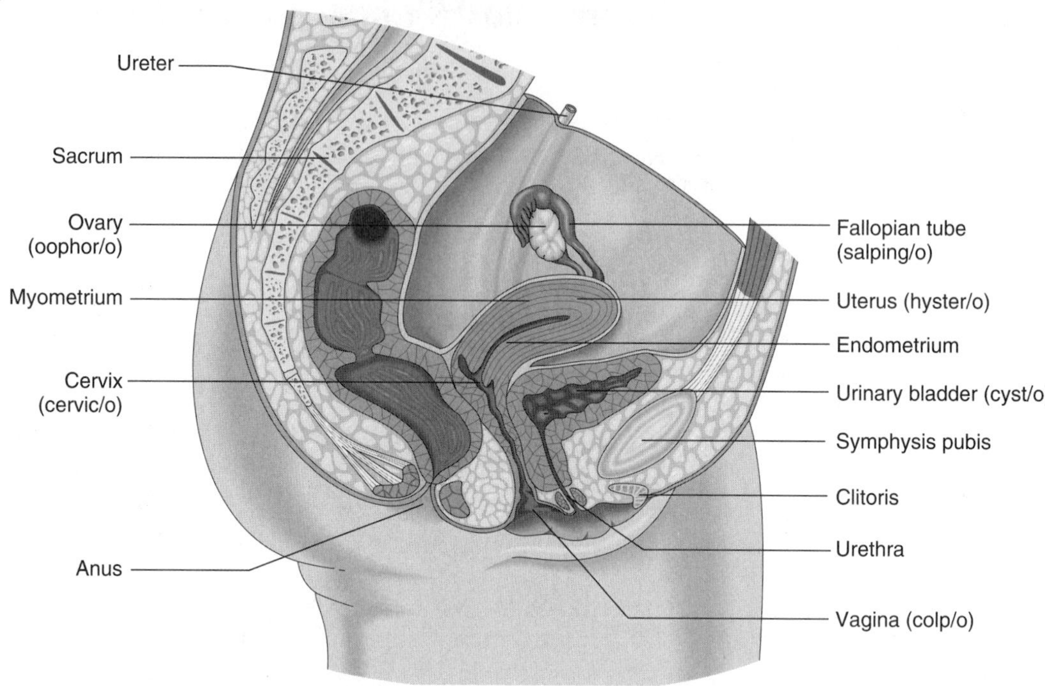

6–3 FEMALE REPRODUCTIVE SYSTEM

Obstetrics/Gynecology Terminology

a

abruptio placentae (ah-brup'-shē-ō pluh-sen'-tuh) – premature detachment of the placenta

amenorrhea (a-men"-ō-rē'-uh) – the complete or abnormal cessation of menstruation

amniocentesis (am"-nē-ō-sen-tē'-sis) – the process whereby the uterus is entered through the abdomen to extract amniotic fluid

amnionitis (am"-nē-ō-nī'-tis) – inflammation of the amnion

amniorrhea (am"-nē-ō-rē'-uh) – the escape of the amniotic fluid

ante partum (an'-tē par'-tum) – the period before the onset of labor

anteflexion of uterus (an-tē-flek'-shun) – condition present when the uterus is abnormally bent forward

antenatal (an"-tē-nā'-tul) – before birth

Apgar score (ap'-gar skōr) – a numerical expression of the condition of a newborn infant, usually determined at one minute and five minutes after birth, being the sum of points gained on assessment of the heart rate, respiratory effort, muscle tone, reflex irritability, and color

autologous ovarian transplantation (aw-tol'-uh-gus ō-vār'-ē-un trans"-plan-tā'-shun) – procedure performed to maintain ovarian function when one is undergoing sterilizing chemotherapy, radiotherapy, or oophorectomy; a strip of the patient's own cortical ovarian tissue is transplanted somewhere under her subcutaneous tissue

b

ballottement (bah-lot'-ment) – the use of a finger to push sharply against the uterus and detect the presence or position of a fetus

bartholinitis (bar"-tō-lin-ī'-tis) – inflammation of Bartholin glands

betamethasone (bā"-tuh-meth'-uh-sōn) – a semisynthetic glucocorticoid that has anti-inflammatory effects and toxicity similar to those of cortisol; trade name is Celestone

c

Candida vaginitis (kan'-dih-duh vaj"-ih-nī'-tis) – an infection of the vagina caused by a yeast-like fungus of the genus Candida

catamenia (kat"-uh-mē'-nē-uh) – the condition of monthly discharge of blood from the uterus

cauterize (kaw"-ter-īz) – to destroy tissue with heat, electric current, or a caustic substance

cephalopelvic disproportion (sef"-uh-lō-pel'-vik dis"-prō-por'-shun) – condition where the head of the fetus is too large for the mother's pelvis

cerclage (sar-klahzh') – encircling of a part with a ring or loop, such as encirclement of the incompetent cervix uteri

cervicectomy (ser"-vih-sek'-tuh-mē) – excision of the cervix uteri

cervix – the narrow passage at the lower end of the uterus that connects with the vagina

cesarean section (sē-zā'-rē-un sek'-shun) – incision through the abdominal and uterine walls for delivery of a fetus

chorioamnionitis (kaw"-rē-ō-am"-nē-ō-nī'-tis) – inflammation of the fetal membranes

chorion (kaw'-rē-ahn) – the outer membrane enclosing the embryo

chorionic villi (kaw"-rē-ahn'-ik vil'-ī) – one of the thread-like projections growing in tufts on the external surface of the chorion

clitoris (klī'-tō-ris) – a small, pea-shaped organ composed of erectile tissue similar in sensitivity to the penis in the male

clonus (klō'-nus) – alternate muscular contraction and relaxation in rapid succession

coitus (kō'-ē-tus) – the act of intercourse

colostrum (kō-lah'-strum) – the thin, yellow, milky fluid secreted by the mammary gland a few days before or after childbirth

colpectomy (kahl-pek'-tuh-mē) – excision of the vagina

colpoperineoplasty (kahl"-pō-pār"-ih-nē'-ō-plas"-tē) – surgical repair of the vagina and perineum

colpoperineorrhaphy (kahl"-pō-pār"-ih-nē-or'-uh-fē) – suture of the ruptured vagina and perineum

colporrhaphy (kahl-pōr'-uh-fē) – the operation of suturing the vagina; the operation of denuding and suturing the vaginal wall for the purpose of narrowing the vagina

colpotomy (kahl-pot'-uh-mē) – incision into the wall of the vagina

copulation (kahp"-yoo-lā'-shun) – sexual union between male and female; usually used in reference to animals lower than humans

culdocentesis (kul"-dō-sen-tē'-sis) – aspiration of fluid from the rectouterine excavation by puncture of the vaginal wall

d

decidua (dē-sid'-yoo-uh) – the mucous lining of the uterus that comes off after childbirth

defervesced (dē"-fer-vest') – fever decreased

descensus uteri (dē-sen'-sus yoo'-ter-ī) – prolapse of the uterus

douglasectomy (dug"-lus-ek'-tuh-mē) – the only definitive laparoscopic procedure for restoring normal anatomy of the pelvic floor as the result of painful uterine retroversion; involves resection of the cul-de-sac of Douglas

dysmenorrhea (diz"-men-ō-rē'-uh) – painful menstruation

dyspareunia (dis"-puh-roo'-nē-uh) – painful or difficult intercourse

dystocia (dis-tō'-sē-uh) – abnormal labor or childbirth

e

eclampsia (ē-klamp'-sē-uh) – convulsions and coma, rarely coma alone, occurring in a pregnant or puerperal woman, associated with hypertension, edema, and/or proteinuria

eclamptic toxemia (ē-klamp'-tik tok-sē'-mē-uh) – toxemia during pregnancy

endocervical (en"-dō-ser'-vih-kul) – pertaining to the interior of the cervix uteri

endocervicitis (en"-dō-ser"-vih-sī'-tis) – inflammation of the mucous membrane of the cervix uteri

endometrioma (en"-dō-mē"-trē-ō'-muh) – a tumor containing shreds of ectopic endometrium

endometriosis (en"-dō-mē"-trē-ō'-sis) – a condition where endometrial tissue occurs in various sites in the abdominal or pelvic cavity

endometrium (en-dō-mē'-trē-um) – the mucous membrane of the uterus, the thickness and structure of which vary with the phase of the menstrual cycle

episiotomy (ē-piz"-ē-ot'-uh-mē) – surgical incision of the vulvar orifice for obstetrical purposes

epithelium (ep"-ih-thē'-lē-um) – – the covering of internal and external surfaces of the body, including the lining of vessels and other small cavities

eutocia (yoo-tō'-sē-uh) – the condition of a good, normal childbirth

f

fornix (fōr'-niks) – a vaulted space

fundus (fun'-dus) – the small rounded part of the uterus above where the fallopian tubes enter

g

gamete intrafallopian transfer (GIFT) (gam'-ēt in"-truh-fah-lō'-pē-an trans'-fur) – a procedure that places the sperm and eggs directly in the fimbriated end of the fallopian tube via a laparoscope

Gelfoam pack (jel'-fōm pak) – an absorbable gelatin sponge

gravid (grav'-id) – pregnant

gravida (grav'-ih-duh) – a pregnant woman

h

Hegar dilator (hā'-gar dī'-lā-tur) – a slender, flexible instrument used for dilating the cervix

hematosalpinx (hēm"-uh-tō-sal'-pinks) – a collection of blood in the fallopian tube that may be associated with tubal pregnancy

High-McCall suspension (hī'-muh-kol" sus-pen'-shun) – a procedure to repair the vaginal vault

hirsutism (hēr'-soo-tizm) – abnormal hairiness, especially in women

hydatid of Morgagni (hī'-dah-tid uv mōr-gahn'-yē) – a cyst-like remnant of the mullerian duct attached to a testis or to the oviduct

hyperemesis gravidarum (hī"-per-em'-ē-sis grav"-ih-dah'-rum) – excessive vomiting during pregnancy

i

introitus (in-trō'-ih-tus) – a general term for the entrance to a cavity or space

ischiorectal (is"-kē-ō-rek'-tul) – pertaining to the ischium and rectum

l

labia majora (lā'-bē-uh mah-jō'-ruh) – two folds of skin that extend backward or downward to the perineum; the outer surfaces are covered with hair

labia minora (lā'-bē-uh mē-nō'-ruh) – two folds of skin-like lips located within the labia majora

Lembert's suture (lahm-bārz' soo-tyoor) – a type of suture used in a cesarean section

leukorrhea (loo"-kō-rē'-uh) – a whitish, viscid discharge from the vagina and uterine cavity

lochia (lō'-kē-uh) – the vaginal discharge that occurs during the first week or two after childbirth

Lunelle™ (loo-nel') – a once-a-month injectable drug for pregnancy prevention

m

mastitis (mass-tī'-tis) – inflammation of the breast

menarche (meh-nar'-kē) – the beginning of the menstrual function

menometrorrhagia (men"-ō-meh"-trō-rā'-jē-uh) – excessive uterine bleeding occurring both during the menses and at irregular intervals

menorrhagia (men"-ō-rā'-jē-uh) – excessive uterine bleeding during the menstrual period

menorrhea (men"-ō-rē'-uh) – normal monthly flow

metrorrhagia (meh"-trō-rā'-jē-uh) – uterine bleeding, usually of normal amount, occurring at completely irregular intervals, the period of flow sometimes being prolonged

mittelschmerz (mit'-el-shmārtz) – intermenstrual pain that occurs during ovulation

Monilia vaginitis (mō-nil'-ē-uh vaj"-ih-nī'-tis) – an inflammation of the vagina caused by a fungus of the genus Moniliaceae

multigravida (mul"-tī-grav'-ih-duh) – woman who has been pregnant several times

multiparity (mul"-tī-par'-ih-tē) – the condition of having two or more pregnancies that resulted in viable fetuses

myoma (mī-o'-muh) – a common tumor of the uterus made up of muscular elements

myometritis (mī"-o-meh-trī'-tis) – inflammation of the muscular substance, or myometrium, of the uterus

myometrium (mī-ō-mē'-trē-um) – the smooth muscle coat of the uterus that forms the main mass of the organ

n

nabothian cyst (nah-bō'-thē-un sist) – cyst-like formation caused by occlusion of the lumina of glands in the mucosa of the uterine cervix, causing them to be distended with retained secretion

Nuck's canal (nuks kuh-nal') – an anomalous peritoneal pouch extending into the labium of the external female genitalia

nulliparous (nuh-lip'-uh-rus) – having never given birth to a viable infant

NuvaRing® (noo'-vuh-ring) – a monthly vaginal ring for birth control

o

oligomenorrhea (ol"-ih-gō-men"-ō-rē'-uh) – markedly diminished menstrual flow; relative amenorrhea

oogenesis (ō"-ō-jen'-eh-sis) – formation of the ovum

oophorectomy (ō"-ō-fōr-ek'-tuh-mē) – the removal of an ovary or ovaries

oophoritis (ō"-ō-fōr-ī'-tis) – inflammation of an ovary

P

panhysterectomy (pan"-his-ter-ek'-tuh-mē) – complete removal of the uterus and cervix; total hysterectomy

Papanicolaou's stain (Pap smear) (pap"-uh-nik"-ō-lā'-ooz stān, smēr) – routine cancer detection test

parturition (par"-tyoo-rish'-un) – the act of giving birth

pelvimetry (pel-vim'-eh-trē) – the measurement of the dimensions and capacity of the pelvis

perimetrium (pār-ih-mē'-trē-um) – the serous coat of the uterus

perineum (pār"-ih-nē'-um) – the pelvic floor and the associated structures occupying the pelvic outlet

peritoneum (pār"-ih-tō-nē'-um) – the serous membrane lining the abdominopelvic walls

Pfannenstiel's incision (fan'-en-stēlz in-sih'-zhun) – a curved abdominal incision named for Hermann Johann Pfannenstiel, a gynecologist in Breslau

placenta praevia (plah-sen'-tuh prē'-vē-uh) – a placenta that develops in the lower uterine segment, so that it obstructs the internal opening of the cervix

polyhydramnios (pol"-ē-hī-dram'-nē-ōs) – too much amniotic fluid

polymenorrhea (pol"-ē-men"-ō-rē'-uh) – abnormally frequent menstruation

preeclampsia (prē"-ē-klamp'-sē-uh) – a toxemia of late pregnancy, characterized by hypertension, albuminuria, and edema

primigravida (prī"-mih-grav'-ih-duh) – a woman who is pregnant for the first time

procidentia (prō"-sih-den'-shē-uh) – condition present when the uterus falls to the degree that the cervix protrudes from the vagina

progesterone (prō-jes'-ter-ōn) – a female hormone that prepares the uterus for the reception and development of the fertilized ovum by inducing secretion in the proliferated glands

prolapse uteri (prō-laps' yoo'-ter-ī) – protrusion of the uterus through the vaginal orifice

pruritus vulvae (proo-rī'-tus vul'-vuh) – intense itching of the external genitals of the female

pseudocyesis (soo"-dō-sī-ē'-sis) – a false pregnancy

pudendal (pu-den'-dul) – pertaining to the female genitalia

pudendal block (pu-den'-dul blahk) – a type of anesthesia used in childbirth

pyometritis (pī"-ō-me-trī'-tis) – purulent inflammation of the uterus

R

retroflexion (reh"-trō-flek'-shun) – the bending backward of the body of the uterus toward the cervix

Retzius's space (ret'-zē-us spās) – space in lower portion of abdomen between bladder and pubic bones and bounded superiorly by peritoneum

S

salpingectomy (sal"-pin-jek'-tuh-mē) – surgical removal of the uterine tube

salpingitis (sal"-pin-jī'-tis) – inflammation of the uterine tube

salpingo (sal-ping'-gō) – a combining form denoting relationship to a tube, specifically to the uterine or to the auditory tube

salpingo-oophorectomy (sal-ping"-gō-ō"-ō-fōr-ek'-tuh-mē) – surgical removal of a uterine tube and ovary

secundines (sek'-un-dīnz) – the afterbirth

Stein-Leventhal syndrome (stīn-lev'-en-thahl sin'-drōm) – a clinical symptom complex characterized by secondary amenorrhea and anovulation (hence sterility), and regularly associated with bilateral polycystic ovaries

subinvolution (sub"-in-vō-loo'-shun) – failure of a part to return to its normal size and condition after enlargement due to functional activity

suprapubic (soo"-pruh-pyoo'-bik) – situated or performed above the pubic arch

symphysis pubis (sim'-fih-sis pyoo'-bis) – the joint formed by union of the bodies of the pubic bones in the median plane by a thick mass of fibrocartilage

T

tenaculum (tē-nak'-yoo-lum) – a hook-like instrument for seizing and holding tissues

tocolysis (tō-kahl'-ī-sis) – inhibition of uterine contractions

toxemia (tok-sē'-mē-uh) – a general intoxication sometimes due to the absorption of bacterial products (toxins) formed in local source of infection

Trichomonas (trih-kō"-mō'-nus) – parasitic protozoa that cause urogenital infection

U

ultrasound (ul'-trah-sownd) – mechanical radiant energy, with a frequency greater than 20,000 cycles per second

utero-ovarian (yoo"-ter-ō-ō-vār'-ē-un) – pertaining to the uterus and ovary

uterosacral ligament (yoo"-ter-ō-sā'-krul lig'-uh-ment) – a part of the thickening of the visceral pelvic fascia beside the cervix and vagina, passing posteriorly in the rectouterine fold to attach to the front of the sacrum

uterovesical (yoo"-ter-ō-vess'-ih-kul) – pertaining to the uterus and bladder

V

vesicouterine (ves"-ih-kō-yoo'-ter-in) – pertaining to or communicating with the urinary bladder and the uterus

vesicovaginal (ves"-ih-kō-vaj'-ih-nul) – pertaining to the urinary bladder and vagina

vulva (vul'-vuh) – the external aspect of the female genitalia

vulvectomy (vul-vek'-tuh-mē) – excision of the vulva

Z

zygote (zī'-gōt) – the fertilized ovum

Transcription Tips

When transcribing obstetrics/gynecology dictation, you should be familiar with the organs of the female reproductive system, their locations, and their functions.

The female reproductive organs comprise the vulva, including the labia majora, labia minora, and clitoris; the vagina; the uterus; two fallopian tubes; and two ovaries. The purpose of these organs is to produce ova, to nurture them after fertilization during their nine-month development period, and then to give them birth. This part of the genitourinary system also secretes certain hormones for the maintenance of secondary sexual characteristics in the female.

Confusing Terms

gland – aggregation of cells specialized to secrete or excrete materials not related to their ordinary metabolic needs

glans – a general term for a small rounded mass

perineal – pertaining to the perineum

peritoneal – pertaining to the peritoneum

perineum – the pelvic floor

peritoneum – the serous membrane lining the abdominopelvic walls and investing the viscera

urethra – the membranous canal that conveys urine from the bladder to the exterior of the body

ureter – the fibromuscular tube that conveys the urine from the kidney to the bladder

vesicle – a small bladder or sac containing liquid

vessel – any channel for carrying a fluid

Roots and/or Combining Forms

Root	Meaning	Root	Meaning
abdomino	abdomen	lyso	breaking down, dissolution
adeno, aden	gland	mammo	breast
carcino	carcinoma	masto, mast	breast
celio	abdomen	myo, my	muscle
cephalo, cephal	head	oophoro	ovary
chordo	cord	pathy	disease
colpo, colp	vagina	poly	many, excessive
cysto, cyst, cysti, cystido	sac, bladder	procto, proct	rectum
		py, pyo	pus
episio	vulva	recto	rectum
gyneco, gyn, gyne, gyno	woman	salpingo, salping	tube, uterine
		splanchno	viscera
hem, hema, hemo, hemat, hemato	blood	spleno, splen	spleen
		steno	narrowed
hydro, hydr	water	uretero	ureter
hystero	uterus, hysteria	urethro	urethra
ileo	ileum	utero	uterus
ilio	ilium, flank	vaso	vessel
laparo	flank, abdomen	veno	vein
leuco, leuko	white		

Remember, combining forms are always found in conjunction with a prefix, suffix, another combining form, or any combination of these.

Terms Used in Reference to the Person Experiencing Parturition (Labor)

parturient – the woman in labor

parous – having given birth, vaginally or abdominally, at or beyond 20 weeks of gestation

parity – refers to the number of parous deliveries, whether live birth, single or multiple, stillbirth, vaginal, or cesarean section

nullipara – a woman who has had no deliveries at or beyond 20 weeks of gestation

primipara – a woman who has had one delivery at or beyond 20 weeks of gestation

multipara – a woman who has had more than one delivery at or beyond 20 weeks of gestation

Supportive Web Sites

www.centerwatch.com
Under "Patient and General Resources," select "Drug Directories"; then click on "Drugs Newly Approved by the FDA." Select "Obstetrics/Gynecology" for a particular year to see drugs approved for this specialty during that year.

www.fda.gov
Select "Site Map"; then "Information for Specific Audiences—Women."

www.mayoclinic.com
Under "Find information fast," select the initial letter of a disease or condition in which you are interested (i.e., "e" for "endometriosis"); then click on the word for more information.

www.merck.com
Click on "The Merck Manuals"; select The Merck Manual of Diagnosis and Therapy; go to Table of Contents; click on "Section 18: Gynecology/Obstetrics," then on topic of interest.

www.my.webmd.com
Select "Diseases and Conditions" link under "Medical Info"; then "Women's Health"; then "search" for topics of interest (such as endometriosis, fibroids, STDs, pregnancy, etc.).

www.nlm.nih.gov
Click on "Health Information", then MEDLINEplus. On the MEDLINEplus page, "search" for obstetrics, gynecology, or other related topics of interest.

Index of Obstetrics/Gynecology Reports

(see table of contents for audio information)

Exercise #	*Patient Name*	*Report/Procedure*
TE#1	Zin, Daboo	Abdominal hysterectomy, bilateral salpingo-oophorectomy, pelvic lymphadenectomy, total omentectomy
TE#2	Zin, Daboo	Discharge summary
TE#3	Linton, Sonya	Cone biopsy of cervix
TE#4	Byrd, Debbie	Vaginal hysterectomy, cystotomy, and repair
TE#5	Shelley, Annie	Abdominal hysterectomy with bilateral salpingo-oophorectomy
TE#6	Hatten, Cheryl	Cesarean section
TE#7	Holloway, Elaine	Suction curettage
TE#8	Pierce, Barbara	Postpartum tubal ligation
TE#9	Yuen, Judi	Vaginal hysterectomy, salpingo-oophorectomy, uterosacral plication

CHAPTER 7

ORTHOPEDICS

Introduction

Orthopedics is the branch of medicine concerned with the preservation and restoration of the function of the *musculoskeletal system* and the treatment of muscular and skeletal diseases such as *poliomyelitis* and *muscular dystrophy.* Disorders of vertebral *disks, fractures, joint injuries,* correction of *deformities,* and diseases such as *arthritis* are also concerns of orthopedics.

The human body is made up of about 40 to 50 percent muscle and 206 bones. In the body, bones perform three major functions: they form the support framework, provide protection for internal organs, and make movement possible with the help of muscles. Bones are made up of approximately 50 percent water and 50 percent solid matter called *osseous tissue.*

Bones are classified into long, short, flat, irregular, and sesamoid. Features found in all bones include compact bone, periosteum, epiphysis, diaphysis, endosteum, medullary canal, and cancellous or spongy bone.

The *vertebral column* is made up of 26 separate bones called vertebrae, grouped in five segments from the base of the skull to the tailbone. The *spinal column* consists of 7 cervical, 12 thoracic, and 5 lumbar vertebrae. The *sacrum* is one fused vertebra, and the *coccyx,* or tailbone, is the last bone in the vertebral column. When the vertebral column is not aligned properly, three curvatures may occur—*scoliosis, lordosis,* and *kyphosis.*

A very serious bone abnormality is *osteoporosis,* caused by a decrease in bone mass. This serious condition affects more than 25 million Americans. More women than men are affected by this disease process.

The muscles are connected to the bones, ligaments, cartilage, and skin either directly or through the intervention of fibrous structures called *tendons* or *fascia,* sometimes called *aponeuroses.*

Common operative procedures performed by orthopedists are hip replacements; knee replacements; open reductions and internal fixations (ORIFs); arthroscopy of the knee, shoulder, and joints (e.g., ankle, elbow, wrist); and amputations. *Arthroscopies* are the most common orthopedic procedure performed in the United States today. Orthopedic surgeons are now able to perform ligament reconstructions, meniscal repairs, and tendon repairs with the aid of an arthroscope.

Critical Thinking Exercise

You are transcribing a knee replacement procedure and the physician has dictated "right knee" in both the preop and postop diagnoses—but in describing the procedure, he says "left knee."

What would you do to determine which knee was actually operated on?

Orthopedics Abbreviations

AC	acromioclavicular
ADL	activities of daily living
AE	above elbow
AK	above knee
AO	anterior oblique
AP	anteroposterior
Arth.	arthrotomy
AVN	avascular necrosis
BE	below elbow
BK	below knee

C1	cervical vertebra, first
C2	cervical vertebra, second
C3	cervical vertebra, third
Ca	calcium
CDH	congenital dislocation of hip
CPM	continuous passive motion
CPPD	calcium pyrophosphate deposition disease
CTR	carpal tunnel release
CVA	costovertebral angle
DIPJ	distal interphalangeal joint
DJD	degenerative joint disease
DP	dorsalis pedis
DTR	deep tendon reflex
DVT	deep venous thrombosis
EMG	electromyography
FCE	functional capacity examination
Fx	fracture
FROM	full range of motion
FWB	full weightbearing
HD	hip disarticulation
HNP	herniated nucleus pulposus
HP	hemipelvectomy
IDK	internal derangement of the knee
IM	intramuscular
IPJ	interphalangeal joint
IT	iliotibial
JRA	juvenile rheumatoid arthritis
jt	joint
KB	knee bearing
KD	knee disarticulation
KJ	knee jerk
L1	lumbar vertebra, first
L2	lumbar vertebra, second
L3	lumbar vertebra, third
LAC	long arm cast
lig	ligament
LDH	lactic dehydrogenase
LLC	long leg cast
LLCC	long leg cylinder case
LOM	limitation or loss of motion
MPJ	metacarpophalangeal joint
MS	musculoskeletal
NSAID	nonsteroidal anti-inflammatory drug
NWB	nonweightbearing
OA	osteoarthritis
ORIF	open reduction internal fixation
orth	orthopedics
PEMFS	pulsing electromagnetic fields
PIPJ	proximal interphalangeal joint
PMR	physical medicine and rehabilitation
psi	pounds per square inch
PVS	pigmented villonodular synovitis
PWB	partial weight bearing
RA	rheumatoid arthritis
ROM	range of motion
SAC	short arm cast
SCFE	slipped capital femoral epiphysis
SD	shoulder disarticulation
SLC	short leg cast
SLR	straight leg raising
T1	thoracic vertebra, first
T2	thoracic vertebra, second
T3	thoracic vertebra, third
TBW	total body weight
TENS	transcutaneous electrical nerve stimulation
THR	total hip replacement
TJ	triceps jerk
Tx	traction
Wt	weight

Anatomic Illustrations

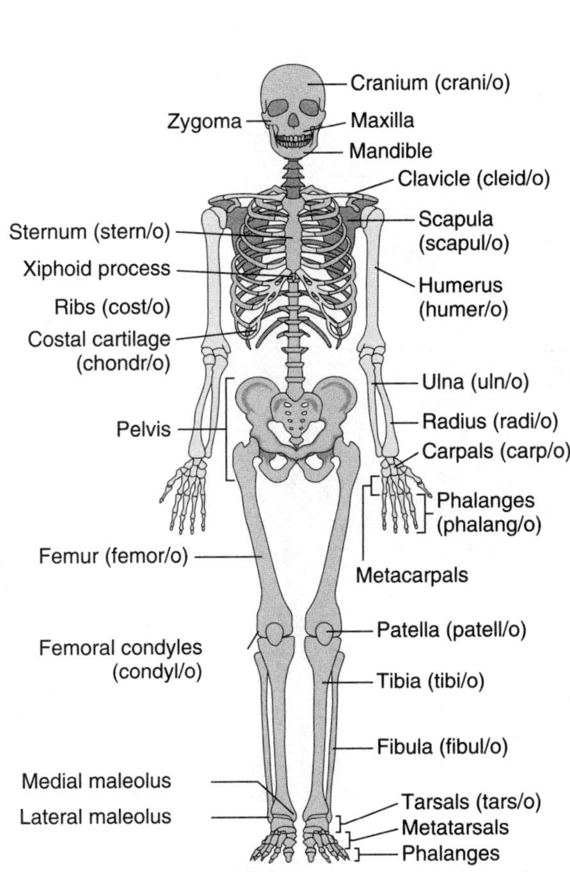

7–1 SKELETAL SYSTEM

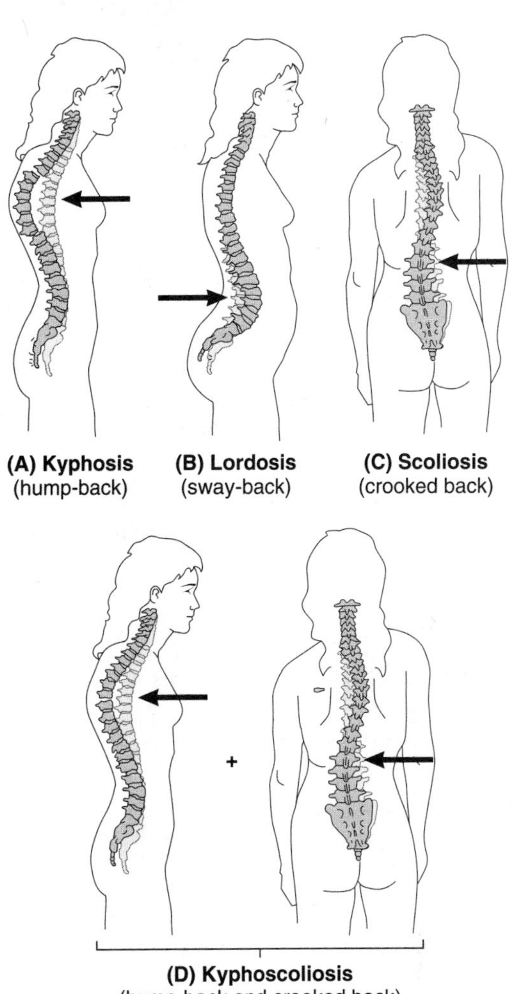

7–2 ABNORMAL CURVATURES OF THE VERTEBRAL COLUMN

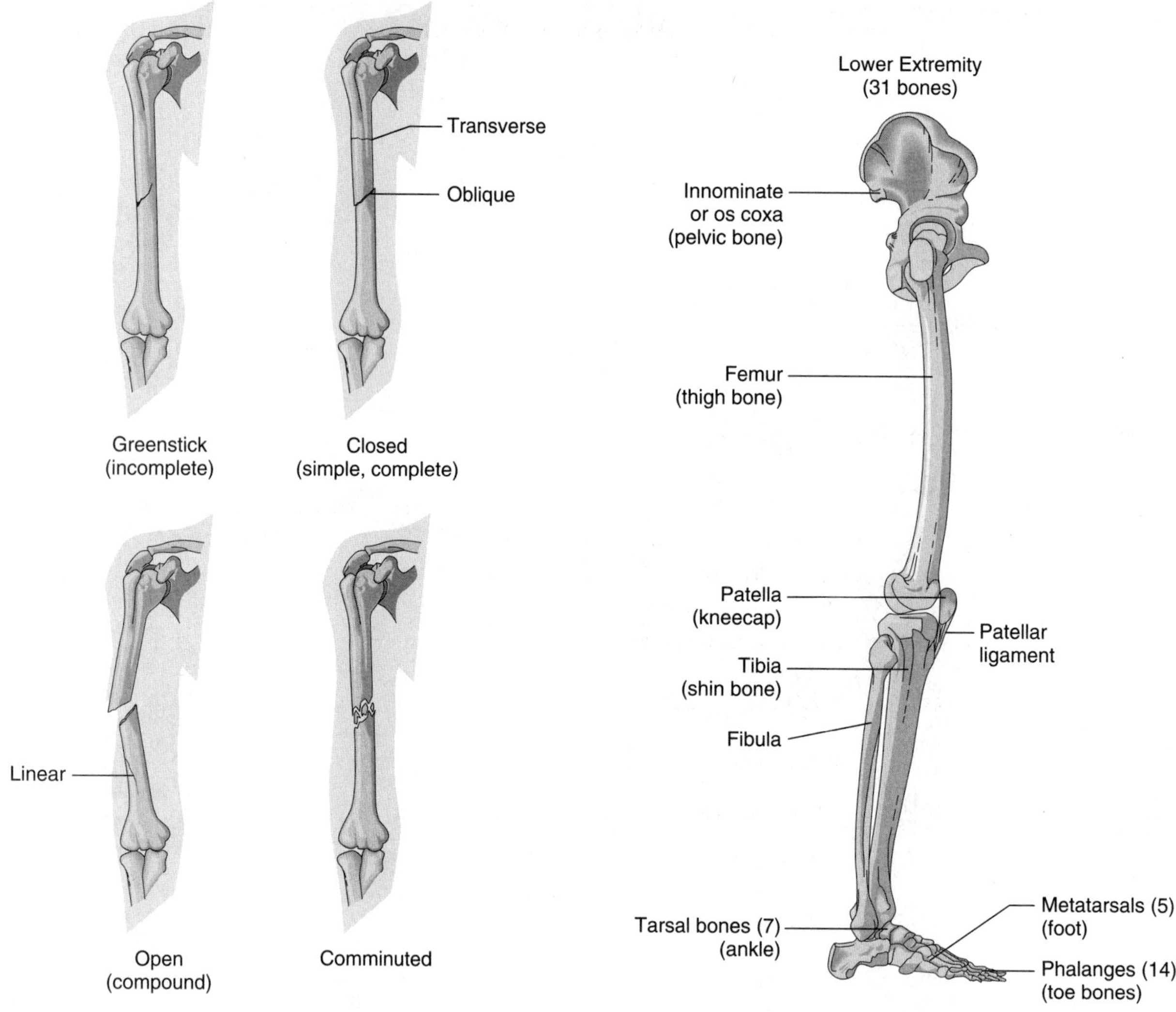

7–3 TYPES OF BONE FRACTURES

7–4 LOWER EXTREMITY (31 BONES)

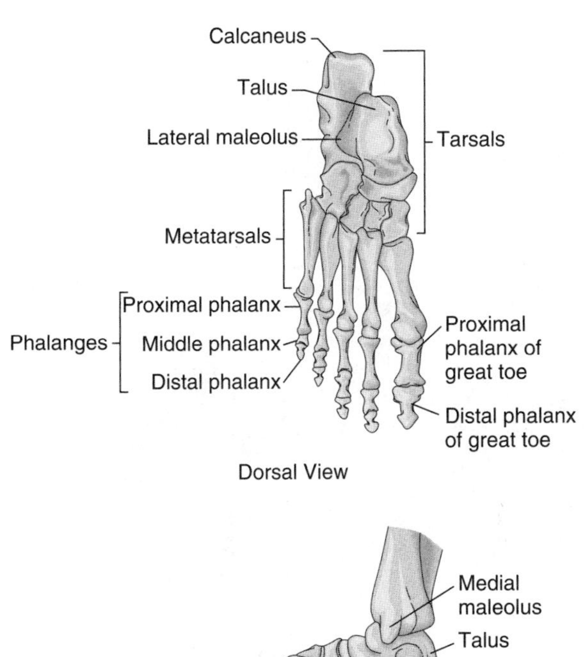

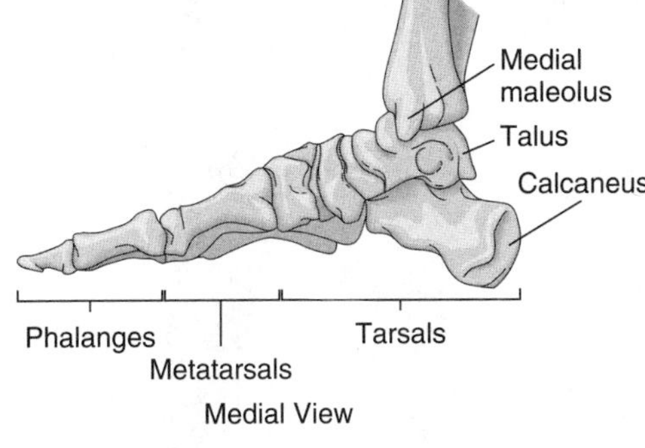

7–5 BONES OF THE RIGHT FOOT

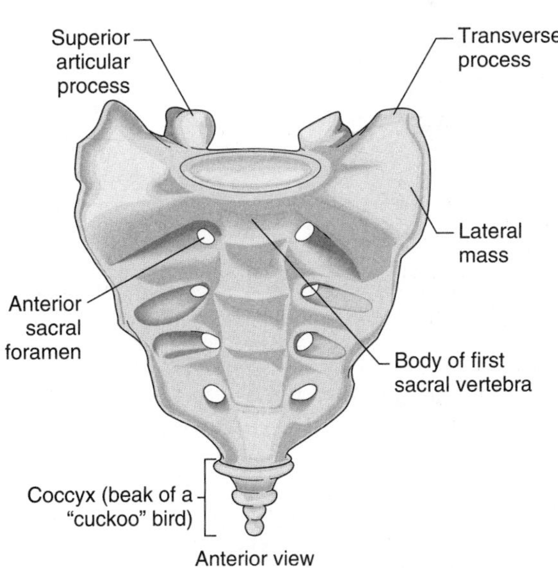

(A) The Sacrum and Coccyx

7–6 THE SACRUM AND COCCYX (ANTERIOR VIEW)

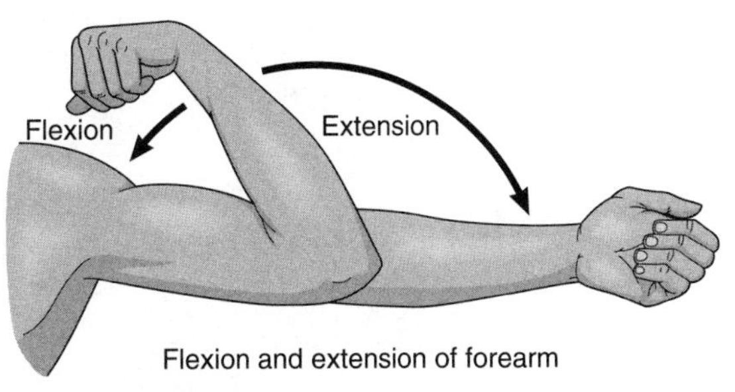

Flexion and extension of forearm

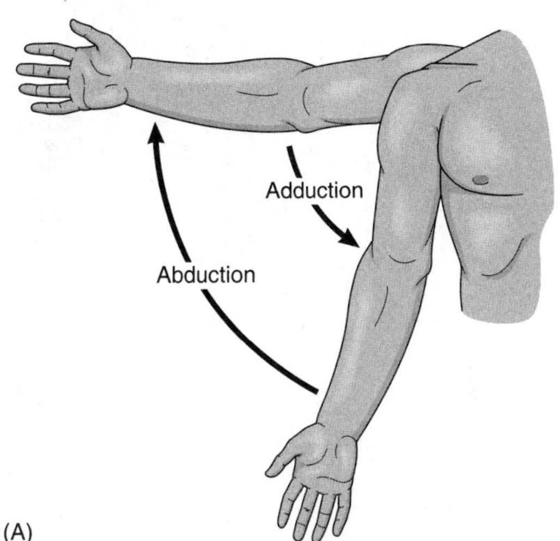

Vertical adduction and abduction of arm

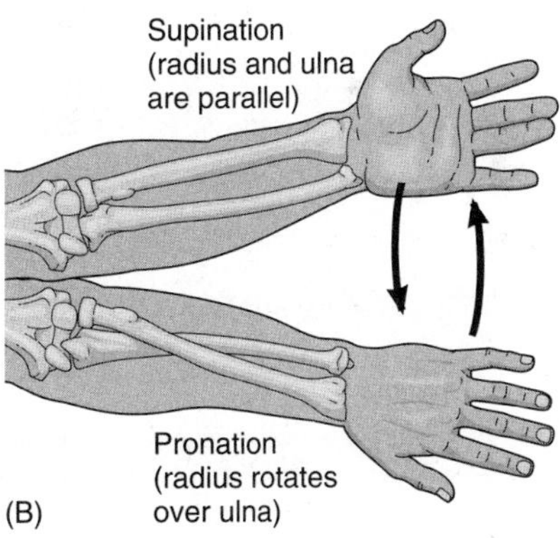

Pronation and supination of the hand

7–7 (A) VERTICAL ADDUCTION AND ABDUCTION OF THE ARM; (B) PRONATION AND SUPINATION OF THE HAND

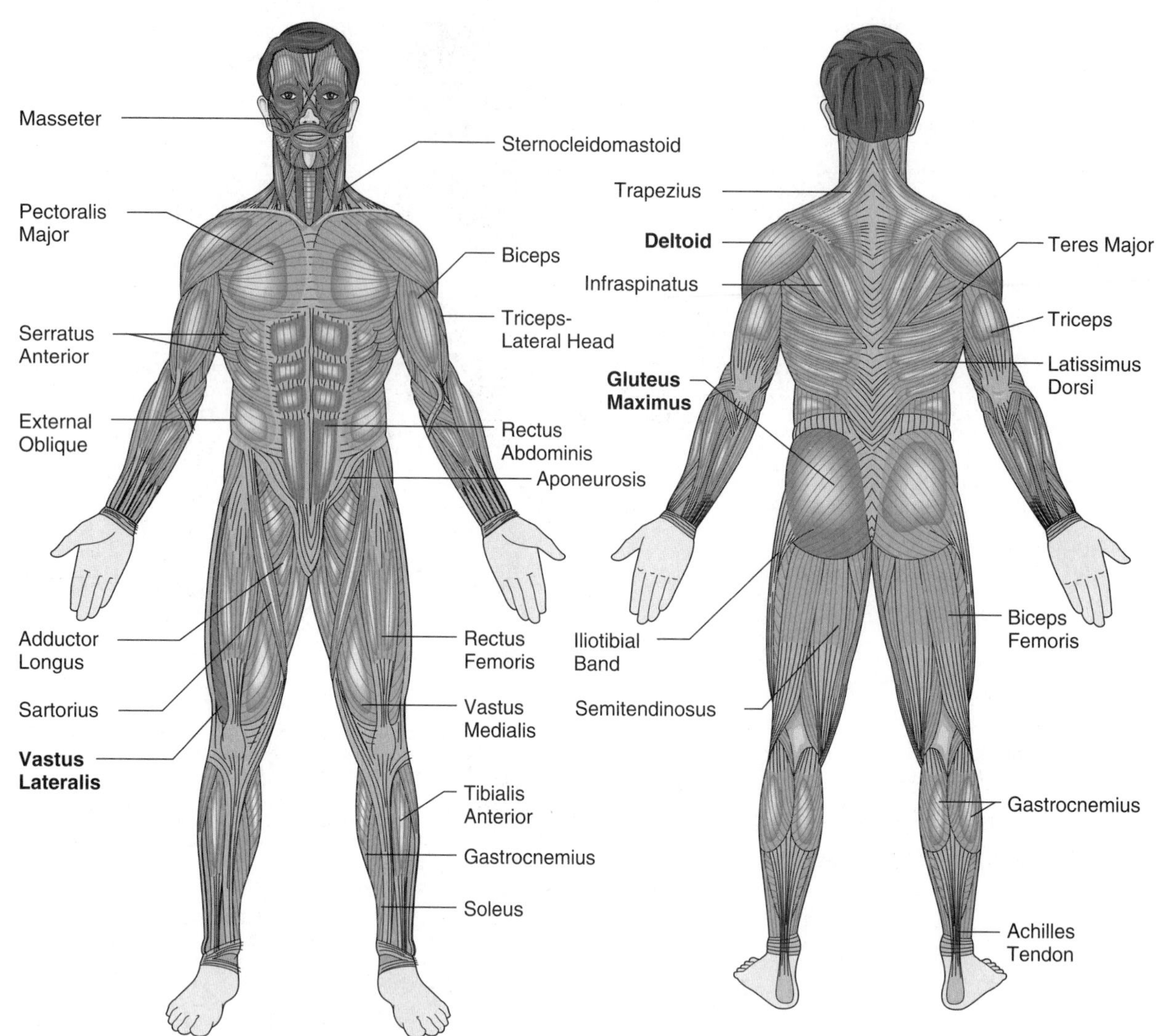

7–8 POSTERIOR AND ANTERIOR VIEWS OF THE MUSCLES

Orthopedics Terminology

a

acetabulum (as"-eh-tab'-yoo-lum) – a cup-shaped bony recess in the ilium that holds the head of the femur

achondroplasia (ā-kon"-drō-plā'-zē-uh) – a hereditary, congenital disturbance of epiphyseal chondroblastic growth and maturation, causing inadequate enchondral bone formation and resulting in a peculiar form of dwarfism with short limbs, normal trunk, small face, normal vault, lordosis, and trident hand

acromial (a-krō'-mē-ul) – pertaining to the lateral extension of the spine of the scapula, projecting over the shoulder joint and forming the highest point of the shoulder (the acromion process)

AlloAnchor RC (al'-ō-ang'-ker) – a graft of tissue (allograft) machined from cortical bone and used in soft tissue reattachment for rotator cuff repair

ankylosing spondylitis (ang'-kih-lō-sing spon"-dih-lī'-tis) – the form of rheumatoid arthritis that affects the spine

antalgic gait (ant-al'-jik gāt) – a limp characteristic of recovered cases of coxalgia, noted by avoidance of weight bearing on the affected side

aponeurosis (ā"-pō-nyoo-rō'-sis) – the end of a muscle where it becomes a tendon; the tendon attaches the muscle to bone

arthroclasia (ar"-thrō-klā'-zē-uh) – the surgical breaking down of an ankylosis in order to secure free movement in a joint

arthrodesis (ar"-thrō-dē'-sis) – the surgical fixation of a joint by a procedure designed to accomplish fusion of the joint surfaces by promoting the proliferation of bone cells

arthrogryposis (ar"-thrō-grī-pō'-sis) – persistent flexure or contracture of a joint

astragalus (uh-strag'-uh-lus) – the ankle bone (talus)

Austin-Moore prosthesis (aws'-tin moor prahs-thē'-sis) – artificial device used for hip fractures

b

brachiocrural (brak"-ē-ō-kroo'-rul) – pertaining to the arm and leg

bursa (pl. bursae) (ber'-suh, ber'-sē) – a sac or sac-like cavity filled with a viscid fluid and situated at places in the tissues at which friction would otherwise develop

c

C-arm fluoroscopy (sē'-arm floo"-ur-os'-kuh-pē) – x-ray equipment that can be rotated over or under a patient without moving the patient; provides a constant view of the bone

calcaneoapophysitis (kal-ka'-nē-ō-uh-pof"-ih-zī'-tis) – a diseased condition of the posterior part of the calcaneus marked by pain at the point of insertion of the Achilles tendon with swelling of the soft parts

calvaria (kal-vā'-rē-uh) – the dome-like superior portion of the cranium

capitellum (kap"-ih-tel'-um) – an eminence on the distal end of the lateral epicondyle of the humerus for articulation with the head of the radius

capsuloplasty (kap'-syoo-lō-plas"-tē) – a plastic operation on a joint capsule

carpometacarpal (kar"-pō-met"-uh-kar'-pul) – pertaining to the carpus and metacarpus

chemonucleolysis (kē"-mō-noo'-klē-ō-lī'-sis) – the enzymatic dissolution of the nucleus pulposus by injection of chymopapain; this procedure is used in the treatment of intervertebral disk lesions

chondrolysis (kahn-drahl'-ih-sis) – the degeneration of cartilage cells that occurs in the process of intracartilaginous ossification

chondromalacia (kahn"-drō-muh-lā'-shē-uh) – softening of the articular cartilage, most frequently in the patella

chymopapain (kī"-mō-puh-pā'-in) – an enzyme from the latex of a chiefly tropical tree

coccydynia (syn. coccygodynia) (kok"-sē-dī'-nē-uh, kok"-sē-gō-dī'-nē-uh) – pain in the coccyx and neighboring region

coccyx (kok'-siks) – the terminal bony complex of the caudal end of the vertebral column composed of three to five fused bones

condyle (kahn'-dīl) – a rounded projection on a bone

coracoacromial (kor"-uh-kō-ā-krō'-mē-ul) – pertaining to the coracoid and acromion processes

coracoclavicular (kor"-uh-kō-klah-vik'-yoo-lur) – pertaining to the coracoid process and the clavicle

CorIS interference screw (kōr'-iss in"-ter-fēr'-ens skroo) – a device machined from allograft cortical bone and designed to reattach soft tissue grafts to bone in the knee

costovertebral (kos"-tō-ver'-tē-bral) – pertaining to a rib and a vertebra

coxalgia (koks-al'-jē-uh) – hip-joint disease; pain in the hip

crepitation (krep"-ih-tā'-shun) – the noise made by the rubbing together of the ends of a fractured bone

d

de Quervain tenosynovitis (duh-kwor'-van ten"-ō-sin"-ō-vī'-tis) – inflammation caused by narrowness of common tendon sheath of abductor pollicis longus and extensor pollicis brevis

deossification (dē-ahs"-ih-fih-kā'-shun) – loss of or removal of the mineral elements of bone

diaphysis (dī-af'-ih-sis) – the long, narrow shaft of the bone

diastasis (dī-as'-tuh-sis) – a form of dislocation in which there is separation of two bones normally attached to each other without the existence of a true joint, as in separation of the pubic symphysis

diskectomy (dis-kek'-tuh-mē) – surgical removal of a herniated intervertebral disk

diskogram (dis'-kō-gram) – an x-ray of the intervertebral disk

Dupuytren's contracture (doo-pwē-truhnz' kun-trak'-tyoor) – shortening, thickening, and fibrosis of the palmar fascia, producing a flexion deformity of a finger

e

enarthrosis (en"-ar-thrō'-sis) – a joint in which the globular head of one bone is received into a socket in another, as in the hip joint

enchondromatosis (en-kahn"-drō-muh-tō'-sis) – a condition characterized by hamartomatous proliferation of cartilage cells within the metaphysis of several bones causing thinning of the overlying cortex and distortion of the growth in length

epicondyle (ep"-ī-kahn'-dīl) – an eminence upon a bone above its condyle

epiphyseal (ep"-ī-fiz'-ē-ul) – pertaining to or of the nature of an epiphysis

epiphysis (ē-pih'-fih-sis) – the knob-like end of a long bone

exarticulation (eks"-ar-tik-yoo-lā'-shun) – amputation at a joint; removal of a portion of a joint

exostosis (ek"-sō-stō'-sis) – a benign bony growth projecting outward from the surface of a bone, characteristically capped by cartilage

f

fasciculation (fah-sik"-yoo-lā'-shun) – the formation of a small bundle of nerve, muscle, or tendon fibers

fasciotomy (fash"-ē-ot'-uh-mē) – a surgical incision or transection of fascia

g

genu valgum (jē'-noo val'-gum) – a deformity in which the knees are abnormally close together and the space between the ankles is increased; known also as knock-knee

glenohumeral (glē"-nō-hyoo'-mer-ul) – pertaining to the glenoid cavity and to the humerus

h

hallux (hal'-uks) – the great toe, or first digit of the foot

hallux valgus (hal'-uks val'-gus) – everted foot; displacement of the great toe toward the other toes

hallux varus (hal'-uks vā'-rus) – displacement of the great toe away from the other toes

humeroradial (hyoo"-mer-ō-rā'-dē-ul) – pertaining to the humerus and the radius

humeroscapular (hyoo"-mer-ō-skap'-yoo-lur) – pertaining to the humerus and the scapula

hydrarthrosis (hī"-drar-thrō'-sis) – an accumulation of watery fluid in the cavity of a joint

i

IDET procedure (i'-det prō-se'-jur) – a minimally invasive outpatient surgical procedure for treatment of patients with chronic low back pain caused by tears or small herniations of the lumbar disks

iliotibial (il"-ē-ō-tib'-ē-ul) – pertaining to or extending between the ilium and tibia

ilium (il'-ē-um) – the expansive superior portion of the hip bone

Ilizarov external fixator (ihl"-ih-zahr'-ahv eks'-ter-nul fiks'-ā-tur – device used externally to hold broken bones in place until they have healed

interosseous (in"-ter-os'-ē-us) – between bones

intertrochanteric (in"-ter-trō"-kan-tār'-ik) – situated in or pertaining to the space between the greater and the lesser trochanter

intramedullary (in"-truh-med'-yoo-lār"-ē) – within the spinal cord, marrow cavity of a bone, or within the medulla oblongata of the brain

ischium (is'-kē-um) – the inferior dorsal part of the hip bone

k

kyphoplasty (kī'-fō-plas"-tē) – the vertebroplasty procedure

kyphoscoliosis (kī"-fō-skō"-lē-ō'-sis) – backward and lateral curvature of the spinal column, as in vertebral osteochondrosis

kyphosis (kī-fō'-sis) – outward curvature of the upper portion of the spine; also known as hunchback

l

LactoSorb copolymer (lak'-tō-sōrb kō-pahl'-ē-mer) – resorbable bone material

laminectomy (lam"-ih-nek'-tuh-mē) – excision of the posterior arch of a vertebra

latissimus (lah-tis'-ih-mus) – a general term denoting a broad structure, as a muscle

m

malleolus (mah-lē'-ō-lus) – a rounded process, such as the protuberance on each side of the ankle joint

Marie-Strumpell disease (mah-rē'-strim'-pel dih-zēz) – rheumatoid spondylitis

McMurray test (mik-mur'-ē tehst) – test for cartilage injury

meniscectomy (men"-ih-sek'-tuh-mē) – removal of the meniscus

meniscus (meh-nis'-kus) – a disc of fibrocartilage found in certain joints

metaphysis (meh-taf'-ih-sis) – the wider part at the extremity of the shaft of a long bone, adjacent to the epiphyseal disk

methyl methacrylate bone cement (meth'-il meth-ak'-rih-lāt" bōn sih-ment) – glue used to hold artificial prostheses in place (total hip, etc.)

myasthenia (mī"-as-thē'-nē-uh) – muscular debility

myelomeningocele (mī"-ē-lō-meh-ning'-gō-sēl) – hernial protrusion of the cord and its meninges through a defect in the vertebral canal

myesthesia (mī"-es-thē'-zē-uh) – muscle sensibility; consciousness of muscle contraction

myositis ossificans (mī"-ō-sī'-tis ah-sif'-ih-kanz) – a condition in which the healing lesion creates new bone formed in the muscle; may occur as the result of repeated injury or severe injury to a muscle

n

Navitrack system (nav'-ih–trak sis'-tum) – computer-assisted surgery system that provides real-time three-dimensional visualizaton for navigation during orthopedic surgery; used in total hip and knee replacements, anterior cruciate ligament procedures, and spinal surgeries

o

olecranon (ō-lek'-ruh-non) – the proximal bony projection of the ulna at the elbow; also known as the "funny bone"

ossification (ah"-sih-fih-kā'-shun) – the conversion of muscle into a bony substance

osteoarthritis (ah"-stē-ō-ar-thrī'-tis) – chronic arthritis of noninflammatory character

osteoarthrotomy (ah"-stē-ō-ar-throt'-uh-mē) – excision of an articular end of a bone

osteochondritis (ah"-stē-ō-kon-drī'-tis) – inflammation of both bone and cartilage

osteoclasia (ah"-stē-ō-klā'-zē-uh) – the absorption and destruction of bony tissue; surgical fracture of a bone done to correct a deformity

osteodystrophy (ah"-stē-ō-dis'-truh-fē) – defective bone formation

osteomyelitis (ah"-stē-ō-mī"-eh-lī'-tis) – inflammation of bone and bone marrow usually caused by a pus-forming bacteria

osteoporosis (ah"-stē-ō-pō-rō'-sis) – a disease characterized by an abnormal absorption of bone

osteotomy (ah"-stē-ot'-uh-mē) – cutting or transecting bone

p

Paget's disease (paj'-etz dih-zēz') – a degenerative disease of bone, cause unknown, with associated inflammation and resultant deformity

patellofemoral (pah-tel"-ō-fem'-ur-ul) – concerning the patella and femur

perichondrium (pār"-ih-kahn'-drē-um) – the layer of dense fibrous connective tissue that surrounds all cartilage except the articular cartilage of synovial joints

periosteum (pār"-ē-os'-tē-um) – a tough fibrous membrane that covers the outside of the diaphysis

Perthes' disease (per'-tēz dih-zēz') – osteochondrosis of the capital femoral epiphysis

polydactylism (pol-ē-dak'-til-izm) – a developmental anomaly characterized by the presence of too many fingers or toes on the hands or feet

polymyositis (pol"-ē-mī"-ō-sī'-tis) – inflammation of several or many muscles at once

porosis (pō-rō'-sis) – the formation of the callus in the repair of a fractured bone

pseudoarthrosis (soo"-dō-ar-thrō'-sis) – a false joint

psoas (sō'-az) – a muscle in the back wall of the abdomen

Pulsavac lavage debridement system (pul'-suh-vak lah-vahzh' dā-brēd'-mawn sis'-tum) – system used to irrigate operative wounds with pulsation-type action

r

rachitis (rah-kī'-tis) – inflammatory disease of the vertebral column

rhabdomyoma (rab"-dō-mī-ō'-muh) – a benign tumor of striated muscle

rongeur (raw-zhur') – an instrument used for cutting tissue, particularly bone

s

sarcolemma (sar"-kō-lem'-uh) – the delicate plasma membrane that surrounds every striated muscle fiber

Scheuermann's disease (kyphosis) (shoy'-er-munz dih-zēz' (kī-fō'-sis)) – osteochondrosis of vertebral epiphyses in juveniles

sciatica (sī-at'-ih-kuh) – a syndrome characterized by pain radiating from the back into the buttock and into the lower extremity along its posterior or lateral aspect; also used to refer to pain anywhere along the course of the sciatic nerve

scoliosis (skō"-lē-ō'-sis) – a lateral or sideways curvature of the spinal column

sequestrectomy (sē"-kwes-trek'-tuh-mē) – surgical removal of dead bone

sequestrum (sē-kwes'-trum) – a piece of dead bone that has become separated from the healthy or living bone during the process of necrosis

sesamoid (ses'-uh-moyd) – denoting a small nodular bone embedded in a tendon or joint capsule

sphenoid (sfē'-noyd) – designating a very irregular wedge-shaped bone at the base of the skull

spina bifida (spī'-nuh bif'-ih-duh) – a developmental anomaly characterized by defective closure of the bony encasement of the spinal cord through which the cord and meninges may or may not protrude

spondylitis (spahn"-dih-lī'-tis) – inflammation of the vertebrae

spondylitis rhizomelica (spahn"-dih-lī'-tis rī-zō-mel'-ih-kuh) – the form of rheumatoid arthritis that affects the spine

spondylodesis (spahn"-dih-lahd'-eh-sis) – the operation of fusing vertebrae

spondylolisthesis (spahn"-dih-lō-lis"-thē'-sis) – forward subluxation of the body of one of the lower lumbar vertebrae on the vertebra below it or on the sacrum

supracondylar (soo"-pruh-kahn'-dih-lur) – situated above a condyle or condyles

supraspinous (soo"-pruh-spī'-nus) – situated above a spine or a spinous process

sural nerve (soo'-rul) – the nerve in the skin on the back of the leg and skin and joints on the lateral side of the heel and foot

Suretac system (shoor'-tak sis'-tum) – method for fracture fixation

symphysis joint (sim'-fih-sis) – permits slight movement

synchondrosis (sin"-kahn-drō'-sis) – a type of cartilaginous joint that is usually temporary; the intervening hyaline cartilage is ordinarily converted into bone before adulthood

syndactylia (sin"-dak-til'-ē-uh) – the most common congenital anomaly of the hand, marked by persistence of the webbing between adjacent digits so they are more or less completely attached

syndesmosis (sin"-des-mō'-sis) – a type of fibrous joint in which the intervening fibrous connective tissue forms as interosseous membrane or ligament

synovium (sih-nō'-vē-um) – a synovial membrane; a membrane that secretes a transparent alkaline viscid fluid resembling the white of an egg

t

talipes (tal'-ih-pēz) – a congenital deformity of the foot, which is twisted out of shape or position

tendinitis (ten"-dih-ni'-tis) – inflammation of tendons and of tendon-muscle attachments

tendolysis (ten-dol'-ih-sis – the operation of freeing a tendon from its adhesions

tenodesis (ten-od'-eh-sis) – tendon fixation; suturing the end of a tendon to a bone

tibiofibular (tib"-ē-ō-fib'-yoo-lur) – pertaining to the tibia and the fibula

torticollis (tor"-tih-kol'-is) – wryneck; a contracted state of the cervical muscles, producing twisting of the neck and an unnatural position of the head

v

valgus (val'-gus) – bent outward, twisted; the term is an adjective and should be used only with the noun it describes, as talipes valgus, genu valgum, etc.

varus (vā'-rus) – bent inward; the term is an adjective and should be used only with the noun it describes, as talipes varus, genu varum, etc.

vertebra (ver'-teh-bruh) – any of the 33 bones of the spinal column

vertebroplasty (ver"-teh-brō-plass'-tē) – a nonsurgical method for the repair of back fractures caused by osteoporosis

X

Xia spinal system (zē'-uh spī'-nul sis'-tum) – a comprehensive system of implants and instruments for stabilization of the spine in the thoracic, lumbar, and sacral regions

xiphoid process (zī'-foyd) – the pointed bottom part of the sternum or breastbone

Transcription Tips

When transcribing orthopedics dictation, you should be familiar with the location and names of the major bones, joints, and muscles of the musculoskeletal system. Acquiring the knowledge to evaluate the combining forms, prefixes, and suffixes used to describe bones, joints, and muscles will enhance the accuracy of your transcription skills.

The following information relates to confusing words; combining forms and/or roots; glossaries of the skeletal system, muscular system, and body movements; classifications of bone fractures; and types of joints. Finally, a list of helpful Web sites is provided to guide further research or study.

Confusing Terms

abduction – drawing away from

subduction – drawing downward

abductor – that which draws away from

adductor – that which draws toward

arthropathy – any joint disease

arthroplasty – plastic surgery of a joint

epiphysis – a center for formation of bone substance at each extremity of long bones

apophysis – outgrowth or swelling

exostosis – a bony growth that emanates from the surface of a bone

enostosis – an osseous tumor within the cavity of a bone

immobilization – rendering immovable

mobilization – the process of rendering a fixed or ankylosed part movable

Roots and/or Combining Forms

Root	Meaning	Root	Meaning
acro	extremity	myo, my	muscle
arterio	artery	necro	death
arthro, arthr	joint	neo	new
chondro, chondr	cartilage	neuro, neur	nerve
costo	rib	ortho	straight, normal, correct
cranio	cranium, skull	osteo, oste	bone
fibro	fibers	patho	disease
ganglio, gangli	ganglion	pedo	foot, child
hydro, hydr	water	poly	many, excessive
kerato	horny tissue	sclero, scler	hard
lipo	fat	steno	narrowed
lyso	breaking down	sterno	sternum
macro	large, long	thoraco	chest
malaco	softening	veno	vein
myelo, myel	bone marrow, spinal cord		

Glossary of the Skeletal System

articulation – joint

brachial – pertaining to the arm

carpus – wrist

clavicle – collarbone

coccyx – tailbone

femur – thigh bone

fibula – calf bone

frontal bone – forehead

humerus – upper arm bone

ilium – upper hip bone

ischium – lower hip bone

malar – cheekbone

mandible – lower jawbone

maxilla – upper jawbone

metacarpus – the part of the skeleton between the wrist and the finger

Glossary of the Skeletal System

metatarsus – the part of the skeleton between the ankle and the toes

occipital bone – the base of the skull

parietal bones – the two bones forming upper sides of the skull

patella – kneecap

periosteum – the membrane around the bones

phalanx – one of the bones of a finger or toe

radius – the bone of the forearm located on the thumb side

sacrum – the bone just below the lumbar vertebrae and above the coccyx

scapula – the shoulder blade

scoliosis – abnormal lateral curvature of the spine

sternum – the breast bone

symphysis pubis – the junction of the pubic bones

tarsus – the ankle

temporal bones – the two bones forming part of the lateral surfaces and base of the skull

tibia – the shin bone

ulna – the larger bone of the forearm located opposite the thumb side

vertebra – a bone of the spinal column

Whereas the skeletal system provides a frame for the body and the flexibility of the joints, the muscular system gives a new dimension to the mobility of the skeleton.

Glossary of the Muscular System

active movement – voluntary movement involving the contraction of muscles with energy supplied by the patient

ambulation – walking

antagonist – a muscle that opposes the action of another muscle

asthenia – weakness

contracture – a shortened or distorted muscle

deltoid – the triangular muscle that invests the shoulder

fascia – a band of tissue enveloping muscles and certain organs of the body

flaccid – limp

gastrocnemius – the calf muscle

gluteus – the buttock muscle

involuntary muscle – a muscle that is not controlled by the patient

ligament – a strong band of fibrous tissue that holds bones to bones or supports large organs

muscle – an organ that produces movement by contracting

myodiastasis – separation of a muscle

myoedema – swelling or edema of a muscle

myogelosis – hardening of a muscle

myotasis – stretching of muscle

passive movement – any movement involving the contraction of muscles with the energy to do so supplied from an outside source

pectoralis major and pectoralis minor – chest muscles

popliteus – muscle posterior to the knee

spasm – an involuntary contraction of a muscle

sphincter – a ring-like band of muscle fibers that closes a natural orifice

synergist – a muscle that acts together with another

tendon – a strong, fibrous band of tissue that attaches muscle to bone

tone, tonus – slight, continuous contraction of muscle

voluntary muscle – a muscle that is controlled by the patient

Glossary of Body Movements

abduction – drawing away from the midline

adduction – drawing toward the midline

circumduction – circular movement

extension – straightening

flexion – bending

hyperextension – extreme or excessive straightening

lateral rotation – turning away from the midline

medial rotation – turning toward the midline

pronation – the act of turning the palm or sole of the foot backward or downward

supination – the act of turning the palm or sole of the foot forward or upward

Classifications of Bone Fractures

Colles – a break in the distal part of the radius

comminuted – a fracture where the bone is shattered into fragments

compound, or open – a fracture where bone protrudes through the skin

compression – a fracture occurring in vertebrae, generally caused by falling on the tailbone

epiphyseal – occurs where the matrix is calcifying and chondrocytes are dying and fractures occur through this growth plate

greenstick – a fracture where one side of the bone is broken and the other side bent

Potts – a break in the ankle that affects both bones of the lower leg

simple, or closed – the fracture where bone does not protrude through the skin

spiral – a fracture, caused by twisting stresses, that extends along the length of the bone

stress—micro-cracks that occur in the bone as a result of the body not producing enough bone

transverse – the fracture occurring when a shaft bone breaks across its long axis

Types of Joints

amphiarthrosis – allows only slight movement, as in the vertebrae

diarthrosis – permits free movement in many directions, such as in the hip, knee, wrist, foot, and elbow

synarthrosis – does not allow movement, such as in the cranial sutures

Types of Splints (Selected)

acrylic
AirFlex carpal tunnel
airplane (also aeroplane)
aluminum bridge, fence, or finger-cot
anterior acute-flexion elbow
Aquaplast
baseball or baseball finger
birdcage
Brooke Army Hospital
buddy
Bunnell hand, finger, or knuckle-bender
calibrated clubfoot
Colles
Curry walking
Darco toe alignment
Denis Browne clubfoot or talipes hobble
dental
Denver nasal
DePuy open-thimble or rocking-leg
drop foot
elephant-ear clavicle
eZY WRAP

Types of Splints (Selected)

Flexisplint flexed-arm board
hand cock-up
Hirschtick utility shoulder
INRO surgical nail
Kanavel cock-up
Kirschner-wire
Magnuson abduction humerus
O'Donaghue knee or stirrup
Ortho Tech cock-up wrist
outrigger
Radstat wrist
Rolyan Gel Shell
Slattery-McGrouther dynamic flexion
synergistic wrist motion
T-finger
talipes hobble
Teare arm sling
Thumz'Up functional thumb
U-splint
utility shoulder
Velcro
von Rosen hip
Versi-Splint
wraparound
Xomed Silastic
Zim-Trac traction

Supportive Web Sites

http://chorus.rad.mcw.edu/
Select "Musculoskeletal system" to get an extensive list of terminology links.

www.howmedica.com/
Choose "Stryker Corporation Website" and click on "Products and Services" under "Company Information" for information on various orthopedic products.

www.mtdesk.com/
Under "MT Desk Index," select "Sample Operative Reports by Specialty" for sample orthopedic reports; choose other links of interest as desired.

www.orthoguide.com/
Click on links of interest here; you can also click on "more" for a more comprehensive orthopedics site.

Index of Orthopedic Reports

(see table of contents for audio information)

Exercise #	Patient Name	Report/Procedure
TE#1	Dickson, Mark	Left fifth ray amputation
TE#2	Mistretta, Robin	Hemiarthroplasty of right shoulder
TE#3	Tule, Keith	ACL repair and Baker's cyst
TE#4	Jiminez, Christa	Total ankle arthroplasty
TE#5	Overmier, Daniel	Rotator cuff repair
TE#6	Horton, Burt	Total hip replacement
TE#7	Graham, Wanda	ORIF involving lateral malleolus; diastasis closed reduction
TE#8	Legette, Gary	Biopsy of left sural nerve and gastrocnemius muscle
TE#9	Parks, Yvonne	Tendon sheath incision for trigger finger
TE#10	DeJean, Wallace	Insertion of olive wire into femur
TE#11	Sutton, Elizabeth	ORIF with hip compression screw
TE#12	Wilkins, Judy	Arthroscopy, partial medial meniscectomy
TE#13	LaFleur, Clifford	Above-knee amputation

CHAPTER 8

GASTROENTEROLOGY

Introduction

Gastroenterology, a subspecialty of internal medicine, is the branch of medical science concerned with the study of the physiology and pathology of the *stomach, intestines,* and related structures such as the *esophagus, liver, gallbladder,* and *pancreas.* The liver, gallbladder, and pancreas contribute hormones, enzymes, and bile vital to digestion. All these components make up the digestive system.

The main functions of this digestive system are the *digestion, absorption,* and *elimination* of food. These processes occur in the gastrointestinal tract, or alimentary canal, which is a tube approximately 30 feet long in adults; it begins at the mouth and ends at the anus.

When food is taken into the mouth, it travels through the pharynx into the esophagus. Next it goes into the stomach, where the digestive process begins. Gastric juices and hydrochloric acid break the food down into a semiliquid state (called *chyme*), and in this state the food passes into the small intestine in stages. The small intestine is composed of the *duodenum,* the *jejunum,* and the *ileum.* While in the small intestine, the food is mixed with bile from the liver and gallbladder and juice from the pancreas.

After nutrients have been absorbed by tiny capillaries and lymph vessels, the food passes into the large intestine where the digestive and absorption process continues.

Components of the large intestine are the *cecum,* the *colon,* the *rectum,* and the *anal canal.* The waste products of digestion are expelled from the body through the rectum and anus.

Physicians who treat diseases of the gastrointestinal tract are known as *gastroenterologists.* Among the procedures performed by gastroenterologists are *esophagogastroduodenoscopy* (EGD), *endoscopic biopsy, small bowel biopsy, esophageal dilatations, esophageal* and *rectal manometry, laparoscopy, endoscopic retrograde cholangiopancreatography* (ERCP), and *endoscopic removal of foreign bodies.*

Critical Thinking Exercise

You work in the transcription department of a medium-sized clinic. One day just before closing time, you find yourself left to close the department. The telephone rings, and on the other end is an irate physician who demands to speak with your supervisor. You tell the doctor that the supervisor became ill and had to leave early in the afternoon, but that you'll be glad to relay a message to her in the morning. The doctor says, "No, I must speak to someone in authority this minute. Whoever transcribed an operative report I dictated last month did it all wrong, and now I'm in hot water with the administration."

What would you do?

Gastroenterology Abbreviations

a.c.	before meals
ACBE	air contrast barium enema
A/G	albumin/globulin (ratio)
ALP/ alk phos	alkaline phosphatase
ALT/SGPT	alanine transaminase, serum glutamic pyruvic transaminase (enzyme tests of liver function)
ANA	antinuclear antibodies
AST/SGOT	aspartic acid transaminase, serum glutamic oxaloacetic transaminase (enzyme tests of liver function)

Ba	barium
BAO	basil acid output
BE	barium enema
BMR	basic metabolic rate
BRBPR	bright red blood per (through) rectum
BS	bowel sounds
Bx	biopsy
CCK	cholecystokinin
CEA	carcinoembryonic antigen
CHO	carbohydrate
chol	cholesterol
CPK	creatine phosphokinase
CRC	colorectal cancer
CUC	chronic ulcerative colitis
E. coli	Escherichia coli
EGD	esophagogastroduodenoscopy
ERCP	endoscopic retrograde cholangiopancreatography
ESR	erythrocytic sedimentation rate
FBS	fasting blood sugar
FOBT	fecal occult blood test
GB	gallbladder
GFR	glomerular filtration rate
GGT	gamma-glutamyl transpeptidase
GI	gastrointestinal
GTT	glucose tolerance test
HAA	hepatitis-associated antigen
HAV	hepatitis A virus
Hb A	hemoglobin adult
Hb F	hemoglobin fetal
Hb S	hemoglobin sickle-cell
HBIG	hepatitis B immune globulin
HBV	hepatitis B virus
H&H	hematocrit and hemoglobin
HH	hiatal hernia
IBD	inflammatory bowel disease
IBS	irritable bowel syndrome
IPPB	intermittent positive pressure breathing
IVC	intravenous cholangiography
KCl	potassium chloride
KVO	keep vein open
LDH	lactic dehydrogenase
LES	lower esophageal sphincter
LFTs	liver function tests; alk phos, bilirubin, AST (SGOT), ALT (SGPT)
Lh	luteinizing hormone
MCV	mean clinical value or mean corpuscular volume
N&V	nausea and vomiting
NANBH	non-A, non-B hepatitis (virus)
NG	nasogastric (tube)
NH_4	ammonia
NPO	nothing by mouth
O&P	ova and parasites
OCG	oral cholecystography
OCP	ova, cysts, parasites
p.c.	after meals
PEG	percutaneous endoscopic gastrostomy
PKU	phenylketonuria
PND	paroxysmal nocturnal dyspnea
PO	by mouth (per os)
PP	postprandial (after meals)
PT	prothrombin time
PTC	percutaneous transhepatic cholangiography
PTT	partial thromboplastin time
PUD	peptic ulcer disease
RDA	recommended dietary or daily allowance
TPN	total parenteral nutrition
UGI	upper gastrointestinal

Anatomic Illustrations

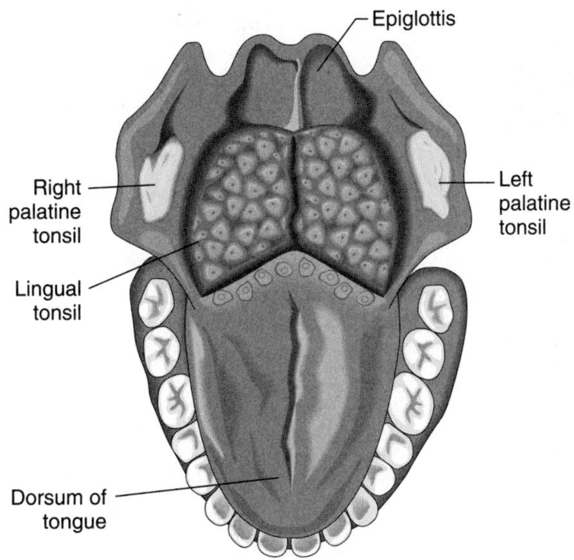

8–1 THE TONSILS

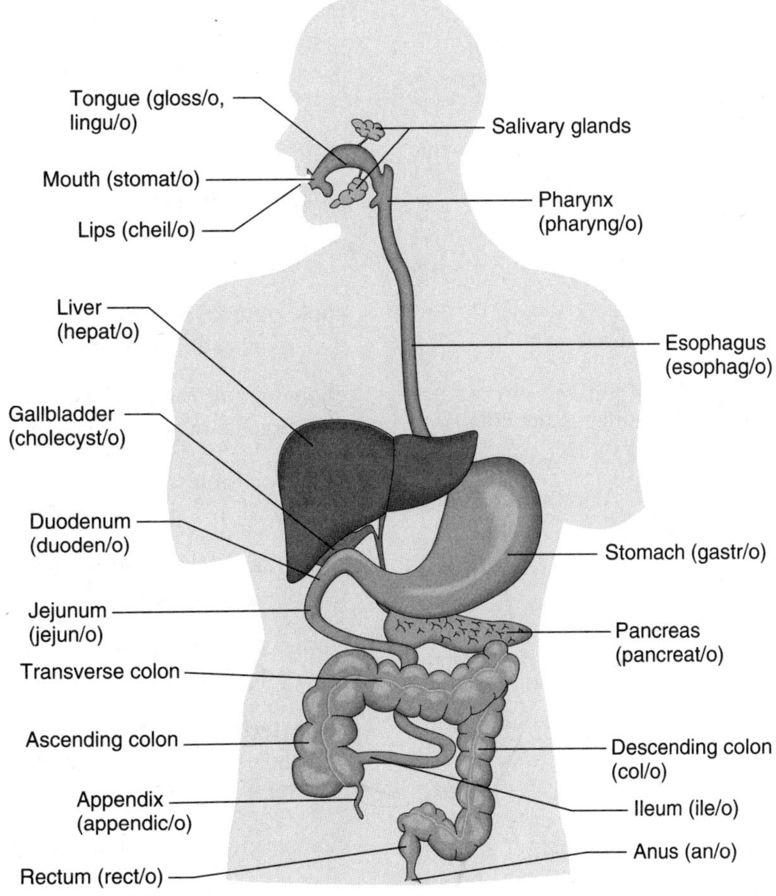

Digestive System

8–2 THE DIGESTIVE SYSTEM

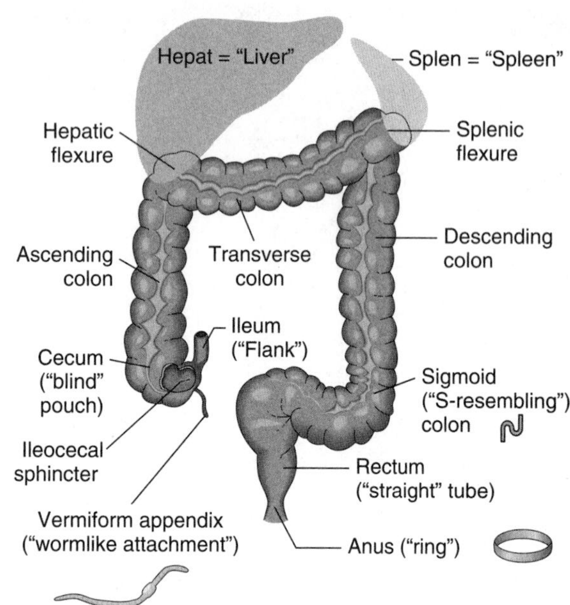

8–3 THE COLON AND ASSOCIATED STRUCTURES

Gastroenterology Terminology

achalasia (ā"-kuh-lā'-zē-uh) – a failure to relax of the smooth muscle fibers of the gastrointestinal tract at any point of junction of one part with another

achlorhydria (ā"-klōr-hī'-drē-uh) – absence of hydrochloric acid in the gastric juice

achylia (ā-kī'-lē-uh) – absence of gastric juice

adenomatous polyp (ad"-ē-nō'-muh-tus pahl'-ip) – a grape-shaped growth on the lining of the colon and rectum; can become cancerous

aerophagia (ā"-er-ō-fā'-jē-uh) – spasmodic swallowing of air followed by eructations

alimentary canal (āl"-ih-men'-tuh-rē kuh-nal') – the digestive tract

amebiasis (am"-ē-bī'-uh-sis) – the state of being infected with ameba

amylase (am'-ih-lāss) – one of the three digestive enzymes produced by the pancreas

amylasuria (am"-ih-lāss-yoo'-rē-uh) – an excess of amylase in the urine; a sign of pancreatitis

ancylostomiasis (an"-sih-lō-stō-mī'-uh-sis) – hookworm disease

anhidrosis (an"-hī-drō'-sis) – an abnormal deficiency of sweat

apepsinia (ā"-pep-sin'-ē-uh) – total absence or lack of secretion of pepsinogen by the stomach

aperistalsis (ā"-per-ih-stal'-sis) – absence of peristaltic action

appendix (uh-pen'-diks) – the worm-like appendage attached to the cecum

ascites (uh-sī'-tēz) – an accumulation of fluid in the abdominal cavity

bacteremia (bak-ter"-ē'-mē-uh) – the presence of bacteria in the blood

bile (bīl) – a digestive fluid secreted by the liver

carcinoid (kar'-sih-noyd) – a yellow circumscribed tumor occurring in the small intestine, appendix, stomach, or colon

cardia (kar'-dē-uh) – the opening of the esophagus into the stomach

catecholamines (kat"-eh-kō'-luh-mēnz) – the chemical substances secreted by the adrenal gland in the urine excreted; in relatively constant amounts in conditions of good health

cecum (sē'-kum) – the first segment of the large intestine

cholangiolitis (kō-lan"-jē-ō-lī'-tis) – inflammation of the cholangioles, the fine terminal elements of the bile duct system

cholecystogastric (kō"-leh-sis"-tō-gas'-trik) – referring to the gallbladder and stomach

choledocholithotomy (kō-led"-ō-kō-lih-thot'-uh-mē) – removal of stone from the bile duct

choledochoplasty (kō-led"-ō-kō-plass'-tē) – plastic repair or reconstruction of the bile duct

cholemia (kō-lē'-mē-uh) – the occurrence of bile or bile pigment in the blood

cholestasis (kō"-leh-stā'-sis) – stoppage or suppression of the flow of bile

cholesterosis (kō-les"-ter-ō'-sis) – a condition in which cholesterol is deposited in tissues in abnormal quantities

chyme (kīm) – the mixture of gastric juices with food

cirrhosis (sir-rō'-sis) – a degenerative disease of the liver

colon (kō'-lun) – segment of the large intestine that extends from the cecum to the rectum

colostomy (kuh-lahss'-tuh-mē) – surgical procedure that creates an opening from the colon through the abdominal wall, to allow waste products to move out of the body

Crohn's disease (krōnz dih-zēz') – inflammation of the colon and lower part of the small intestine; can increase the risk for colorectal cancer

Cruveilhier-Baumgarten syndrome (kroo-vāl-yā'-bom'-gar-ten sin'-drōm) – cirrhosis of the liver with portal hypertension, associated with congenital patency of the umbilical or paraumbilical veins

cystadenocarcinoma (sis-tad"-eh-nō-kar"-sih-nō'-muh) – carcinoma and cystadenoma

d

defecation (def"-eh-kā'-shun) – the passage of stool

deglutition (dē"-gloo-tih'-shun) – swallowing

dehydrogenase (dē-hī"-drah'-jen-āz) – an enzyme

diverticulum (dī"-ver-tik'-yoo-lum) – a pouch opening from a tubular organ, such as the esophagus or intestine

duodenitis (doo"-ahd-eh-nī'-tis) – inflammation of the duodenum

duodenoduodenostomy (doo"-ō-dē'-nō-doo"-ō-deh-nahs'-tuh-mē) – operative formation of an artificial opening between two segments of the duodenum

duodenoileostomy (doo"-o-dē'-nō-il"-ē-ahs'-tuh-mē) – operative formation of an artificial opening between the duodenum and ileum

duodenojejunostomy (doo"-ō-dēh'-nō-jeh"-joo-nahs'-tuh-mē) – operative formation of an artificial opening between the duodenum and jejunum

duodenum (doo"-ō-dē'-num OR doo-ahd'-eh-num) – the first part of the small intestine

dysentery (dis'-en-ter"-ē) – an intestinal disease characterized by inflammation of the mucous membrane

dyspepsia (dis-pep'-sē-uh) – indigestion

e

emesis (em'-eh-sis) – vomiting

EndoCinch suturing system (en'-dō-sinch" soo'-tyoo-ring sis'-tum) – method used to treat symptomatic gastroesophageal reflux disease

enzyme (en'-zīm) – a chemical that speeds up a reaction between substances

eructation (ē-ruk-tā'-shun) – the act of belching

esophagoscope (ē-sof'-uh-gō-skōp) – an endoscope for examination of the esophagus

f

fecal impaction (fē'-kul ī-pak'-shun) – feces firmly lodged in the rectum

fecalith (fe'-kah-lth) – a fecal concretion

flatus (flā'-tus) – gas in the stomach or intestines

fundoplication (fun"-dō-plih-kā'-shun) – operative procedure to relieve gastroesophageal reflux of large amounts of acid-peptic juice and to restore gastroesophageal competence

g

galactosemia (guh-lak"-tō-sē'-mē-uh) – a hereditary disorder of galactose metabolism

gastrectomy (gas-trek'-tuh-mē) – excision of all or part of the stomach

gastrojejunostomy (gas"-trō-jē-joo-nahs'-tuh-mē) – surgical creation of an anastomosis between the stomach and jejunum

gastrorrhea (gas"-trō-rē'-uh) – excessive secretion of mucus or gastric juice in the stomach

gastrosuccorrhea (gas"-trō-suk"-ō-rē'-uh) – excessive and continuous secretion of gastric juice

Given Diagnostic Imaging System (giv'-un dī-ug-nahs'-tik ih'-muh-jing sis'-tum) – diagnostic technique for endoscopic procedures that uses an imaging capsule that is swallowed by the patient

h

hemochromatosis (hē"-mō-krō"-muh-tō'-sis) – an excess of iron absorption and the presence of iron-containing deposits in the liver, pancreas, kidneys, adrenals, and heart

hemorrhoid (hem'-uh-royd) – a large distorted vein within the rectum

hepatomalacia (hep"-uh-tō-muh-lā'-shē-uh) – softening of the liver

hepatomegaly (hep"-uh-tō-meg'-uh-lē) – enlargement of the liver

hepatorrhea (hep"-uh-tō-rē'-uh) – a morbidly excessive secretion of bile; any morbid flow from the liver

hiatal hernia (hī-ā'-tul her'-nē-uh) – produced when the hiatus weakens and stretches so that part of the stomach and/or esophagus intrudes into the chest cavity

Hirschsprung's disease (hersh'-sprungz dih-zēz') – excessive enlargement of the colon associated with an absence of ganglion cells in the narrowed bowel wall distally

hyperalimentation (hī"-per-al"-ih-men-tā'-shun) – the ingestion or administration of a greater-than-optimal amount of nutrients

hyperinsulinism (hī"-per-in'-suh-lin-izm") – excessive secretion of insulin by the pancreas, resulting in hypoglycemia; insulin shock

hypochlorhydria (hī"-pō-klōr-hī'-drē-uh) – deficiency of hydrochloric acid in the gastric juice

icterus (ik'-ter-us) – jaundice

ileitis (il"-ē-ī'-tis) – inflammation of the ileum

ileocolitis (il"-ē-ō-kō-lī'-tis) – inflammation of the ileum and colon

ileum (il'-ē-um) – the third part of the small intestine

ileus (il'-ē-us) – obstruction of the intestines

jejunum (jē-joo'-num) – the second part of the small intestine

kalemia (kah-lē'-mē-uh) – the presence of potassium in the blood

Laennec's cirrhosis (lā"-en-neks' sih-rō'-sis) – cirrhosis of the liver closely associated with chronic excessive alcohol ingestion

leukocytosis (loo"-kō-sī-tō'-sis) – a transient increase in the number of leukocytes in the blood, resulting from various causes

leukopenia (loo"-kō-pē'-nē-uh) – reduction in the number of leukocytes in the blood

lingua (ling'-gwuh) – the tongue

lipase (lip'-āz OR lī'-pāz) – one of the three digestive enzymes produced by the pancreas

lipomatosis (lip"-ō-muh-tō'-sis) – a condition characterized by abnormal localized, or tumor-like, accumulations of fat in the tissues

liver (lih-vur) – the largest gland of the body; it secretes bile

lymphangioma (lim-fan"-jē-ō'-muh) – a tumor composed of new-formed lymph spaces and channels

M2A Swallowable Imaging Capsule (em-too-ā' swal'-ō-uh-bul kap'-sul) – a capsule containing a camera; after the patient swallows it (like a regular pill), the camera transmits images of the GI tract to an external device worn on a belt

maduromycosis (mad-yoor"-ō-mī-kō'-sis) – a chronic disease caused by a variety of fungi or actinomycetes, affecting the foot, hand, legs, or other parts, including the internal organs

mastication (mas"-tih-kā'-shun) – the act of chewing

megacolon (meg"-uh-kō'-lun) – abnormally large or dilated colon

melena (meh-lē'-nuh OR mel'-eh-nuh) – black feces caused by the action of intestinal juices on blood

mononucleosis (mon"-ō-noo"-klē-ō'-sis) – the presence of an abnormally large number of mononuclear leukocytes in the blood

neutropenia (noo"-trō-pē'-nē-uh) – a decrease in the number of neutrophilic leukocytes in the blood

oxyuriasis (ok"-sē-yoo-rī'-uh-sis) – pinworm

paralytic ileus (pār"-uh-lit'-ik il'-ē-us) – paralysis of the intestines that causes distention and symptoms of acute obstruction and prostration

parenteral (puh-ren'-ter-ul) – outside the alimentary tract

pellagra (peh-lag'-ruh) – a clinical deficiency syndrome due to deficiency of niacin

peristalsis (pār"-ih-stahl'-sis) – the rhythmic-like contractions of the tubes of the alimentary tract and other tubular structures

peritoneum (pār"-ih-to-nē'-um) – the serous membrane lining the abdominal cavity and covering its organs

peritonitis (pār"-ih-tō-nī'-tis) – inflammation of the peritoneum

pharynx (fār'-inks) – the throat

polydipsia (pol"-ē-dip'-sē-uh) – excessive thirst

polypectomy (pol"-ih-pek'-tuh-mē) – excision of a polyp

polyposis (pol"-ē-pō'-sis) – a condition in which the colon is lined with many polyps

polyserositis (pol"-ē-sē-rō-sī'-tis) – general inflammation of serous membranes with serous effusion

postprandial (post-pran'-dē-ul) – occurring after dinner or after a meal

psychogenic (sī"-kō-jen'-ik) – having an emotional or psychologic origin

ptyalocele (tī-al'-ō-sēl) – cystic tumor of a salivary gland

pylorectomy (pī"-lōr-ek'-tuh-mē) – excision of the pylorus

pyloric sphincter (pī-lōr'-ik sfingk'-ter) – the ring of muscle at the distal region of the stomach

pyloroplasty (pī-lōr'-ō-plas"-te) – a surgical operation to relieve pyloric obstruction or to accelerate gastric emptying

pyrosis (pī-rō'-sis) – heartburn

r

rugae (roo'-jē) – irregular folds of the mucous membrane of the stomach in which gastric glands are embedded

s

salivary gland (sal'-ih-vār-ē gland) – a gland that secretes saliva

sialaden (sī-al'-ah-den) – a salivary gland

sialoadenectomy (sī"-ul-ō-ad"-ē-nek'-tuh-mē) – excision of a salivary gland

sialozemia (sī"-ul-ō-zē'-mē-uh) – involuntary flow of saliva

sideropenia (sid"-er-ō-pē'-nē-uh) – iron deficiency

sigmoid colon (sig'-moyd kō'-lun) – the S-shaped segment of the colon between the descending colon and the rectum

singultus (sing-gul'-tus) – hiccup due to a nervous state of the stomach

stomatitis (stō-muh-tī'-tis) – inflammation of the oral mucosa, due to local or systemic factors, which may involve the buccal and labial mucosa, palate, tongue, floor of the mouth, and the gingivae

Stretta procedure (streh'-tuh prō-cē-jur) – outpatient, nonsurgical procedure for treatment of gastroesophageal reflux disease; uses electrosurgical coagulation

t

toxicosis (tok"-sih-kō'-sis) – any disease condition due to poisoning

triglycerides (trī-glih'-sir-īdz) – large fat molecules

trypsin (trip'-sin) – one of the three digestive enzymes produced by the pancreas

u

ulcerative colitis (ul'-ser-ā"-tiv kō-lī'-tis) – an inflammatory process of the inner lining of the large intestine

uvula (yoo'-vyoo-luh) – the small fleshy mass hanging from the soft palate

v

volvulus (vol'-vyoo-lus) – intestinal obstruction due to a knotting and twisting of the bowel

Transcription Tips

You will find transcription in gastroenterology easier if you are familiar with the names of the organs of the digestive system, can locate them on a chart, and can describe their functions. Knowledge of the digestive hormones and enzymes, confusing terms, roots and/or combining forms, and diagnostic and laboratory tests also make the transcription process easier.

Organs of the Digestive System

The digestive system is composed of the mouth, pharynx, esophagus, stomach, and intestines. The accessory organs are the teeth, salivary glands, liver, gallbladder, and pancreas.

The gastrointestinal tract, or alimentary canal, has three functions: the digestion and absorption of food and the excretion of the waste products of digestion from the large intestine.

Digestive Hormones

gastrin
gastric inhibitory peptide
villikinin
secretin
pancreozymin
cholecystokinin

Digestive Enzymes

saliva
gastric juice
bile
pancreatic juice
intestinal juice

Confusing Terms

absorption – the uptake of substance into or across tissues such as skin, intestines, and kidney tubules

adsorption – the attachment of one substance to the surface of another

acathexia – the inability to retain bodily secretions

cachexia – a profound and marked state of constitutional disorder

achylia – absence of chyle

acholia – absence of secretion of bile

bile – a fluid secreted by the liver

bowel – the intestine

colonic – pertaining to the colon

clonic – pertaining to muscular contractions and relaxations that alternate in rapid succession

dysphagia – difficulty in swallowing

dysphasia – impairment of speech

ileum – the segment of the small intestine between the jejunum and the cecum

ilium – the hip bone

Roots and/or Combining Forms

Root	Meaning	Root	Meaning
abdomino	abdomen	lipo	fat
adeno, aden	gland	litho, lith	stone, calculus
aero, aer	air, gas	melano	black
angio, angi	vessel	necro	death
carcino	carcinoma	neo	new
celio	abdomen	oligo	few, deficient
chole, chol, cholo	bile	oro	mouth
duodeno	duodenum	phago	eating
entero, enter	intestines	pharyngo	pharynx
erythro	red	phlebo, phleb	vein
eu	normal	poly	many, excessive
fibro	fibers	procto, proct	rectum
glosso, gloss	tongue	py, pyo	pus
gluco	glucose	recto	rectum
glyco	sugar	sclero, scler	hard
hem, hema, hemo, hemat, hemo	blood	splanchno	viscera
		spleno, splen	spleen
hepato, hepat	liver	steno	narrowed
hydro, hydr	water	thrombo	clot
ileo	ileum	tracheo	trachea
jejuno	jejunum	tropho	nourishment
laparo	flank, abdomen		

Diagnostic and Laboratory Tests

alcohol toxicology – test performed on blood serum or plasma to calculate levels of alcohol

ammonia – test conducted on plasma to determine the level of ammonia

barium enema – test performed by administering barium through the rectum and viewing via x-ray to ascertain the condition of the colon

bilirubin blood test – test performed on blood serum to discover if bilirubin is conjugated and excreted in the bile

carcinoembryonic antigen (CEA) – test done on whole blood or plasma to discover the presence of antigens originally segregated from colon tumors

cholangiography – x-ray examination of the common bile duct, cystic duct, and hepatic ducts to assess presence of obstruction, stones, and tumors

cholecystography – x-ray examination of the gallbladder

colonoscopy – test performed using a flexible colonoscopy to view the colon; a fiberoptic colonoscopy

endoscopic retrograde cholangiopancreatography (ERCP) – x-ray exam of the biliary and pancreatic ducts to assess presence of such things as cysts, stones, fibrosis, or pancreatitis; uses a flexible endoscope

esophagogastroduodenoscopy – an endoscopic exam of the esophagus, stomach, and small intestine

fecal occult blood test (FOBT) – test for detection of blood in the stool

gamma-glutamyl tranferase (GGT) – test conducted on blood serum to determine the level of GGT, an enzyme found in the liver, kidney, prostate, heart, and spleen

gastric analysis – test performed to assess quality of secretion, amount of free and combined HCl, and absence or presence of blood, bacteria, bile, and fatty acids

gastrointestinal (GI) series – fluoroscopic examination (following ingestion of barium) of the esophagus, stomach, and small intestine

Hemoccult test – a quantitative assay test that detects heme (the iron-containing portion of hemoglobin) in the stool

hepatic antigen (HAA) – test conducted to assess the presence of the hepatitis B virus

liver biopsy – a microscopic exam of liver tissue

occult blood – test done on feces to determine GI bleeding that is invisible

ova and parasites (O&P) – test conducted on stool to identify ova and parasites

stool culture – test done on stool to determine the presence of organisms

ultrasonography, gallbladder – a test performed to image the gallbladder by using high-frequency sound waves

ultrasonography, liver – test done to image the liver by using high-frequency sound waves

upper gastrointestinal fiberoscopy – use of a flexible fiberscope to see the gastric mucosa

Supportive Web Sites

www.acg.gi.org/
Under "Patient Information," click on "Common GI Problems" and other links of interest.

www.gastro.com
In the introductory paragraph, click on the "gastroenterology," "liver disease," and "endoscopes" links for helpful information. Explore each of these links further by clicking on other links of interest.

www.gastromd.com
Click on "Medications and Prescriptions," "Liver Function Tests," "Radiographic Studies," and other links of interest.

www.mayoclinic.com
Click on the "Diseases and Conditions" link and then on related gastroenterology links; "search" on the home page for "gastroenterology" and then on links of interest.

www.medmark.org
Click on "Gastroenterology" and items of interest under the "For Consumers" link.

www.mtdesk.com
Click on "WORD LISTS (by specialty)," then on "Digestive/Gastroenterology terms".

www.my.webmd.com
Click on the "Diseases and Conditions" link and then select links of interest; "search" for gastroenterology and/or specific conditions and select links of interest.

Index of Gastroenterology Reports

(see table of contents for audio information)

Exercise #	***Patient Name***	***Report/Procedure***
TE#1	Dentler, Sherri Lynn	Esophagogastroduodenoscopy with Maloney dilatation
TE#2	Dimartino, Frank Joe	Flexible sigmoidoscopy
TE#3	Desilva, Austin	Endoscopic retrograde cholangiopancreatography
TE#4	LeBlance, Joseph	Colonoscopy, polypectomy, and biopsy note
TE#5	Almond, Misty	Esophagogastroduodenoscopy and PEG
TE#6	Dill, Judy	Colonoscopy
TE#7	Darensburg, Charlotte	Esophagogastroduodenoscopy and biopsy
TE#8	Cobb, Lisa Marie	Consultation
TE#9	Blouin, Desire	Discharge summary

CHAPTER 9

RESPIRATORY/ PULMONARY MEDICINE

Introduction

Physicians specializing in *respiratory/pulmonary medicine* treat diseases of the *respiratory system.* This system embraces all the structures concerned with the exchange of carbon dioxide and oxygen between the blood and the atmosphere. Components of the respiratory system include the *lung tissue,* where this gaseous exchange takes place; and the *respiratory tract,* a system of tubes that carry air to and from the lungs.

The respiratory system is divided into upper and lower tracts. The *upper tract* consists of the *nose, mouth, nasopharynx, oropharynx, laryngopharynx,* and *larynx.* The *lower tract* is subdivided into the *conducting airways (trachea, primary bronchi, lobar,* and *segmental bronchi)* and the *acinus,* which is the area of gas exchange (respiratory *bronchioles, alveolar ducts,* and *alveoli*).

Air travels over the following pathway from the nose to capillaries of the lungs:

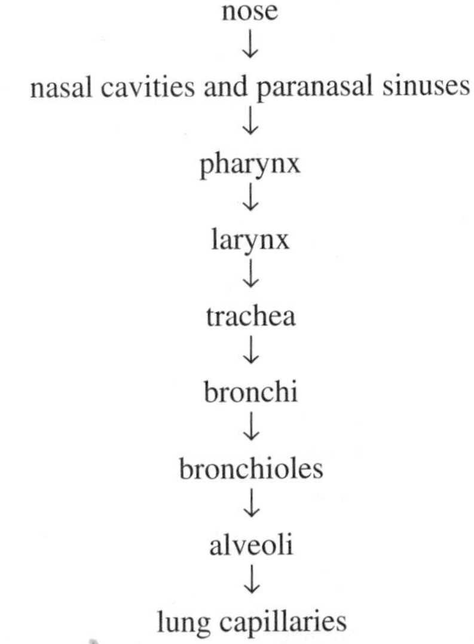

The *lungs* and accessory structures—*pleura, thoracic cavity,* and *mediastinum*—form significant parts of the respiratory system. Straddling the heart, the cone-shaped lungs fill the thoracic cavity. The right lung is shorter and broader than the left. Above and behind the heart lies the *hilum,* the opening through which pass the lung's root structures—primary *bronchus, pulmonary* and *bronchial blood vessels, lymphatics,* and *nerves.*

The *pleura* totally encloses the lungs and is composed of a *visceral* layer and a *parietal* layer. The *thoracic cavity* is the area within the chest wall; it is bounded below by the *diaphragm,* above by the *scalene muscles* and the fascia of the neck, and circumferentially by the *ribs, intercostal muscles, vertebrae, sternum,* and *ligaments.*

The *mediastinum* is the space between the lungs, which includes the heart; the thoracic aorta, pulmonary artery, and veins; the vena cavae and azygos veins; the thymus, lymph nodes, and vessels; the trachea, esophagus, and thoracic duct; and the vagus, cardiac, and phrenic nerves.

Physicians concerned with the treatment of the respiratory system treat such conditions as *bronchitis, pneumonia, asthma, emphysema, cystic fibrosis, tuberculosis, asbestosis, pleurisy,* and *cancerous conditions* that occur throughout the respiratory tract.

Critical Thinking Exercise

You have been asked to speak to a newly formed transcription group on the topic of becoming a CMT. What information do you think the audience will need? Prepare the outline you would use and share the appropriate information with class members.

Respiratory/Pulmonary Medicine Abbreviations

ABG	arterial blood gas
AFB	acid-fast bacillus
ARD	acute respiratory disease
ARDS	adult (or acute) respiratory distress syndrome
BOOP	bronchitis obliterans—organizing pneumonia
Bronch	bronchoscopy
CF	cystic fibrosis
COLD	chronic obstructive lung disease
COPD	chronic obstructive pulmonary disease
CPR	cardiopulmonary resuscitation
CT	computer tomography scan
CTA	clear to auscultation
CVD	cerebrovascular disease
CXR	chest x-ray
DIP	desquamative interstitial pneumonitis
DLCO	diffusing capacity for carbon monoxide
DPT	diphtheria, pertussis, tetanus
ERV	expiratory reserve volume
ET	endotracheal
FEF	forced expiratory flow
FEV	forced expiratory volume
FEV_1	FEV in 1 second
FIF	forced inspiratory flow
FVC	forced vital capacity
HBOT	hyperbaric oxygen therapy
HMD	hyaline membrane disease
HPS	Hantavirus pulmonary syndrome
HRCT	high-resolution CT scan
IC	inspiratory capacity
IMV	intermittent mandatory ventilation
IPF	idiopathic pulmonary fibrosis
IPPB	intermittent positive-pressure breathing
IRDS	infant respiratory distress syndrome
IRV	inspiratory reserve volume
JVD	jugular vein distention
KOH	potassium hydroxide
L	lymphangioleiomyomatosis
LL	left lung
LLL	left lower lobe
LUL	left upper lobe
MBC	maximal breathing capacity
MUGA	multiple gated acquisition (scan)
MV	minute volume
MVV	maximum voluntary ventilation
$PaCO_2$, pCO_2	carbon dioxide partial pressure
PaO_2, pO_2	oxygen partial pressure
PCP	Pneumocystis carinii pneumonia
PE	pulmonary embolism
PEEP	positive end expiratory pressure
PEFR	peak expiratory flow rate
PET	position emission tomography
PFT	pulmonary function test
PND	paroxysmal nocturnal dyspnea; postnasal drip
PPD	purified protein derivative
PPH	primary pulmonary hypertension
PPY	packs per year
R	respiration
RAD	reactive airways disease (bronchial asthma)
RD	respiratory disease
RDS	respiratory distress syndrome
RLL	right lower lobe
RUL	right upper lobe
RV	residual volume

SIDS	sudden infant death syndrome
SOB	shortness of breath
TB	tuberculosis
TINA	transthoracic needle aspiration biopsy
TLC	total lung capacity
TV	tidal volume
URI	upper respiratory infection
VC	vital capacity
V/Q scan	ventilation-perfusion scan

Anatomic Illustrations

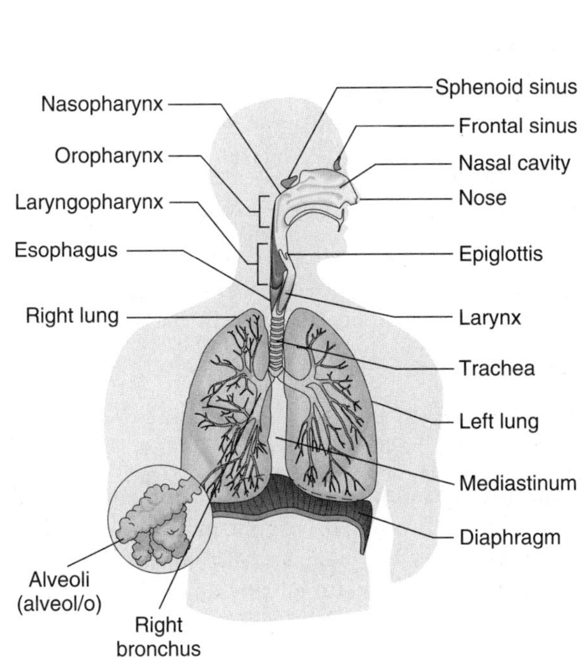

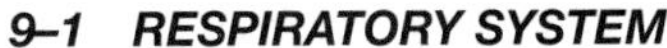
9–1 RESPIRATORY SYSTEM

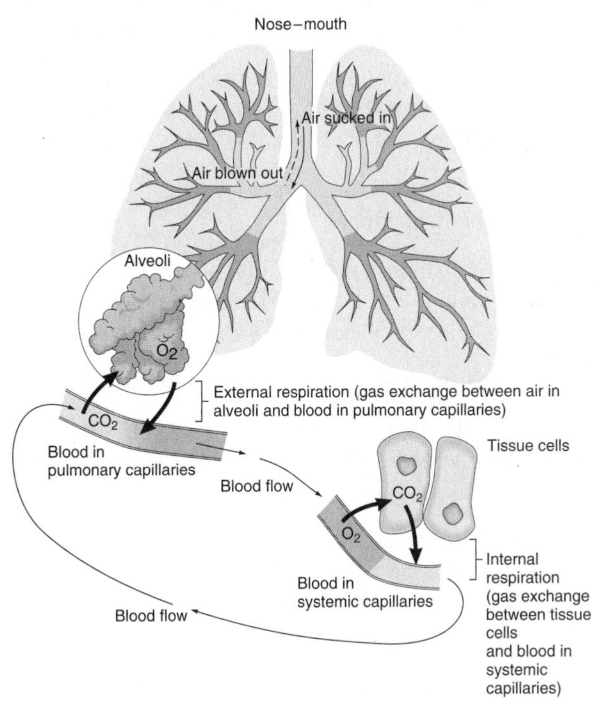

9–2 RESPIRATION VS. VENTILATION

Respiratory/Pulmonary Medicine Terminology

a

alveolus (pl. alveoli) (al-vē'-ō-lus, al-vē'-o-lī) – an air sac in the lung

anoxia (uh-nok'-sē-uh) – absence, or lack of, oxygen

apical (ā'-pih-kul, ap'-ih-kul) – pertaining to the apex, the uppermost portion of the lung

asbestosis (as"-beh-stō'-sis) – pneumoconiosis due to inhalation of asbestos particles

asphyxia (as-fik'-sē-uh) – suffocation

atelectasis (at"-eh-lek'-tuh-sis) – loss of air space as a result of collapse of lung tissue

b

bronchial asthma (brong'-kē-ul az'-muh) – a condition of the lungs characterized by narrowing of airways throughout the lungs; results in dyspnea and wheezing due to spasmodic contraction of the bronchi

bronchiectasis (brong"-kē-ek'-tuh-sis) – chronic dilatation of the bronchi as a result of inflammatory disease or obstruction; irreversible lung disease

bronchiole (brong'-kē-ōl) – one of the smallest branches of the bronchial tubes

bronchiolitis (brong"-kē-ō-lī'-tis) – inflammation of the bronchioles, often associated with bronchopneumonia and caused by a virus

bronchiolus (brong-kī'-ō-lus) – one of the smaller subdivisions of the bronchial tree

bronchitis (brong-kī'-tis) – inflammation of the mucous membrane of the bronchial tubes

bronchogenic carcinoma (brong-kō-jen'-ik kar"-sih-nō'-muh) – the principal malignancy of the lung; lung cancer

bronchoscopy (brong-kos'-kuh-pē) – examination of the interior of the tracheobronchial tree through a bronchoscope

bronchus (pl. bronchi) (brong'-kus, brong'-kī) – any of the larger air passages of the lungs

c

Cheyne-Stokes respiration (chān'-stōks res"-pih-rā'-shun) – a common and bizarre breathing pattern characterized by a period of apnea lasting 10 to 60 seconds followed by gradually increasing depth and frequency of respirations

cilia (sil'-ē-uh) – thin hairs attached to the mucous membrane epithelium lining the respiratory tract

coccidioidomycosis (kok-sid"-ē-oyd"-ō-mī-kō'-sis) – infection caused by breathing in spores of a fungus, Coccidioides immitis, found in desert regions

cor pulmonale (kōr pul'-mō-nāl) – failure of the right side of the heart to pump a sufficient amount of blood to the lungs

cystic fibrosis (sis'-tik fī-brō'-sis) – a congenital disorder of exocrine glands affecting the sweat glands and pancreatic acini as well as the lungs, in which abnormally thick mucus plugs the bronchioles, causing a chronic inflammatory reaction and leading to collapse and consolidation of alveoli

d

diaphragm (dī'-uh-fram) – the muscle separating the chest and the abdomen

e

emphysema (em"-fih-sē'-muh) – overinflation of the lungs with enlargement of air spaces due to a breakdown of alveolar septa

empyema (em"-pī-ē'-muh) – a pocket of pus between visceral and parietal pleura

expectoration (ek-spek"-tō-rā'-shun) – the process of coughing up and spitting out sputum from the lungs

h

Hantavirus pulmonary syndrome (hahn"-tuh-vī'-rus pul'-mō-nār"-ē sin'-drōm) – a potentially deadly disease carried by rodents, especially the deer mouse

hemithorax (hem"-ē-thō'-raks) – one side of the chest

hemoptysis (hē-mop'-tī-sis) – the spitting of blood derived from the lungs or bronchial tubes

i

idiopathic pulmonary fibrosis (id"-ē-ō-path'-ik pul'-mō-nār"-ē fī-brō'-sis) – an inflammatory lung disorder characterized by abnormal formation of fibrous tissue (fibrosis) between tiny air sacs (alveoli) or ducts in the lungs

l

laryngostasis (lah"-ring-gos'-tuh-sis) – croup

Legionella pneumonia (lē"-jun-el'-uh noo-mō'-nē-uh) – an acute infectious disease with flu-like symptoms and a rapidly rising high fever, followed by severe pneumonia; Legionnaires' disease

leukoplakia (loo"-kō-plā'-kē-uh) – a disease characterized by the development of white, thickened patches on the mucous membrane of the cheeks or tongue that cannot be rubbed off

lobectomy (lō-bek'-tuh-mē) – excision of a lobe of the thyroid, liver, brain, or lung

lymphangioleiomyomatosis (lim-fan"-jē-ō-lī"-ō-mī"-ō-muh-tō'-sis) – a rare lung disease characterized by an unusual type of muscle cell that invades the tissue of the lungs

m

mediastinoscopy (mē"-dē-as"-tih-nahs'-kuh-pē) – a visual examination of the mediastinum via a surgical procedure

mediastinum (mē"-dē-as-tī'-num) – the region between the lungs in the chest cavity

mesothelioma (mez"-ō-thē"-lē-ō'-muh) – a malignant tumor arising in the pleura

mycoplasmal pneumonia (mī"-kō-plaz'-mul noo-mō'-nē-uh) – the most common form of primary atypical pneumonia; occurs most frequently in young adults

n

naris (pl. nares) (nā'-ris, nā'-rēz) – nostril

o

orthopnea (or"-thop'-nē-uh) – difficult breathing except in an upright position

oximetry (ok-sim'-eh-trē) – measurement with an oximeter of the oxygen saturation of hemoglobin in a sample of blood

p

pleura (ploor'-uh) – the double-folded membrane surrounding each lung

pleural effusion (ploor'-ul ē-fyoo'-zhun) – escape of fluid into the pleural cavity

pleural rub (ploor'-ul rub) – the grating sound produced by the motion of pleural surfaces rubbing each other

pleurodesis (ploor"-ō-dē'-sis) – surgical creation of a fibrous adhesion between the visceral and parietal layers of the pleura

pneumoconiosis (noo"-mō-kō"-nē-ō'-sis) – inflammation commonly related to fibrosis of the lungs due to irritation from inhalation of dust incident to an occupation

pneumonectomy (noo"-mō-nek'-tuh-mē) – the excision of lung tissue, particularly of the entire lung

pneumothorax (noo"-mō-thor'-aks) – air in the pleural cavity

psittacosis (sit-uh-kō'-sis) – a disease caused by a strain of Chlamydia psittaci; usually takes the form of a pneumonia

pulmonary parenchyma (pul'-mō-nār"-ē pah-reng'-kih-muh) – the key cells of the lung, those performing its main function; the air sacs and small bronchioles

pulmonary tuberculosis (pul'-mō-nār"-ē too-ber"-kyoo-lō'-sis) – tuberculosis of the lungs

r

rhonchi (rong'-kī) – abnormal, rumbling sounds heard during expiration

s

sarcoidosis (sar"-koy-dō'-sis) – a systemic granulomatous disease of unknown cause, especially involving the lungs with resulting fibrosis

silicosis (sil"-ih-kō'-sis) – pneumoconiosis due to the inhalation of silica dust, with formation of generalized nodular fibrotic changes in both lungs

supraglottic (soo"-pruh-glot'-ik) – located above the glottis

t

thoracentesis (thor"-uh-sen-tē'-sis) – thoracocentesis; surgical puncture of the chest wall for drainage of fluid

thoracostomy (thor"-uh-kos'-tuh-mē) – surgical creation of an opening in the chest cavity for the purpose of drainage

thoracotomy (thor"-uh-kot'-uh-mē) – incision into the chest wall

tracheobronchial tree (trā"-kē-ō-brong'-kē-ul) – pertaining to the trachea and bronchi

tracheostomy (trā"-kē-os'-tuh-mē) – the creation of an opening into the trachea through the neck and insertion of a tube to create an airway

turbinate (tur'-bih-nāt) – shaped like a top, such as a turbinate bone

v

visceral pleura (viss'-er-ul ploor'-uh) – the inner fold of pleura lying closest to the lung tissue

Transcription Tips

You will find it easier to transcribe dictation about the respiratory system if you are familiar with the terms that describe its functions and structures that make respiration possible. A study of information presented in the chapter introduction, the confusing terms that follow, types of drugs commonly used, and lab and diagnostic tests used to delineate disease processes in respiratory/pulmonary medicine will make the task easier.

Confusing Terms

bronchi – plural of bronchus

rhonchi – pertaining to a rattling in the throat or a dry, coarse rale in the bronchial tubes

coarse – not fine

course – the path over which something moves or extends

dysphagia – difficulty in swallowing

dysphasia – impairment of speech

effusion – escape of a fluid into a part

affusion – pouring of water upon the body to reduce temperature

infusion – the steeping of a substance in water for obtaining its constituents

emphysema – a pathological accumulation of air in tissues or organs

empyema – accumulation of pus in a cavity

hyaline – glassy and transparent

hilum – pertaining to the hilus, which is a depression or pit at that part of an organ where the vessels and nerves exit and/or enter

hypertension – persistently high arterial blood pressure

hypotension – abnormally low blood pressure

mucus – the free slime of the mucous membranes

mucous – resembling mucus

perfusion – the act of pouring over or through, especially the passage of a fluid through the vessels of a specific organ

profusion – great quantity

reflux – a backward flow

reflex – an involuntary response to a stimulus

Commonly Used Types of Drugs

antihistamines
antituberculosis agents
antitussives
bronchodilators
corticosteroids
decongestants
expectorants
mucolytics

Lab and Diagnostic Tests

acid-fast bacilli (AFB)
antistreptolysin (ASO)
arterial blood gases (ABGs)
bronchoscopy
laryngoscopy
nasopharyngography
pulmonary function test
rhinoscopy
sputum culture
throat culture

Lung Function Tests

Arterial blood gases – determine the amount of oxygen and carbon dioxide in the bloodstream

Body plethysmography – measures the total amount of air the lungs can hold (total lung volume)

Carbon monoxide diffusing capacity – measures how well the lungs transfer a small amount of carbon monoxide gas into the blood

Gas dilution tests – measure the amount of air that remains in the lungs after complete exhalation (residual volume)

Spirometry – measures how quickly the lungs move air in and out

Common Measurable Lung Function Values	
Diffusing capacity for carbon monoxide (DLCO)	Residual volume (RV)
Forced expiratory volume (FEV)	Tidal volume (TV)
Maximum voluntary ventilation (MVV)	Total lung capacity (TLC)
Peak expiratory flow rate (PEFR)	Vital capacity (VC)

Bronchial Tube Disorders	
asthma	chronic bronchitis
bronchogenic carcinoma	cystic fibrosis

Lung Disorders	
atelectasis	pulmonary abscess
emphysema	pulmonary edema
pneumoconiosis	pulmonary embolism
pneumonia	tuberculosis

Pleural Disorders	
mesothelioma	pleurisy (pleuritis)
pleural effusion	pneumothorax

Supportive Web Sites

http://chorus.rad.mcw.edu/
Click on "Respiratory System" for an extensive terminology list.

www.mayoclinic.com
Search for "respiratory or pulmonary" or under "Find Information Fast"; look up a particular condition or disease by clicking on the initial letter of the word.

www.mtdesk.com
Click on "WORD LISTS (by specialty)," then on "respiratory terms."

www.my.webmd.com
Click on "Diseases and Conditions," then on links of interest.

www.nhlbi.nih.gov
Click on "Health Information," then on "Lung Diseases" or other links of interest.

www.nlm.nih.gov
Click on "Health Information" link, then on "MEDLINEplus." "Search" for "respiratory" and "pulmonary" and select links of interest. You can also click on "Health Topics" and search for different diseases and conditions by clicking on the appropriate letter of the alphabet.

Index of Respiratory/Pulmonary Reports

(see table of contents for audio information)

Exercise #	Patient Name	Report/Procedure
TE#1	Spier, William	Thoracentesis
TE#2	Carter, Brady	Ultrasound-guided right thoracentesis
TE#3	Lemoine, Sammy	Discharge summary
TE#4	Cutrell, Stephen	Death note
TE#5	Hodges, JoAnn	Fiberoptic bronchoscopy with biopsy
TE#6	Foster, Oscar	H&P
TE#7	Long, Ella Mae	Flexible bronchoscopy
TE#8	Taylor, Lillie Mae	Bronchoscopy with radiation catheter placement

CHAPTER 10

UROLOGY/NEPHROLOGY

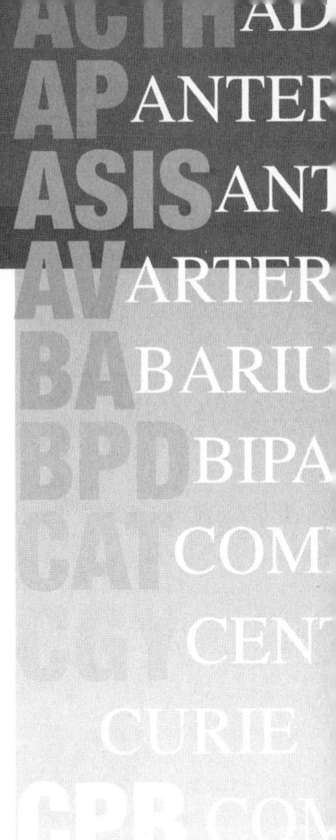

Introduction

Urology is the study of the urinary tract in the male and female as well as the reproductive system in the male; *nephrology* is the study of the kidneys, their anatomy, physiology, pathology, and disorders.

The urinary system is made up of two *kidneys,* which form and excrete urine, thereby removing various poisons from the body; two *ureters,* which carry urine from the kidneys down to the bladder; the urinary *bladder,* which serves as a collecting reservoir for urine; and the *urethra,* which transports the urine to the outside of the body. Other terms by which the urinary system may be identified are the genitourinary system, the excretory system, the renal-urologic system, and the urogenital system.

A *urologist* is a surgeon who treats *surgical disorders* of the kidneys, ureter, bladder, and male reproductive system. In addition, he or she treats such disorders as kidney stones, hematuria, cystitis, and prostate and impotence problems in men. A physician who treats only kidney disorders is called a *nephrologist.*

Critical Thinking Exercise

A friend recently confided in you that her husband is experiencing erectile dysfunction, as a result of diabetes mellitus. Because of your familiarity with medical resources, she asked you to get information for her on penile implants.

Where would you obtain such information? Identify some Web sites you could direct her to for more information.

Urology/Nephrology Abbreviations

AA	amino acid
ACTH	adrenocorticotropic hormone
ADH	antidiuretic hormone
A/G	albumin/globulin ratio
AGN	acute glomerulonephritis
ANA	antinuclear antibody
ARF	acute renal failure
ATN	acute tubular necrosis
AV	arteriovenous
BNO	bladder neck obstruction
BPH	benign prostatic hypertrophy
BUN	blood urea nitrogen
CAPD	continuous ambulatory peritoneal dialysis
CC	clean catch
CFR	glomerular filtration rate
CGN	chronic glomerulonephritis
CMG	cystometrogram
CRF	chronic renal failure
C&S	culture and sensitivity
cysto	cystoscopic exam

ECF	extracellular fluid
ESRD	end-stage renal disease
ESWL	extracorporeal shockwave lithotripsy
FEP	free erythrocyte protoporphyrin
FSH	follicle-stimulating hormone
GBM	glomerular basement membrane
GFR	glomerular filtration rate
GU	genitourinary
G6PD	a red cell enzyme; also a lab test
HD	hemodialysis
HPF	high-power field
I&O	intake and output
IPD	intermittent peritoneal dialysis
IVP	intravenous pyelogram
KUB	kidneys, ureters, bladder
LDH	lactic dehydrogenase (enzyme in blood and tissues)
LH	luteinizing hormone
LPF	low-power field
MRI	magnetic resonance imaging
PD	peritoneal dialysis
pH	potential of hydrogen
PKU	phenylketonuria
PSA	prostate-specific antigen
PSP	phenolsulfonphthalein
PUL	percutaneous ultrasonic lithotripsy
PVC	postvoiding cystogram
RP	retrograde pyelogram
TUE	transurethral extraction
TUR	transurethral resection
TURB	transurethral resection, bladder
TURP	transurethral resection, prostate
UA	urinalysis
UPJ	ureteropelvic junction
UTI	urinary tract infection
UVJ	ureterovesical junction
VCUG	voiding cystourethrogram; vesicoureterogram
XC	excretory cystogram
XU	excretory urogram

Anatomic Illustrations

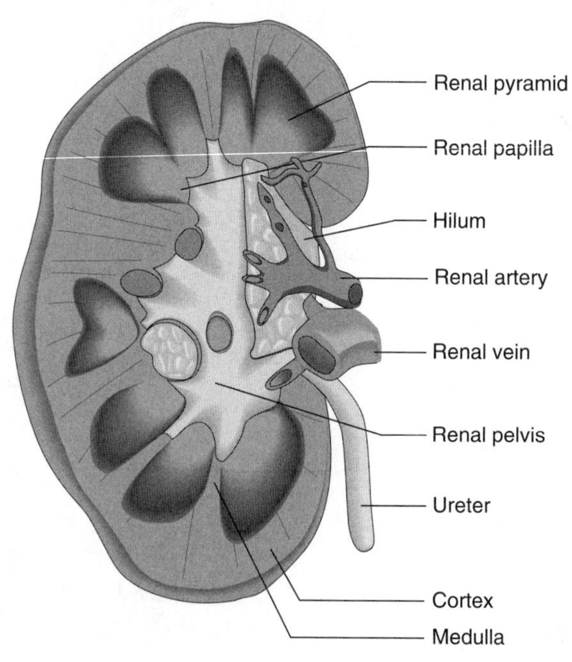

10–1 THE KIDNEY

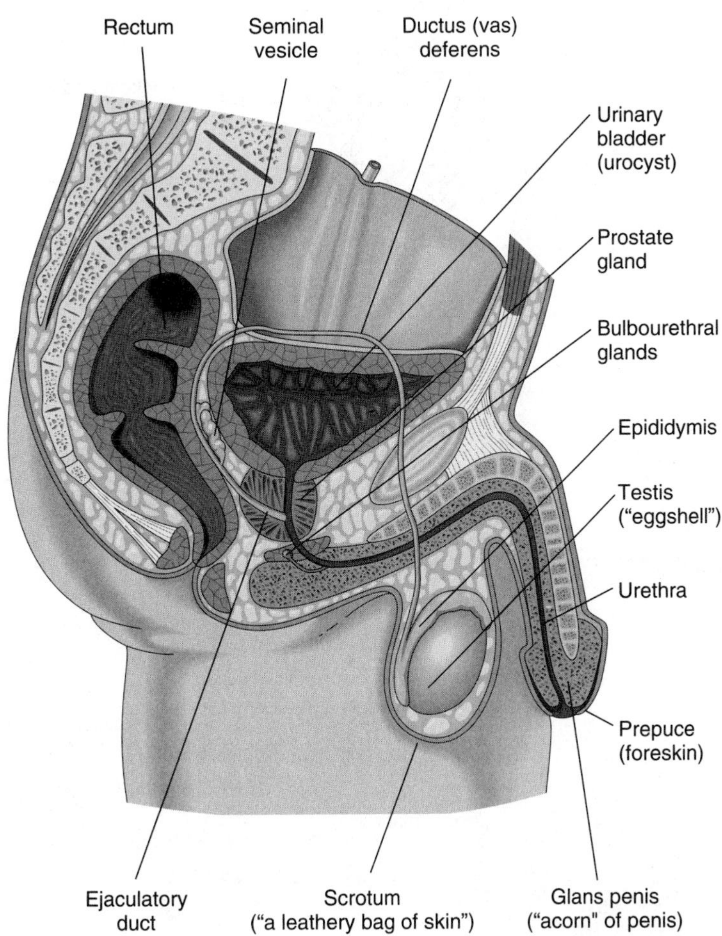

10–2 MALE REPRODUCTIVE ORGANS

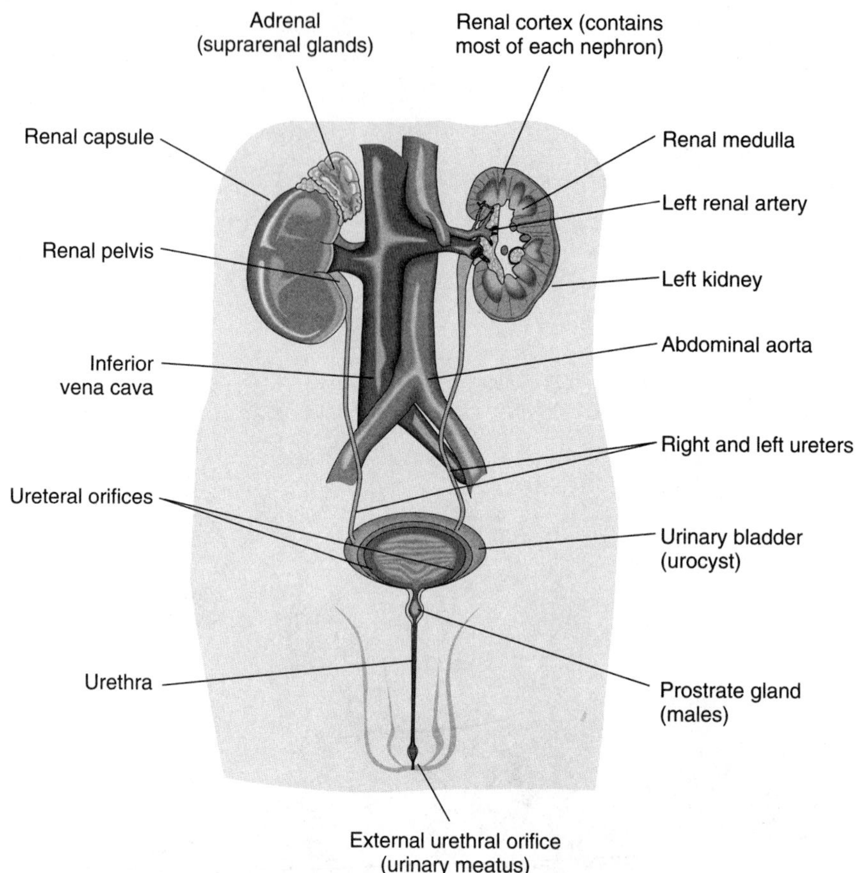

10–3 GROSS ANATOMY OF THE URINARY SYSTEM

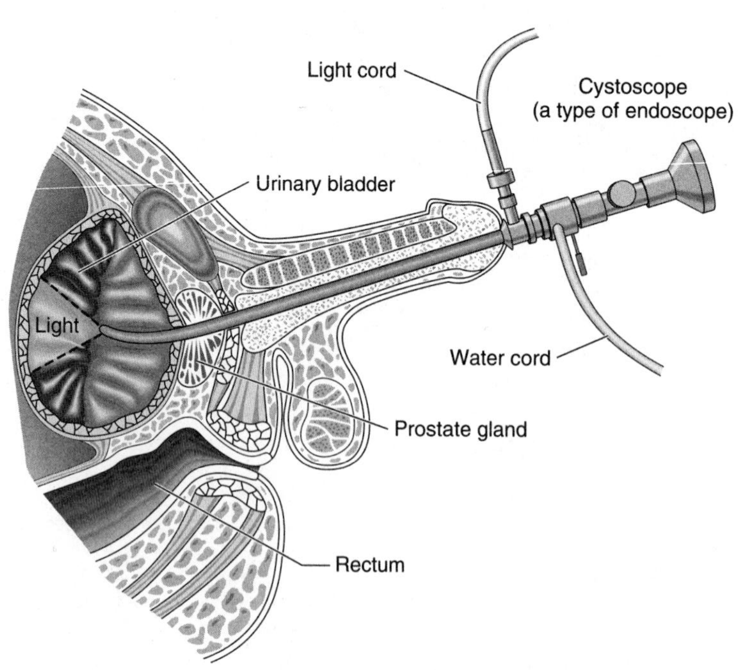

10–4 ENDOSCOPY OF THE URINARY BLADDER

Urology/Nephrology Terminology

a

albuminuria (al"-byoo-mih-nyoo'-rē-uh) – presence in the urine of serum albumin

aminoaciduria (ah-mē"-nō-as"-ih-dyoo'-rē-uh) – an excess of amino acids in the urine

anorchism (an-or'-kizm) – congenital absence of the testis, which may occur unilaterally or bilaterally

antidiuretic (an"-tī-dī"-yoo-ret'-ik) – agent used to suppress the rate of urine formation

anuria (ah-nyoo'-rē-uh) – absence of excretion of urine from the body

aspermia (ā-sper'-mē-uh) – failure of formation or emission of semen

athrocytosis (ath"-rō-sī-tō'-sis) – absorption of macromolecules from the lumen of the renal tubules by renal tubular cells, by means of a process similar to phagocytosis

azoospermia (ā-zō"-ō-sper'-mē-uh) – the absence of living sperm

b

bacteriuria (bak-tēr"-ē-yoo'-rē-uh – the presence of bacteria in the urine

balanitis (bal"-uh-nī'-tis) – inflammation of the glans penis

Bence Jones protein (behns jōnz prō-tēn) – an abnormal urinary protein found almost exclusively in multiple myeloma; constitutes the light-chain component of myeloma globulin

brachytherapy (brak"-ē-thăr'-uh-pē) – a procedure used to permanently implant tiny radioactive "seeds" into cancerous prostate glands; the seeds emit low-level radiation for several months

bulbourethral (bul"-bō-yoo-rē'-thrul) – pertaining to the bulb of the urethra

c

calculus (kal'-kyoo-lus) – an abnormal concretion occurring within the body and usually composed of mineral salts

caliectasis (syn. calicectasis) (kal"-ē-ek'-tuh-sis, kal"-ih-sek'-tuh-sis) – dilatation of a calix of a kidney

calyx (syn. calix) (kā'-liks) – a cup-shaped organ or cavity

capsulectomy (kap"-suh-lek'-tuh-mē) – excision of a capsule

capsulotomy (kap"-suh-lot'-uh-mē) – the incision of a capsule

chyluria (kī-loo'-rē-uh) – the presence of chyle in the urine, giving it a milky appearance

cloaca (klō-ā'-kuh) – the terminal end of the hindgut before division into the rectum, bladder, and genital primordia

creatinine (krē-at'-ih-nēn) – a basic substance, creatine anhydride, procurable from creatine and from urine

cryptorchidism (krip-tōr'-kih-dizm) – a developmental defect characterized by failure of the testes to descend into the scrotum

crystalluria (kris-tuh-loo'-rē-uh) – the excretion of crystals in the urine, causing renal irritation

cystinosis (Fanconi's syndrome) (sis"-tih-nō'-sis, fan-kō'-nēz sin'-drōm) – a congenital hereditary disease

cystinuria (sis"-tih-nyoo'-rē-uh) – the occurrence of cystine in the urine

cystitis (sis-tī'-tis) – inflammation of the bladder

cystogram (sis'-tuh-gram) – x-ray of the bladder

cystolithectomy (sis"-tō-lih-thek'-tuh-mē) – the removal of a calculus by cutting into the urinary bladder

cystoplasty (sis'-tō-plas"-tē) – surgical repair of the bladder

cystorrhagia (sis"-tō-rā'-jē-uh) – condition of blood bursting forth from the bladder

cystoscope (sis'-tō-skōp") – instrument used for examining the bladder

cystoureteritis (sis"-tō-yoo-rē"-ter-ī'-tis) – inflammation involving the urinary bladder and ureters

cystoureterolithotomy (sis"-tō-yoo-rē"-ter-ō-lih-thot'-uh-mē) – cystoscopy and ureterolithotomy for removal of calculus

cystourethroscopy (sis"-tō-yoo"-rē-thrah'-skuh-pē) – examination of the bladder and posterior urethra

d

dartos (syn. tunica dartos) (dar'-tōs, too'-nih-kuh dar'-tōs) – a layer of smooth muscle fibers situated in the superficial fascia of the scrotum

Denonvilliers' fascia (deh-nawn-vēl-yāz' fā'-shē-uh) – a membranous partition separating the rectum from the prostate and urinary bladder

descensus testis (dē-sen'-sus tes'-tis) – the descent of the testis from its fetal position in the abdominal cavity to the scrotum

dialysis (dī-al'-ih-sis) – the process of separating crystalloids and colloids in solution by the difference in their rates of diffusion through a semipermeable membrane

diuresis (dī"-yoo-rē'-sis) – increased secretion of urine

dysuria (dis-yoo'-rē-uh) – painful or difficult urination

e

elephantiasis (el"-eh-fan-tī'-uh-sis) – a chronic filarial disease due to infection of the lymphatic channels; characterized by inflammation and obstruction of the lymphatics and hypertrophy of the skin and subcutaneous tissues; the legs and external genitals are mainly affected

endopelvic (en"-dō-pel'-vik) – within the pelvis

enuresis (en"-yoo-rē'-sis) – involuntary discharge of the urine; bed-wetting

epididymis (ep"-ih-did'-ih-mis) – a set of coiled tubes that lie alongside and connect the testes to the vas deferens

epididymitis (ep"-ih-did"-ih-mī'-tis) – inflammation of the epididymis

epispadias (ep"-ih-spā'-dē-us) – a congenital defect in which the urethra opens on the dorsum of the penis

f

Foroblique (for"-ō-blēk') – trademark for an obliquely forward visual telescopic system used in certain cystoscopes

funiculitis (fyoo-nik"-yoo-lī'-tis) – inflammation of the spermatic cord

g

glomerular (glō-mer'-yoo-lar) – pertaining to or of the nature of a glomerulus, especially a renal glomerulus

glomerulitis (glō-mer"-yoo-lī'-tis) – inflammation of the glomeruli of the kidney, with proliferative or necrotizing changes of the endothelial or epithelial cells or thickening of the basement membrane

glomerulonephritis (glō-mer"-yoo-lō-neh-frī'-tis) – a variety of nephritis characterized by inflammation of the capillary loops in the glomeruli of the kidney

glomerulosclerosis (glō-mer"-yoo-lō-skleh-rō'-sis) – fibrosis and scarring, which result in senescence of the renal glomeruli

glomerulus (glō-mer'-yoo-lus) – a tuft or cluster; often used alone to designate one of the glomeruli of the kidney

glycosuria (glī"-kō-syoo'-rē-uh) – the presence of an abnormal amount of glucose in the urine; especially the excretion of an abnormally large amount of sugar (glucose) in the urine

gonadectomy (gō"-nah-dek'-tuh-mē) – removal of an ovary or a testis

gonococcal (gon"-ō-kok'-ul) – pertaining to gonococci, an individual microorganism of the species Neisseria gonorrhoeae, the organism causing gonorrhea

gonorrhea (gon"-ō-rē'-uh) – infection due to Neisseria gonorrhoeae; transmitted venereally in most cases

h

hematuria (hēm"-ah-tyoo'-rē-uh) – blood in the urine

hemoglobinuria (hē"-mō-glō"-bih-nyoo'-rē-uh) – the presence of free hemoglobin in the urine

hemorrhagic (hem"-ō-raj'-ik) – pertaining to or characterized by hemorrhage; descriptive of any tissue into which bleeding has occurred

hermaphroditism (her-maf'-rō-dih-tizm") – a condition characterized by the presence of both male and female sex organs

Hesselbach's triangle (hes'-ul-boks trī'-ang-gul) – the area on the inferoanterior abdominal wall bounded by the rectus abdominis muscle, the inguinal ligament, and the inferior epigastric vessels

hydrocele (hī'-drō-sēl) – a collection of fluid in the membranes surrounding the testes

hydronephrosis (hī"-drō-neh-frō'-sis) – distention of the pelvis and calices of the kidney with urine, as a result of obstruction of the ureter, with accompanying atrophy of the parenchyma of the organ

hypercalciuria (hī"-per-kal"-sē-yoo'-rē-uh) – an excess of calcium in the urine

hyperkalemia (hī"-per-kuh-lē'-mē-uh) – abnormally high potassium concentration in the blood, most often due to defective renal excretion

hyperoxaluria (hī"-per-oks"-ah-loo'-rē-uh) – the excretion of an excessive amount of oxalate in the urine

hyperuricuria (hī"-per-yoo"-rih-kyoo'-rē-uh) – excess of uric acid in the urine

hypocitruria (hī"-pō-sih-troo'-rē-uh)—low levels of citric acid in the urine

hypospadias (hī"-pō-spa'-dē-us) – a developmental anomaly in the male in which the urethra opens on the underside of the penis or on the perineum

i

intrarenal (in"-truh-rē'-nul) – within the kidney

isoimmunization (ī"-sō-im"-yoo-nih-zā'-shun) – development of antibodies against an antigen derived from a genetically dissimilar individual of the same species

k

kraurosis (kraw-rō'-sis) – a dry, shriveled condition of a part, especially of the vulva

l

leukocyturia (lyoo"-kō-sī-tyoo'-rē-uh) – the discharge of leukocytes in the urine

lipiduria (lip"-ih-dyoo'-rē-uh) – the presence of lipids in the urine

lithiasis (lih-thī'-uh-sis) – a condition characterized by the formation of calculi and concretions

litholapaxy (lih-thol'-uh-pak"-sē) – the crushing of a calculus in the bladder, followed at once by the washing out of the fragments

m

Marshall-Marchetti technique (mar'-shul-mar-shet'-ē tek-nēk') – operation for stress incontinence in a female

meatotomy (mē"-uh-tot'-uh-mē) – incision made into the urinary meatus to enlarge it

micturition (mik"-tyoo-rih'-shun) – the passage of urine; urination

myoglobinuria (mī"-ō-glō"-bih-nyoo'-rē-uh) – the presence of myoglobin in the urine

n

neocystostomy (nē"-ō-sis-tos'-tuh-mē) – recent cystostomy

nephrectomy (neh-frek'-tuh-mē) – excision of a kidney

nephritis (neh-frī'-tis) – inflammation of a kidney

nephroblastoma (neh"-frō-blas-tō'-muh) – Wilms' tumor

nephrocalcinosis (neh"-frō-kal"-sih-nō'-sis) – a condition characterized by precipitation of calcium phosphate in the tubules of the kidney, with resultant renal insufficiency

nephrocystitis (neh"-frō-sis-tī'-tis) – inflammation of the kidney and bladder

nephrolithiasis (neh"-frō-lih-thī'-uh-sis) – a condition marked by the presence of renal calculi

nephrolithotomy (neh"-frō-lih-thot'-uh-mē) – the removal of renal calculi by cutting through the body of the kidney

nephrology (neh-frahl'-uh-jē) – scientific study of the kidney, its anatomy, physiology, and pathology

nephropathy (neh-frahp'-uh-thē) – disease of the kidneys

nephropexy (neh'-frō-pek"-sē) – the fixation or suspension of a floating kidney

nephrosclerosis (neh"-frō-skleh-rō'-sis) – hardening of the kidney; the condition of the kidney caused by renovascular disease

nephrosis (neh-frō'-sis) – any disease of the kidney

nephroureterectomy (neh"-frō-yoo"-rē-ter-ek'-tuh-mē) – excision of a kidney and a whole or part of the ureter

o

oligospermia (ō"-lih-gō-sper'-mē-uh) – deficiency in the number of spermatozoa in the semen

oliguria (ō"-lih-gyoo'-rē-uh) – secretion of a diminished amount of urine in relation to fluid intake

orchialgia (or"-kē-al'-jē-uh) – pain in a testis

orchiopexy (or"-kē-ō-pek'-sē) – surgical fixation in the scrotum of an undescended testis

orchitis (or-kī'-tis) – inflammation of a testis

p

paraphymosis (pār"-uh-fī-mō'-sis) – condition in which the foreskin is stuck behind the head of the penis and cannot be pulled back down to a normal position

pelviolithotomy (pel"-vē-ō-lih-thot'-uh-mē) – the operation in which a renal calculus is excised from the pelvis of the kidney

penectomy (peh-nek'-tuh-mē) – surgical removal of the penis

penoscrotal (pē'-nō-skrō'-tul) – relating to the penis and the scrotum

percutaneous ultrasonic lithotripsy (per"-kyoo-tā'-nē-us ul'-truh-sah'-nik lith'-ō-trip"-sē) – the use of ultrasound to crush a kidney stone

peritoneal dialysis (pār"-ih-tō-nē'-ul dī-al'-ih-sis) – use of a peritoneal catheter and dialysis to separate waste from the blood

periurethral (pār"-ē-yoo-rē'-thrul) – occurring around the urethra

Peyronie's disease (pā-rō-nēz' dih-zēz') – penile deformation characterized by a plaque or hard lump that develops on the upper or lower side of the penis in the layers containing erectile tissue

phalloplasty (fal'-ō-plas"-tē) – plastic surgery of the penis

phallus (fal'-us) – the penis

pheochromocytoma (fē-ō-krō"-mō-sī-tō'-muh) – a tumor of chromaffin tissue, most commonly of the adrenal medulla; can be lethal

phimosis (fī-mō'-sis) – tightness of the foreskin, so that it cannot be drawn back from over the glans

polyuria (pol"-ē-yoo'-rē-uh) – the passage of a large volume of urine in a given period, a characteristic of diabetes

prevesical (prē-veh'-sih-kul) – situated in front of the bladder

priapism (prī'-uh-pihzm) – persistent abnormal erection of the penis, usually without sexual desire, and accompanied by pain and tenderness

prostate gland (prah'-stāt gland) – structure surrounding the ejaculatory ducts that produces some of the components of sperm

prostatectomy (prahs"-tā-tek'-tuh-mē) – surgical removal of the prostate or of a part thereof

proteinuria (prō"-tē-in-yoo'-rē-uh) – the presence of an excess of serum proteins in the urine

pyelectasis (pī"-eh-lek'-tuh-sis) – dilatation of the renal pelvis

pyelitis (pī"-eh-lī'-tis) – inflammation of the pelvis of the kidney

pyelocaliectasis (pī"-eh-lō-kal"-ē-ek'-tuh-sis) – dilatation of the kidney pelvis and calices

pyelonephritis (pī"-eh-lō-neh-frī'-tis) – inflammation of the kidney and its pelvis

pyonephrosis (pī"-ō-neh-frō'-sis) – suppurative destruction of the parenchyma of the kidney, with total or almost complete loss of renal function

pyuria (pī-yoo'-rē-uh) – the presence of pus in the urine

S

scrotum (skrō'-tum) – pouch-like structure containing the testes

seminal vesicles (sem'-ih-nul vess'-ih-kulz) – sac-like structures attaching to the vas deferens that provide fluids to lubricate the duct system and nourish the sperm

seminiferous tubules (seh"-mih-nif'-er-us too'-byoolz) – tiny coiled tubes in the testes that produce sperm

seminoma (seh"-mih-nō'-muh) – a malignant tumor of the testis thought to arise from primitive gonadal cells

smegma (smeg'-muh) – a foul-smelling, pasty accumulation of desquamated epidermal cells and sebum that has collected in moist areas of the genitalia

Sonolith Praktis (sōn'-ō-lihth prak'-tis) – a portable lithotripter used to treat stones in the kidney and ureters

spermaturia (syn. seminuria) (sper"-muh-tyoo'-rē-uh, seh"-mih-nyoo'-rē-uh) – the presence of semen in the urine

synorchism (sin-or'-kizm) – fusion of the two testes into one mass, which may be located in the scrotum or in the abdomen

T

Tenckhoff catheter (tenk'-hawf kath'-eh-tur) – a catheter inserted into the peritoneum for peritoneal dialysis

testicle (tess'-tih-kul) – the structure in males in which sperm are produced

testosterone (tess-tos'-ter-ōn) – the major male sex hormone

transvesical (trans-veh'-sih-kul) – through the bladder

trigonitis (trig"-uh-nī'-tis) – inflammation or localized hyperemia of the trigone of the bladder

U

urea (yoo-rē'-uh) – a white, crystalline substance found in the urine, blood, and lymph

ureterectasis (yoo-rē"-ter-ek'-tuh-sis) – distention of the ureter

ureteritis (yoo"-rē-ter-ī'-tis) – inflammation of a ureter

ureteroenteric (yoo-rē"-ter-ō-en-tār'-ik) – pertaining to or connecting the ureter and the intestine

ureterolithiasis (yoo-rē"-ter-ō-lih-thī'-uh-sis) – the formation of a calculus in the ureter

ureterolithotomy (yoo-rē"-ter-ō-lih-thot'-uh-mē) – the removal of a calculus from the ureter by incision

ureteropelvic (yoo-rē"-ter-ō-pel'-vik) – pertaining to or affecting the ureter and the renal pelvis

ureteroureterostomy (yoo-rē"-ter-ō-yoo-rē"-ter-os'-tuh-mē) – end-to-end anastomosis of the two portions of a transected ureter

urethrovesical (yoo-rē"-thrō-veh'-sih-kul) – pertaining to or communicating with the urethra and the bladder

uriniferous (yoo"-rih-nih'-fer-us) – transporting or conveying the urine

urochrome (yoo'-rō-krōm) – the pigment that makes urine yellow

urostomy (yoo"-rahs'-tuh-mē) – surgical opening in the urinary bladder

urotoxia (yoo"-rō-tok'-sē-uh) – the toxicity of the urine; the toxic substance of the urine

V

varicocele (vār'-ih-kō-sēl") – a varicose condition of the veins of the scrotum

vasectomy (vah-sek'-tuh-mē) – surgical removal of the ductus (vas) deferens, or of a portion of it; done in association with prostatectomy, or to induce infertility

vesicourethropexy (veh"-sih-kō-yoo-rē'-thrō-pek"-sē) – surgical fixation of bladder and urethra for correction of stress incontinence in a female

Transcription Tips

You will find it easier to transcribe dictation in urology/nephrology if you are familiar with the names of the organs of the renal-urologic system, their locations, and their functions. You should also study the confusing terms, the meanings of roots and/or combining forms, prefixes, and suffixes relevant to this system. Knowledge of lab and diagnostic terminology used in this specialty will also be beneficial.

The kidneys constitute the major portion of the renal-urologic system. The lower urinary tract consists of the ureters, the urinary bladder, and the urethra.

Confusing Terms

circumcision – the surgical removal of the end of the prepuce of the penis

circumscribe – to draw a line around; to encircle; to confine within bounds

diuresis – an increased secretion of urine

uresis – the passage of urine

epididymis – the structure attached to the back of the testis

epididymitis – inflammation of the epididymis

micturition – urination or voiding

miction – urination

ureter – the tube that carries urine from the kidney to the bladder

urethra – the tube that carries urine from the bladder to the exterior of the body

vesical – pertaining to the bladder

vesicle – a small bladder or sac containing liquid

Roots and/or Combining Forms

Root	Meaning	Root	Meaning
abdomino	abdomen	necro	death
adeno, aden	gland	neo	new
angio, angi	vessel	nephro, nephr	kidney
arterio	artery	oligo	few, deficient
carcino	carcinoma	orchio, orchi,	testis, testes
celio	abdomen	orchido	
costo	rib	poly	many, excessive
cysto, cyst,	sac, bladder	procto, proct	rectum
cysti, cystido		pyelo, pyel	pelvis of the kidney
hem, hema, hemo,	blood	steno	narrowed
hemat, hemato		uretero	ureter
ilio	ilium, flank	urethro	urethra
lipo	fat	uro, ur	urine
litho, lith	stone, calculus	vaso	vessel
myo, my	muscle	veno	vein

Lab Tests and/or Diagnostic Procedures

blood urea nitrogen (BUN) – blood test to assess amount of urea excreted by the kidneys

creatinine – blood test to determine amount of creatinine present

creatinine clearance – urine test to determine the glomerular filtration rate (GFR)

cystoscopy – visual examination of the bladder and urethra using a lighted cystoscope

intravenous pyelography – test conducted with use of radiopaque substance injected intravenously to see the kidneys, ureters, and bladder

kidney, ureter, bladder (KUB) – x-ray of the abdomen to reveal the size and position of the kidneys, ureters, and bladder

magnetic resonance imaging (MRI) – procedure that uses magnetic waves to make images of the pelvic and retroperitoneal regions

radioisotope studies – pictures taken of kidneys following injection of a radioactive substance (isotope) into the bloodstream

renal biopsy – removal of tissue from the kidney

retrograde pyelography – use of a contrast medium to see the kidneys, ureters, and bladder

ultrasonography of the kidneys – the use of high-frequency sound waves to view the kidneys

urine culture – urine test to determine the presence of microorganisms

voiding cystourethrogram (VCUG) – x-ray of the bladder and urethra as patient expels urine, after the bladder has been filled with contrast material

Other Procedures

dialysis – the separation of waste materials from the bloodstream when the kidneys can no longer function; two types are hemodialysis and peritoneal dialysis

extracorporeal shock wave lithotripsy (ESWL) – procedure where kidney stones are crushed by use of shock waves; fragments can then be passed out with urine

renal transplantation – procedure in which a kidney is transplanted into a patient with renal failure from either an identical twin (isograft) or other individual (allograft)

Disorders Affecting the Male Reproductive System

epididymitis
hydrocele
inguinal hernias
testicular cancer
testicular torsion
testicular trauma
undescended testicles

Penile Disorders

ambiguous genitalia
hypospadias
micropenis
phimosis

Supportive Web Sites

www.atnephrology.com
Click on links of interest.

www.cancer.gov
Click on "Cancer Information," then "Types of Cancer," then links of interest; also search for "urology" or "nephrology."

http://chorus.rad.mcw.edu/
Click on "Genito-Urinary System," then on other related links for an extensive terminology list.

www.my.webmd.com
Under "Medical Info," click on "Diseases and Conditions"; select links of interest.

www.niddk.nih.gov
Click on "Health Information," then on "Kidney and Urologic Diseases" for links of interest concerning urology.

www.nlm.nih.gov
Click on "Health Information," then "MEDLINEplus," then search for "urology"; select links of interest.

www.thekidney.org/
Click on links of interest.

Index of Urology/Nephrology Reports

(see table of contents for audio information)

Exercise #	Patient Name	Report/Procedure
TE#1	Juneau, Brooke	Ureteroscopic stone fragmentation with lithoclast; stent placement
TE#2	Pendergrass, Nathaniel	Radioactive seed implantation to prostate
TE#3	Crumley, Aaron	Extracorporeal shock wave lithotripsy
TE#4	Ely, Eric	Hydrocelectomy and hernia repair
TE#5	Tuten, Nicole	Ureteroscopic basket stone extraction
TE#6	Verberkmoes, Robert	Lymphadenectomy, prostatectomy
TE#7	Wofford, Gareth	Ultrasound-guided seed placement of radioactive seeds
TE#8	Gasparro, Chet	Cystoscopy, pyelogram, stone extraction, and placement of stent
TE#9	Vincent, Henry	Scrotal exploration with replacement of pump

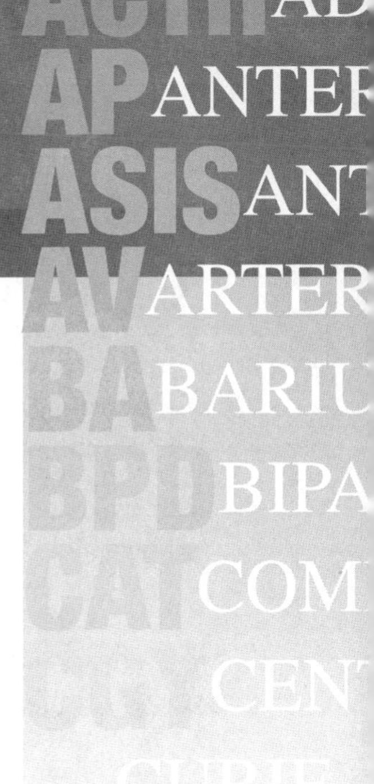

CHAPTER 11

ONCOLOGY

Introduction

Oncology is a word derived from the Greek *onchos,* meaning a lump or tumor. *Oncology* is the study of cancer. An *oncologist* is a physician, surgeon, or radiotherapist who specializes in the diagnosis and treatment of cancer.

Cancer is a proliferation of cells that grow in an uncontrolled manner, invading local tissues and spreading widely through the blood or lymphatics to produce secondary deposits, or *metastases,* in distant parts of the body. The cells composing the tumor grow better than normal cells and have either partially or completely escaped the complex mechanisms of restraint that control growth in normal cells.

More than 200 different types of cancer have been identified; however, these different types can be divided into three main groups based on the tissue from which the tumor cells originate. These three classes are carcinomas, sarcomas, and mixed-tissue tumors.

Carcinomas comprise the largest group and are malignant tumors that arise from the epithelial tissues that line internal and external body surfaces. For example, lung carcinoma arises from the epithelium lining the main airways or bronchi, breast carcinoma develops from the ductal tissue in the breast, and stomach and colon carcinomas originate from their epithelial linings.

Sarcomas develop from supportive and connective tissue such as cartilage, bone, muscle, fat, and bone marrow, as well as from cells of the lymph system. Another word for bone sarcomas is osteosarcomas; fat sarcomas are called liposarcomas. Sarcomas are more commonly seen in children and spread via the bloodstream, whereas carcinomas are more commonly seen in adults and usually spread via the lymphatics.

Mixed-tissue tumors originate in tissue that can separate into both epithelial and connective tissue. When cancer occurs simultaneously in adjacent tissue types, it is known as a mixed-tissue tumor.

The method of classifying tumors involves establishing the tumor's *grade* (degree of maturity) and its *stage* (extent of metastasis) within the body. The aggressiveness of tumor malignancy is classified using the Broders index on a scale of 1 to 4. A *grade 1* tumor indicates the most differentiation and best prognosis, whereas a *grade 4* indicates the least differentiation and poorest prognosis. Other classification systems are used to describe malignancies in different parts of the body; for example, Dukes A, B, and C are used to classify the extent of operable adenocarcinoma of the colon or rectum, and FIGO stages describe gynecologic malignancies, particularly carcinomas of the ovary. FIGO stages are expressed using Roman numerals with the word *stage.*

Although the evolution of a normal cell into a cancerous one is not understood fully, the genetic material deoxyribonucleic acid (DNA) of the cell holds the key. DNA contains genes (codes) that direct the production of new cells. During cell division, DNA replicates itself to pass the same genetic material to two new cells. This process is called *mitosis.* Sometimes during mitosis the process is disrupted because the DNA stops making the codes that allow cells to function normally. Instead, the cells begin to make new signals that cause them to move and invade adjacent tissue and *metastasize* or spread. These are malignant cells. As these malignant cells reproduce, the *mutations* (cell changes) are passed on to the new cells and the process is replicated over and over, leading to malignant growths.

Chemicals, drugs, radiation, and some viruses can cause DNA changes that lead to cancer. Heredity can also predispose a person to certain types of cancer. Although cancer occurs most frequently in older people, it can occur at any age and can affect any body tissue.

Each type of cancer requires a specific type of therapy. The four basic methods used to treat cancer are chemotherapy, surgery, radiation therapy, and biological therapy. At times a combination of these methods is used for the most effective treatment plan.

Chemotherapy employs drugs to treat cancer. Chemotherapeutic agents fall into five classifications: alkylating agents, antibiotics, antimetabolites, plant derivatives, and steroids. *Surgery* removes the cancerous tissue from the body through excision. *Radiation therapy* involves the use of radiation to the tumor tissue; high doses damage DNA. *Biological therapy* uses the body's own immune system to fight tumor cells.

As cancer research continues to be aggressively pursued, new treatment methods emerge. Some of the newer methods are therapies that use interferon, whole body hyperthermia, differentiation or maturation agents, intraoperative radiation, tumor necrosis factor (TNF), cloning, and monoclonal antibodies.

For additional information about cancer classifications, see one of the following references:

Iverson, C., Chair. *The AMA Manual of Style.* Philadelphia: Lippincott Williams & Wilkins; 1998:344–347.

Tessier, C. *The AAMT Book of Style for Medical Transcription.* Modesto, CA: American Association for Medical Transcription; 2002:48–52.

Critical Thinking Exercise

When dictating a discharge summary, the physician omitted the discharge date. What should you do?

Oncology Abbreviations

Adeno-Ca	adenocarcinoma
BMT	bone marrow transplantation
Bx	biopsy
CA	cancer
CEA	carcinoembryonic antigen
chem	chemotherapy
CMF	Cytoxan, methotrexate, 5-fluorouracil (combination chemotherapy)
CML	chronic myelogenous leukemia
CR	complete response
DES	diethylstilbestrol
DNA	deoxyribonucleic acid
ER	estrogen receptors
Ga	gallium
HD	Hodgkin's disease
HTLV	human T-cell leukemia-lymphoma virus
IL-2	interleukin-2
LAK	lymphokine-activated killer (cells)
mets	metastasis
NED	no evidence of disease
NHL	non-Hodgkin's lymphoma
NSCLC	non-small cell lung cancer
PR	partial remission
prot.	protocol
PSA	prostate-specific antigen
RNA	ribonucleic acid
TNF	tumor necrosis factor
TNM	tumor, node, metastasis
VIP	vasoactive intestinal peptides
XRT	radiation therapy

Oncology Terminology

a

adenoacanthoma (ah-de"-nō-ak"-an-thō'-muh) – an adenocarcinoma in which some of the cells exhibit squamous differentiation

adenocarcinoma (ah-dē"-nō-kar"-sih-nō'-muh) – a malignant new growth derived from glandular tissue or in which the tumor cells form recognizable glandular structures

adenomyosarcoma (ah-dē"-nō-mī"-ō-sar-kō'-muh) – a mixed mesodermal tumor in which striated muscle cells are one component

adjuvant therapy (ad'-joo-vent thār'-uh-pe) – the use of drugs (chemotherapy) along with surgery or radiation to attack cancer cells

alkylating agent (al'-kih-lāt"-ing ā'-jent) – a synthetic compound that disrupts the process of DNA synthesis

amelanotic melanoma (ā"-mel-uh-not'-ik mel"-uh-nō'-muh) – an unpigmented malignant melanoma

ameloblastoma (uh-mel"-ō-blas-tō'-muh) – a tumor of the jaw arising from enamel-forming cells

antimetabolites (an"-tī-meh-tab'-uh-lītz) – drugs used in cancer chemotherapy that block the formation of substances necessary to make DNA

apoptosis (ap"-op-tō'-sis) – disintegration of cells into membrane-bound particles that are then ingested by other cells; process may be important in limiting growth of tumors

astrocytoma (ass"-trō-sī-tō'-muh) – a tumor composed of astrocytes

b

basosquamous carcinoma (bā'-zōo skwā'-mus kar"-sih-nō'-muh) – carcinoma that histologically exhibits both basal and squamous elements

Brenner's tumor (bren'-erz too'-mur) – a benign fibroepithelioma of the ovary

bronchogenic carcinoma (brong-kō-jen'-ik kar"-sih-nō'-muh) – carcinoma originating in the bronchus

c

carcinoid (kar'-sih-noyd) – a yellow circumscribed tumor occurring in the small intestine, appendix, stomach, or colon

carcinoma in situ (kar"-sih-nō'-muh in sih'-tyoo) – a condition in which the tumor cells of a neoplastic entity still lie within the epithelium of origin, without invasion of the basement membrane

carcinosarcoma (kar"-sih-nō-sar-kō'-muh) – a malignant tumor composed of carcinomatous and sarcomatous tissues

cellular oncogenes (sel'-yoo-lur ong'-kō-jēnz) – broken or dislocated pieces of human DNA

chondroblastoma (kahn"-drō-blas-tō'-muh) – a benign neoplasm in which the cells resemble cartilage cells and the tumor appears to be cartilage

chondrosarcoma (kahn"-drō-sar-kō'-muh) – a malignant tumor derived from cartilage cells or their precursors

chordoma (kor-dō'-muh) – a rare tumor that occurs any place along the vertebral column

choriocarcinoma (ko"-rē-ō-kar"-sih-nō'-muh) – an extremely rare, very malignant neoplasm, usually of the uterus but sometimes at site of ectopic pregnancy

chronic myelogenous leukemia (krah'-nik mī"-eh-lah'-jeh-nus loo-kē-'mē-uh) – a malignant cancer of the bone marrow

cryosurgery (krī"-ō-sur'-jer-ē) – procedure that uses cold to freeze and destroy cancerous tissue; often used to treat brain and bladder tumors

cystocarcinoma (sis"-tō-kar"-sih-nō'-muh) – carcinoma associated with cysts

d

dermatofibrosarcoma protuberans (der"-muh-tō-fī"-brō-sar-kō'-muh prō-too'-ber-enz) – a fibrosarcoma of the skin

dysgerminoma (dis"-jer-mih-nō'-muh) – a malignant neoplasm of the ovary

e

en bloc resection (awn blahk' rē-sek'-shun) – process whereby a malignant tumor is removed along with a large area of surrounding tissue containing lymph nodes

ependymoma (eh-pen"-dī-mō'-muh) – a tumor arising from fetal inclusion of ependymal elements

epidermoid carcinoma (ep"-ih-der'-moyd) – carcinoma in which the cells tend to differentiate in the same way that the cells of the epidermis do

epithelioma (ep"-ih-thē"-lē-ō'-muh) – a malignant tumor, consisting mainly of epithelial cells, that originates in the epidermis of the skin or in a mucous membrane

Ewing's sarcoma (yoo'-ingz sar-kō'-muh) – a malignant tumor of the bone that always arises in medullary tissue, occurring more often in cylindrical bones; pain, fever, and leukocytosis are prominent symptoms

exenteration (eks-en"-ter-ā'-shun) – process of removing a tumor together with the organ from which it originated and all surrounding tissue in the body space

fibromatosis (fī"-brō-muh-tō'-sis) – the formation of a fibrous, tumor-like nodule arising from the deep fascia, with a tendency to local recurrence

glioblastoma multiforme (glī"-ō-blas-tō'-muh mul"-tih-for'-muh) – a neoplasm of the central nervous systems, especially the cerebrum, consisting of a variety of cellular types

glucagonoma (gloo'-kuh-guh-nō"-muh) – pancreatic tumor that is usually malignant

granulocytic leukemia (gran'-yoo-lō-sit"-ik loo-kē'-mē-uh) – myelocytic leukemia; leukemia arising from myeloid tissue in which the granular, polymorphonuclear leukocytes and their precursors predominate

hemangioblastoma (hē-man"-jē-ō-blas-tō'-muh) – a capillary hemangioma of the brain consisting of proliferated blood vessel cells or angioblasts

hemangiosarcoma (hē-man"-jē-ō-sar-kō'-muh) – a malignant tumor formed by proliferation of endothelial and fibroblastic tissue

hepatoblastoma (hep"-uh-tō-blas-tō'-muh) – a malignant intrahepatic tumor occurring in infants and young children and consisting chiefly of embryonic hepatic tissue

hepatocellular carcinoma (hep"-uh-tō-sel'-yoo-lur kar"-sih-nō'-muh) – a malignant tumor of the liver

hepatoma (hep"-uh-tō'-muh) – a tumor of the liver

Hodgkin's disease (hahj'-kinz dih-zēz') – a disease of unknown etiology producing enlargement of lymphoid tissue, spleen, and liver with invasion of other tissues

human T-cell leukemia-lymphoma virus (HTLV) (hyoo'-mun tē-sel loo-kē'-mē-uh-lim-fō'-muh vī'-rus) – the first virus known to cause cancer in humans

Hürthle cell tumor (her'-tel sel too'-mur) – a tumor of the thyroid and composed of Hurthle cells (large eosinophil-staining cells occasionally present in the thyroid gland)

immunotherapy (ih-myoo"-nō-thār'-uh-pē) – a type of therapy, currently being researched as a treatment for cancer, whereby the body's own immune system is stimulated

interferon (in"-ter-fēr'-on) – substance produced by lymphocytes that either directly blocks tumor growth or stimulates the immune system and other body defenses

interleukin (in"-ter-loo'-kin) – substance that stimulates the immune system to destroy tumors

islet cell carcinoma (ī'-let sel kar"-sih-nō'-muh) – a tumor of the islands of Langerhans; such tumors may result in hyperinsulinism

IsoMed (ī'-sō-med) – an implantable drug pump used to deliver chemotherapy directly to the liver; also used to deliver morphine sulfate

Kaposi's sarcoma (kap'-uh-sēz sar-kō'-muh) – a multifocal, metastasizing, malignant reticulosis with features resembling those of angiosarcoma, mainly involving the skin, most often on the toes or feet, as reddish blue or brownish soft nodules and tumors

Krukenberg's tumor (kroo'-ken-bergz too'-mur) – a special type of carcinoma of the ovary, usually metastatic from cancer of the gastrointestinal tract, especially of the stomach

leiomyosarcoma (lī"-ō-mī"-o-sar-kō'-muh) – a sarcoma containing large spindle cells of smooth muscle, most commonly of the uterus or retroperitoneal region

leukemia (loo-kē'-mē-uh) – cancer of blood-forming tissues

leukocytopenia (loo"-kō-sī"-tō-pē'-nē-uh) – leukopenia; a reduction of the number of leukocytes in the blood to a count of 5,000 or fewer

Leydig's cell tumor (lī'-digz sel too'-mur) – the most common nongerminal tumor of the testis, derived from the Leydig cells of the testis; such tumors are rarely malignant

liposarcoma (lip"-ō-sar-kō'-muh) – a malignant tumor derived from primitive or embryonal lipoblastic cells that exhibit varying degrees of lipoblastic and/or lipomatous differentiation

lymphangiography (lim-fan"-jē-ahg'-ruh-fē) – x-ray of the lymphatic vessels following the injection of a contrast medium

lymphangiosarcoma (lim-fan"-jē-ō-sar-kō'-muh) – a malignant tumor of lymphatic vessels, usually arising in a limb that is the site of chronic lymphedema

lymphosarcoma (lim"-fō-sar-kō'-muh) – a general term applied to malignant neoplastic disorders of lymphoid tissue, but not including Hodgkin's disease

malignant fibrous histiocytoma (muh-lig'-nent fī'-brus his"-tē-ō-sī-tō'-muh) – a malignant fibrous tumor-like nodule of the dermis

malignant schwannoma (muh-lig'-nent shwon-nō'-muh) – a malignant neoplasm of the white substance of Schwann (i.e., of a nerve sheath)

medulloblastoma (meh-dul"-ō-blas-tō'-muh) – a cerebellar tumor composed of undifferentiated neuroepithelial cells

melanoma (mel"-uh-nō'-muh) – a tumor made up of melanin-pigmented cells; when used alone, the term refers to malignant melanoma

meningioma (meh-nin"-jē-ō'-muh) – a hard, slow-growing, usually vascular tumor that originates in the arachnoidal tissue

mesenchymal tumor (mez-eng'-kī-mul too'-mur) – a tumor composed of tissue that resembles mesenchymal cells

mesenchymoma (mez"-eng-kī-mō'-muh) – a neoplasm containing a mixture of mesenchymal and fibrous tissue

mesonephroma (mez"-ō-neh-frō'-muh) – a relatively rare malignant tumor of the female genital tract, most often the ovary

mesothelioma (mez"-ō-thē"-lē-ō'-muh) – a tumor developed from mesothelial tissue

metastasis (meh-tass'-tuh-sis) – the process by which cancer spreads from a primary site to a secondary one

modality (mō-dal'-ih-tē) – method of treatment

morbidity (mōr-bid'-ih-tē) – the condition of being diseased or morbid

mucinous tumor (myoo'-sih-nus too'-mur) – a cyst (open space filled with fluid) containing thick, sticky fluid

multiple myeloma (mul'-tih-pul mī"-eh-lō'-muh) – a malignant tumor of bone marrow

mycosis fungoides (mi-kō'-sis fung-goy'-dēz) – a rare, chronic, malignant, lymphoreticular neoplasm of the skin and, in the late stages, the lymph nodes and viscera

myeloma (mī"-eh-lō'-muh) – a tumor originating in cells of the hematopoietic portion of bone marrow

myosarcoma (mī"-ō-sar-kō'-muh) – cancerous tumor of muscle tissue

n

nephroblastoma (neh"-frō-blas-tō'-muh) – a rapidly developing malignant mixed tumor of the kidneys, made up of embryonal elements (Wilms' tumor); usually affects children before the fifth year

neuroblastoma (nyoo"-rō-blas-tō'-muh) – sarcoma of nervous system origin, composed mainly of neuroblasts and affecting mostly infants and children up to 10 years of age

neuroepithelioma (nyoo"-rō-ep"-ih-thē"-lē-ō'-muh) – a relatively rare tumor of neuroepithelium in a nerve of special sense

neurofibromatosis (nyoo"-rō-fī"-brō-muh-tō'-sis) – a condition in which there are tumors of various sizes on peripheral nerves

o

oligodendroglioma (ol"-ih-gō-den"-drō-glī-ō'-muh) – a malignant tumor occurring mainly in the cerebrum, consisting mostly of neuroglial cells

oncogene (ong'-kō-jēn) – a piece of DNA that has the ability to cause a cell to become malignant

oncogenic (ong"-kō-jen'-ik) – giving rise to tumors, especially malignant tumors

osteoblastoma (ah"-stē-ō-blas-tō'-muh) – a benign, rather vascular tumor of bone characterized by the formation of osteoid tissue and primitive bone

osteogenic sarcoma (ah"-stē-ō-jen'-ik sar-kō'-muh) – a malignant primary tumor of bone composed of a malignant connective tissue stroma with evidence of malignant osteoid, bone, and/or cartilage formation

osteosarcoma (ahss"-tē-ō-sar-kō'-muh) – osteogenic sarcoma

p

Paget's disease (paj'-etz dih-zēz') – an inflammatory cancerous affection of the areola and nipple, usually associated with carcinoma of the lactiferous ducts and deeper structures of the breast; occurs mainly in middle-aged women

palliative (pal'-ē-uh-tiv) – refers to a form of treatment that relieves symptoms without curing

pancytopenia (pan"-sī-tō-pē'-nē-uh) – deficiency of all cell elements of the blood; aplastic anemia

peritoneoscopy (pār"-ih-tō"-nē-ahs'-kuh-pē) – examination of the peritoneal cavity by an instrument inserted through the abdominal wall

pheochromocytoma (fē-ō-krō"-mō-sī-tō'-muh) – a well-encapsulated, lobular, vascular tumor of chromaffin tissue of the adrenal medulla or sympathetic paraganglia

pinealoma (pin"-ē-ul-ō'-muh) – a tumor of the pineal body (glandlike structure in the brain), usually encapsulated

pituitary adenoma (pih-tyoo'-ih-tār"-ē ad"-eh-nō'-muh) – an adenoma of the pituitary gland

pleomorphic (plē"-ō-mōr'-fik) – occurring in various distinct forms

radiocurable tumor (rā"-dē-ō-kyoor'-uh-bul too'-mur) – a tumor that can be completely eliminated by radiation therapy; usually a tumor that has not metastasized

radioresistant tumor (rā"-dē-ō-rē-zis'-tent too'-mur) – a tumor that requires large doses of radiation to kill the malignant cells; the high doses of radiation may kill surrounding healthy cells

radiosensitive tumor (rā"-dē-ō-sen'-sih-tiv too'-mur) – a tumor in which radiation can kill cells without doing serious damage to surrounding healthy tissue

radiosensitizers (rā"-dē-ō-sen"-sih-tī'-zerz) – drugs that boost the sensitivity of tumors to x-rays

reticulosarcoma (reh-tik"-yoo-lō-sar-kō'-muh) – a cancerous tumor of the lymphatic system

retinoblastoma (ret"-ih-nō-blas-tō'-muh) – a cancerous tumor of the retina

rhabdomyoma (rab"-dō-mī-ō'-muh) – a striated muscular tissue tumor

rhabdomyosarcoma (rab"-dō-mī"-ō-sar-kō'-muh) – an extremely malignant neoplasm originating in skeletal muscle

sarcoma (sar-kō'-muh) – cancer arising from connective tissue such as muscle or bone; may affect the bones, bladder, kidneys, liver, lungs, parotids, and spleen

scirrhous carcinoma (skēr'-us kar"-sih-nō'-muh) – a form of cylindrical carcinoma with a firm, hard structure

seminoma (seh"-mih-nō'-muh) – a cancerous tumor of the testis

teratocarcinoma (teh"-rat-tō-kar"-sih-nō'-muh) – a carcinoma thought to originate from primordial germ cells or misplaced blastomeres; contains tissues from all three embryonic layers, such as bone, muscle, cartilage, nerve, tooth buds, and various glands

teratoma (tār"-uh-tō'-muh) – congenital tumor containing one or more of the three primary embryonic germ layers

villous adenoma (vil'-us ad"-eh-nō'-muh) – a large soft papillary polyp on the mucosa of the large intestine

VIPoma (vī-pō-muh) – vasoactive intestinal peptide-producing tumor; pancreatic endocrine tumor

xerostomia (zē"-rō-stō'-mē-uh) – condition of mouth dryness caused by chemotherapy or radiation therapy

Transcription Tips

When transcribing oncology reports, you should be familiar with relevant terminology, root words and/or combining forms, cancer classifications, and treatment procedures and chemotherapeutic drugs employed in treating cancer patients. This chapter includes a list of helpful Web sites to assist you in the transcription process.

The progress of cancer is described in grades or stages. When referring to stages, use roman numerals; with grades, use arabic numerals. The following terms are used to classify cancer in its different stages:

Broders' index – indexes the aggressiveness of cancer using different grades

CIN (cervical intraepithelial neoplasia) grade – used to indicate the progression of cervical cancer; indicated as from grades 1 to 3, with 3 being the most advanced

Clark level – delineates the level of invasion of primary malignant melanoma of the skin; goes from level I through level IV, with IV being the deepest penetration

Dukes classification – categorizes the degree of operable adenocarcinoma of the colon or rectum; uses A, B, C to classify

FAB (French-American-British) classification – utilizes "M" plus numerals 1–6 to classify morphology of acute nonlymphoid leukemia

FIGO (Federation Internationale de Gynecologie et Obstetrique) staging – uses "stage" with roman numerals to classify stages of gynecologic malignancy, particulary ovarian cancer

Gleason score – a system for grading the prognosis of prostate cancer; uses arabic numbers

Jewett classification – uses O, A, B, C, D to describe severity of bladder cancer

TNM classification – a system used for grading malignant tumors. A "T" plus an arabic numeral denotes the size or involvement of the tumor. An "N" plus a numeral indicates the extent of lymph node involvement; an "M" plus a numeral denotes the extent of metastasis

Roots and/or Combining Forms

Root	Meaning	Root	Meaning
adeno	gland	melan	black
alveolo	small sac	mucos	mucus
caco	bad	muta	genetic change
cancer	crab	mutageno	causing genetic change
carcino	cancer, cancerous	myco	fungus
cautero	burn, heat	myel	marrow
chemo	chemical, drug	onco	tumor
chondro	cartilage	papillo	nipple-like
cryo	cold	pharmaco	chemical, drug
cysto	sac of fluid	plaso	formation
cyt	cell	pleo	many, more
fibro	fiber	polypo	polyp
folliculo	small glandular sacs	rhabdo	rod
fungo	fungus, mushroom	sarco	flesh, connective tissue
immuno	safe	scirrho	hard
leio	smooth	semin	seed
lipo	fat	tox	poison
lympho	lymph	trism	grating
medullo	marrow, soft, inner part		

Surgical Procedures Used in Treatment of Cancer

biopsy – a piece of tissue is dissected surgically from the questionable area and sent to a pathology laboratory for diagnostic verification

curative surgery – removal of the primary site of malignancy and any lymph nodes to which the neoplasm has extended; such surgery may be all that is required to rid the patient of cancer

palliative surgery – surgery that attempts to relieve the complications of cancer (e.g., obstruction of the gastrointestinal tract or pain produced by tumor extension into surrounding nerves)

preventive or prophylactic surgery – removal of lesions which, if left in the body, are likely to develop into cancer

surgery combined with radiation, chemotherapy, or immunotherapy – combinations of treatment required to halt the spread of a malignancy

The American Cancer Society identifies the following five main categories of chemotherapy drugs used to fight cancer:

1. *Alkylating agents* – work directly on a cancer cell's DNA to prevent it from replicating; examples are melphalan and busulfan.
2. *Nitrosureas* – work to inhibit the enzymes that a cancer cell needs for DNA repair; examples are carmustine and lomustine.
3. *Antimetabolites* – interfere with a cancer cell's DNA and RNA; methotrexate and 5-fluorouracil are examples.
4. *Antitumor antibiotics* – interfere with a cancer cell's DNA and change its cellular membrane; examples are bleomycin and doxorubicin.
5. *Mitotic inhibitors* – plant alkaloids that restrain the enzymes needed for protein synthesis in cancer cells; docetaxel and vinorelbine are examples.

Typical chemotherapeutic drugs used in the treatment process appear on the following pages. You will note that the trade names are capitalized; generic names are not. For ease of reference, the drugs are listed alphabetically by trade name in Section I and then by generic name in Section II. Many times a combination of drugs is used; examples are given in Section III.

Chemotherapeutic Drugs—Section I			
Trade Names	**Generic Names**	**Trade Names**	**Generic Names**
5-FU	fluorouracil	Genasense	—
6-MP	mercaptopurine	Gleevec	imatinib mesylate
6-TG	thioguanine	GVAX	—
Actiq	fentanyl citrate	Herceptin	trastuzumab
Adriamycin	doxorubicin HCl	Hycamtin	topotecan HCl
Adrucil	fluorouracil	Hydrea	hydroxyurea
Alkeran	melphalan	Idamycin	idarubicin
ara-C	cytarabine	Ifex	ifosfamide
Aredia	pamidronate disodium	Intron A	interferon alfa-2b
Arimidex	anastrozole	Iressa	gefinitub
Aromasin	exemestane	Kytril	granisetron HCl
BCNU	carmustine	Leukeran	chlorambucil
Bexxar	iodine I 131 tositumomab	L-PAM	melphalan
BiCNU	carmustine	Lupron	leuprolide acetate
Blenoxane	bleomycin sulfate	Lysodren	mitotane
Busulfex	busulfan	Matulane	procarbazine HCl
C-225	cituximab	Magace	megestrol acetate
Campath	alemtuzumab	Mexate	methotrexate sodium
Camptosar	irinotecan HCl	Mithracin	plicamycin, mithramycin
CCNU	lomustine	MTX	methotrexate
CeeNU	lomustine	Mustargen	mecholorethamine HCl
Celebrex	celecoxib	Mutalane	procarbazine
Cerubidine	daunorubicin HCl	Mutamycin	mitomycin
Cosmegen	dactinomycin	Myleran	busulfan
CPT-11	irinotecan	Mylotarg	gemtuzumab ozogamicin
Cytadren	aminoglutethimide	Navelbine	vinorelbine tartrate
Cytosar-U, ara-C	cytarabine	Neosar	cyclophosphamide
Cytoxan	cyclophosphamide	Neovastat	—
Deca-Durabolin	nandrolone decanoate	Neumega	oprelvekin
Deltasone	prednisone	Neupogen	filgrastim
DepoCyt	cytarabine, liposomal	Nipent	pentostatin
Depo-Provera	medroxyprogesterone acetate	Nolvadex	tamoxifen citrate
		Novanrone	mitoxantrone HCl
Diflucan	fluconazole	Oncovin	vincristine sulfate
DTIC	dacarbazine	Ontak	denileukin diftitox
DTIC-Dome	dacarbazine	Paraplatin	carboplatin
Efudex	fluorouracil	Photofrin	porfimer sodium
Eldisine	vindesine sulfate	Platinol	cisplatin
Ellence	epirubicin HCl	Proleukin	aldesleukin
Elspan	asparaginase	Purinethol	mercaptopurine
Emcyt	estramustine phosphate sodium	Rituxan	rituximab
		Roferon-A	interferon alfa-2a
Ethyol	amifostine	Rubex	doxorubicin HCl
F-18	fludeoxyglucose	Sodren	mitotane
Femara	letrozole	Stilphostrol	diethylstilbestrol diphosphate
Fludara	fludarabine phosphate		
Fluorodeoxyuridine	gloxuridine	Tarceva	—
Folex PFS	methotrexate sodium	Targretin	bexarotene
FUDR	floxuridine	Taxol	paclitaxel
Gemzar	gemcitabine HCl	Taxotere	docetaxel

Chemotherapeutic Drugs—Section I			
Trade Names	**Generic Names**	**Trade Names**	**Generic Names**
Temodar	temozolomide	Virulizin	(investigative drug)
Tabloid	thioguanine	VP-15	etoposide
Thioplex	thiotepa	VP-16	etoposide
Trelstar Depot	triptorelin pamoate	Vumon	teniposide
Trisenox	arsenic trioxide	Wellcovorin	leucovorin calcium
Uvadex	methoxsaler	Xeloda	capecitabine
Valstar	valrubicin	Zanosar	streptozocin
Velban	vinblastine sulfate	Zinecard	dexrazoxane
VePesid	etoposide	Zofran	ondansetron HCl
Viadur	leuprolide acetate	Zoladex	goserelin acetate

Chemotherapeutic Drugs—Section II			
Trade Names	**Generic Names**	**Trade Names**	**Generic Names**
5-azacytosine	ara-AC	leuprolide	Lupron
6-MP (mercaptopurine)	Purinethol	levamisole	Ergamisol
altretamine	Hexalen	lomustine	CCNU, CeeNU
aminoglutethimide	Cytadren	mechlorethamine	Mustargen, nitrogen mustard
asparaginase	Elspar	medroxy progesterone acetate	Depo-Provera
bleomycin sulfate	Blenoxane	megestrol acetate	Megace
busulfan	Myleran	melphalan	Alkeran, L-PAM
capecitabine	Xeloda	mercaptopurine	Purinethol, 6-MP
carboplatin	Paraplatin	methotrexate oral	Rheumatrex
carmustine	BCNU, BiCNU	methotrexate sodium	Folex PFS, Mexate
chlorambucil	Leukeran	mitomycin	Mutamycin
cisplatin	Platinol	mitotane	Lysodren
cyclophosphamide	Cytoxan, Neosar	mitoxantrone	Novantrone
cytarabine	Cytosar-U, ara-C	paclitaxel	Taxol
dacarbazine	DTIC-Dome	pamidronate	Aredia
dactinomycin	Cosmegen, actinomycin D	pentostatin	Nipent
daunorubicin HCl	Cerubidine	plicamycin	Mithracin, Mithramycin
dexrazoxane	Zinecard	prednisone	Deltasone
docetaxel	Taxotere	procarbazine	Matulane
doxorubicin HCl	Adriamycin, Rubex	rituximab	Rituxan
estramustine phosphate sodium	Emcyt	somatostatin	—
etoposide	VP-16, VePesid	streptozocin	Zanosar
floxuridine	FUDR, fluorodeoxyuridine	tamoxifen	Nolvadex
fludarabine	Fludarax	tamoxifen citrate	Nolvadex
fluorouracil	5-FU, Adrucil	teniposide	Vumon
gemcitabine	Gemzar	thioguanine	6-TG, Thioguanine Tabloid
hydroxyurea	Hydrea	thiotepa	Thioplex
idarubicin	Idamycin	topotecan HCl	Hycamtin
ifosamide	Ifex	vinblastine sulfate	Velban
interferon	Intron-A, Roferon-A	vincristine sulfate	Oncovin
irinotecan	Camptosar, CPT-11	vindesine sulfate	Eldisine
leucovorin calcium	Wellcovorin	vinorelbine	Navelbine

Chemotherapeutic Drugs—Section III			
Trade Names	**Generic Names**	**Trade Names**	**Generic Names**
ABVD	MOPP	CVP	VBP
CHOP	MPL + PRED	CY-VA-DIC	VP-L-asparaginase
CMF	MTX + MP + CTX	FAC	
COPP	VAC	FAM	

Supportive Web Sites

http://cancer.med.upenn.edu/
Click on "Types of Cancer" or "Treatment Options" for helpful information; select other links of interest.

http://content.health.msn.com/
Search on "cancer" or "oncology" for other links of interest.

www.cancer.gov
Click on "Clinical Trials," "Developments," "Newly Approved Cancer Treatments," and other links of interest.

www.canceradvocacy.org/
Click on "Resources," then on "Glossary" for a list of terms.

www.cancerkids.org/
Use this site's Search function for any cancer-related term.

www.mtdesk.com/
For helpful information, select links of interest from the options provided across top of this page.

www.my.webmd.com/
Click on "Disease and Conditions," then on "Cancer" for topics of interest.

www.nlm.nih.gov/
Click on "Health Information," then "MEDLINEplus"; then search for "cancer" or "oncology." You can also search for "cancer drugs" or select the "Guide to Cancer Drugs" link and search by "generic or trade/brand name." Contains an extensive list of chemotherapy drugs.

www.oncology.com/
Select "Cancer Type" or other topic of interest.

www.scitalk.com/
Click on "Breast Cancer," then on "Medications" and/or "Web Sites" for more information on breast cancer.

www.wcn.org/
Under "Quick Links," click on "Cancer Types" or "Topics" for additional links of interest; select other links of interest on the home page.

Index of Oncology Reports

(see table of contents for audio information)

Exercise #	***Patient Name***	***Type of Report***
TE#1	Chiniche, Jin Joo	Op. Rep.—bone-marrow harvest
TE#2	Morales, Monee	Op. Rep.—peripheral blood stem cell transplantation
TE#3	Morris, Andrew	Op. Rep.—colonoscopy to the cecum
TE#4	McLemore, Susie	Op. Rep.—left subclavian Groshong catheter
TE#5	White, Bobby	Discharge Summary
TE#6	Black, Judy	Discharge Summary
TE#7	Smith, James	Discharge Summary
TE#8	Pritchett, Brenda	Op. Rep.—metastatic ovarian cancer
TE#9	Miller, Katherine	Consultation Report
TE#10	Bullock, Carl	Discharge Summary

CHAPTER 12

HEMATOLOGY/INFECTIOUS DISEASES

Introduction

The blood or hematopoietic system in humans consists of several interconnected components: the peripheral blood, the bone marrow, and the lymph-node system. The circulating blood, consisting of some 5 liters in a man (almost 10 percent less in a woman) comprises a fluid component (the *plasma*) and makes up some 55 percent of total blood volume. The plasma contains the three basic cell types: the *erythrocytes* (red cells), the *leukocytes* (white cells), and the *thrombocytes* (platelets).

The *erythrocytes* are largely concerned with oxygen transport; the *leukocytes* play various parts in defense against infection and tissue injury; and the *thrombocytes* are involved in maintaining the integrity of blood vessels and the prevention of blood loss by helping the blood to clot.

Blood serves three main purposes in the body:

1. Maintaining a constant environment for the other living tissues of the body.
2. Acting as a transport medium for hormones as they move from the sites of secretion (in glands) to distant body areas where they regulate growth, reproduction, and energy production.
3. Acting as the repository for proteins, white blood cells that fight infection, and platelets that assist in blood clotting.

An abnormal condition of the blood is called blood *dyscrasia* or disease. Diseases of red and white blood cells, bone marrow, and disorders of blood clotting are examples of blood dyscrasias. *Anemia, hemochromatosis,* and *polycythemia vera* are diseases of red blood cells. Diseases of white blood cells are *leukemia* and *granulocytosis.* Two disorders of blood clotting are *hemophilia* and *purpura.*

Lymph, the other main fluid in the body, does not circulate as does the blood. Lymph travels in one direction through lymph vessels, which drain into large veins of the circulatory system situated in the neck region. Although lymph does not contain erythrocytes or platelets, it does contain *lymphocytes* and *monocytes.*

Lymph capillaries, lymphatic vessels, lymphatic ducts, and lymph nodes form the lymphatic system. This system serves as a drainage medium to transport needed proteins and fluid that have leaked out of the blood capillaries back to the bloodstream via the veins. In addition, the lymphatic vessels absorb *lipids* (fats) from the small intestine and carry them to the bloodstream. The lymphatic system also assists the immune system in protecting the body by producing antibodies or by engulfing and destroying foreign matter.

Though they are not specific parts of the lymphatic system, the *spleen, tonsils,* and *thymus* are closely related to it by virtue of the functions they perform in the body. Of particular importance is the thymus, which manufactures infection-fighting *T cells.* These cells play a very important role in the body's immune response.

T-cell lymphocytes also form in stem cells in the bone marrow. After being processed in the thymus gland, they move to lymph nodes and lymphoid organs. Individuals who have fewer than 200 CD4+ T cells are classified as HIV-infected. *HIV* destroys T-cell helper lymphocytes and thereby affects the body's cell-mediated immune response. Thus, the infected person is vulnerable to infections such as *AIDS* and life-threatening malignancies.

Associated with AIDS are two particular malignancies: *Kaposi's sarcoma,* a cancer arising from the lining cells of capillaries, that produces bluish-red skin nodules (usually at first on the legs and feet); and *lymphoma* (cancer of the lymph nodes).

Because the HIV virus lowers resistance to bacteria and parasites that are easily contained by normal defenses, *opportunistic infections* occur easily. Examples of these infections are candidiasis, herpes simplex, Pneumocystis carinii pneumonia, and toxoplasmosis.

A practicing hematologist or hematological physician spends a great deal of time treating patients suffering from blood malignancies. When people think of blood cancers, they automatically think of acute leukemia, and most regard acute leukemia as being most common in children. In fact, the most common form of blood tumor is lymph-node cancer (*Hodgkin's disease* and *non-Hodgkin's lymphoma*), which accounts for some 200–250 cases out of a caseload of 500. Acute leukemia will account for some 100–120 cases, only one-fifth of which will occur in children below the age of 15. Contrary to popular opinion, most acute leukemia occurs in individuals over the age of 50. Four to six percent of blood cancers occur in children under age 15.

Critical Thinking Exercise

You have just completed transcribing a death summary on an old high-school classmate who died of AIDS. When you attend the class reunion a week later, you are approached by several classmates who ask you whether it is true that Robin died of AIDS. (They know you work in a position where you have access to such information.)

How would you respond to their question?

Hematology/Infectious Diseases Abbreviations

AIDS	acquired immunodeficiency syndrome
AHF	antihemophilic factor
ALL	acute lymphocytic leukemia
AML	acute myelogenous leukemia
ARC	AIDS-related complex
BAC	blood-alcohol concentration
baso	basophils
BMT	bone-marrow transplant
CBC	complete blood count
CFS	chronic fatigue syndrome
CLL	chronic lymphocytic leukemia
CML	chronic myelogenous (myelocytic) leukemia
CMV	cytomegalovirus
diff	differential (count)
EBV	Epstein-Barr virus
ELISA	enzyme-linked immunosorbent assay (AIDS test)
eos	eosinophil(s)
ESR	erythrocyte sedimentation rate
Hct	hematocrit
Hgb, Hg	hemoglobin
HIV	human immunodeficiency virus
Hp	haptoglobin
IgA, IgD IgE, IgG IgM	immunoglobulins
LGV	lymphogranuloma venereum
lymphs	lymphocytes
MCH	mean corpuscular hemoglobin—average amount of hemoglobin per cell
MCHC	mean corpuscular hemoglobin concentration—average concentration of hemoglobin in a single red cell
MCV	mean corpuscular volume—average volume or size of a single red blood cell
mono	monocyte
PCP	Pneumocystis carinii pneumonia
PCV	packed cell volume
PMN, PMNL	polymorphonuclear neutrophil
poly	polymorphonuclear leukocyte
PT	prothrombin time
PTT	partial thromboplastin time
RBC	red blood cell (red blood cell count)
Rh	Rhesus (factor)
RIA	radioimmunoassay
RMSF	Rocky Mountain spotted fever
sed rate	erythrocyte sedimentation rate
segs	segmented, mature white blood cells
WBC	white blood cell (white blood cell count)

Anatomic Illustrations

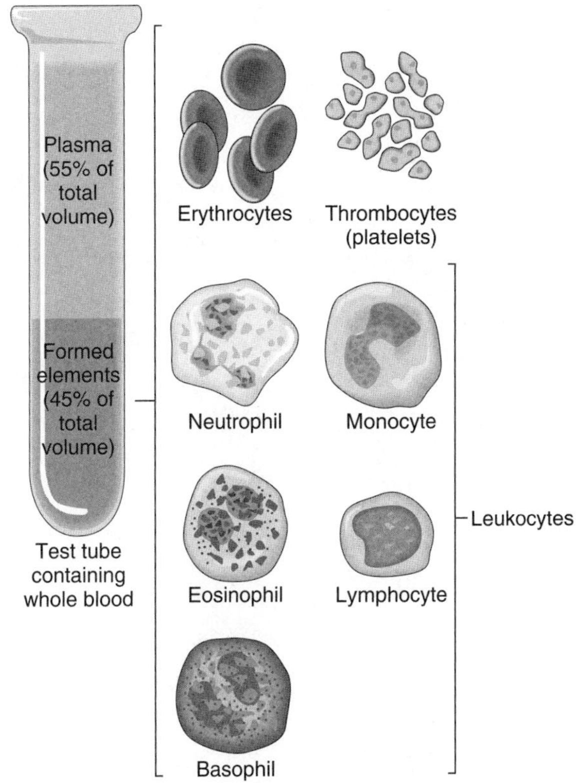

12–1 THE FORMED ELEMENTS IN BLOOD

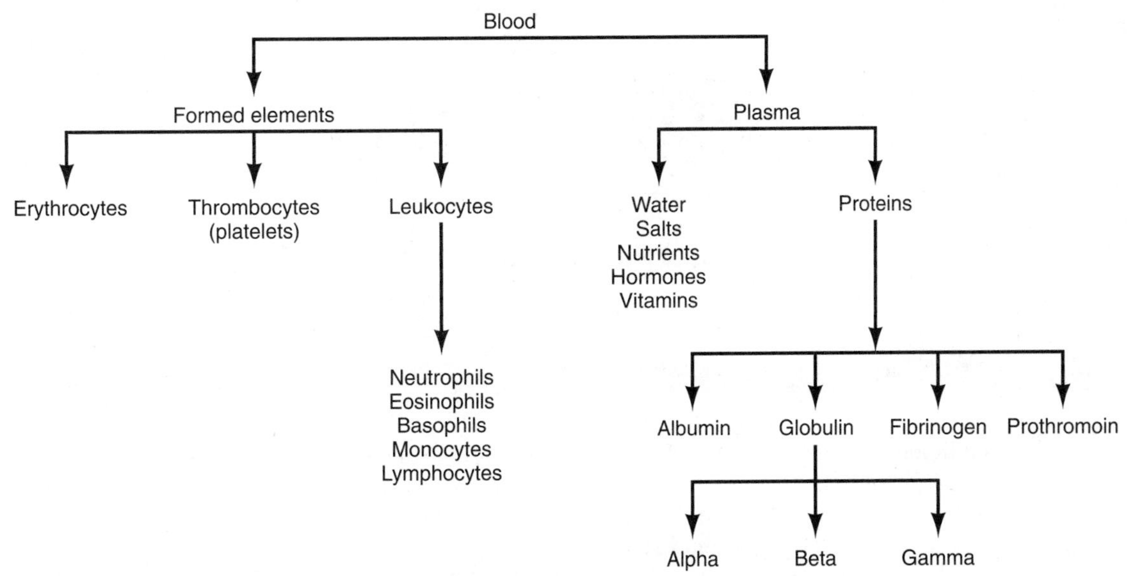

12–2 COMPOSITION OF BLOOD. (REPRINTED FROM CHABNER DE, THE LANGUAGE OF MEDICINE, 5TH ED. PHILADELPHIA: W. B. SAUNDERS COMPANY, P. 436; COPYRIGHT (C) 1996, WITH PERMISSION FROM ELSEVIER SCIENCE.)

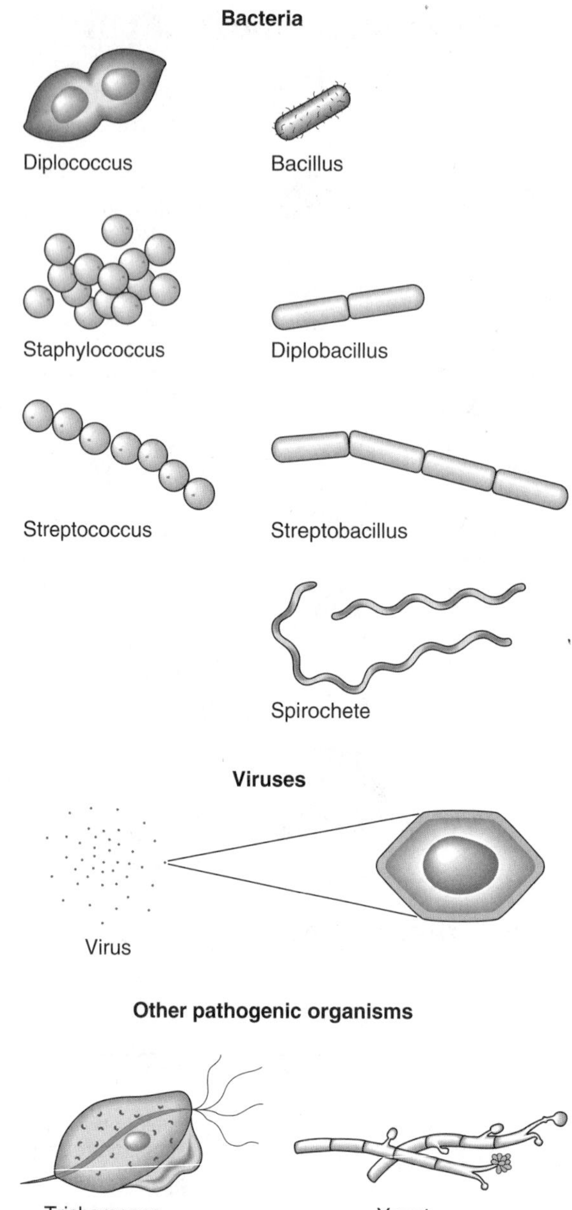

12–3 DISEASE-PRODUCING MICROORGANISMS

Hematology/Infectious Diseases Terminology

a

acquired immunodeficiency syndrome (AIDS) (uh-kwī'-urd ih"-myoo-nō-dē-fish'-en-sē sin'-drōm, ādz) – condition resulting from suppression or deficiency of the immune response, caused by exposure to HIV

agglutination (uh-gloo"-tih-nā'-shun) – the clumping of blood when incompatible blood types are mixed; is fatal to the recipient because it stops the flow of blood

albumin (serum albumin) (al-byoo'-min) – a protein found in blood that maintains the proper amount of water in the blood

anaphylaxis (an"-uh-fih-lak'-sis) – an exaggerated or unusual hypersensitivity to foreign protein or other substances

anemia (uh-nē'-mē-uh) – a deficiency in erythrocytes or hemoglobin; the five types are aplastic, hemolytic, pernicious, sickle cell, and thalassemia

antigens (an'-tih-jens) – foreign materials that cause the production of an antibody

antihemorrhagic (an"-tī-hēm"-ō-raj'-ik) – preventing or stopping hemorrhage

apheresis (af"-er-ē'-sis) – a procedure where blood is separated into its parts

aplastic anemia (ā-plass'-tik uh-nē'-mē-uh) – occurs when blood cell production fails due to lack of formation of bone marrow cells

b

B cells – lymphocytes that change into plasma cells and secrete antibodies

basophil (ba'-zō-fil) – a type of white blood cell containing coarse granules that stain readily with basic dyes

c

CD4+ lymphocytes (sē-dē-fōr-pluhs lim'-fō-sītz) – helper T cells that carry the CD4+ protein antigen on their surface; HIV binds to CD4+ and infects and kills T cells bearing this protein

creatinemia (krē"-ah-tih-nē'-mē-uh) – an excess of creatine in circulating blood

cytomegalovirus (sī"-tō-meg"-uh-lō-vī'-rus) – one member of a group of large herpes-type viruses that can cause many diseases in persons with impaired immunity

cytotoxic cells (sī"-tō-tok'-sik selz) – killer cells (T cells) that promptly kill foreign cells; also called T8 cells

d

dengue (dāng'-ā) – a severe, potentially fatal infection that causes hemorrhagic fever and occurs when someone with immunity to one type of dengue virus is infected by another, different type; spread by certain mosquitoes

e

Ebola virus hemorrhagic fever (ē-bō'-luh vī'-rus hēm"-ō-raj'-ik fē'-vur) – a severe, frequently fatal disease transmitted to humans by infected animals and animal materials

electrophoresis (ē-lek"-trō-fō-rē'-sis) – the method of separating substances by electrical charge

enzyme-linked immunosorbent assay (ELISA) (en'-zīm-lingkt ih"-myoo-nō-sor'-bunt as'-ā, eh-lē'-suh) – test used to screen blood for the antibody to the AIDS virus; because false-positive results can occur with this test, a backup test (Western blot) is used to confirm positive findings

eosinophil (ē"-ō-sin'-ō-fil) – a granular leukocyte that stains readily with the acid stain eosin

erythroblast (ē-rith'-rō-blast) – an immature red blood cell

erythrocytosis (ē-rith"-rō-sī-tō'-sis) – an abnormal condition in which there is an increase in red blood cells

erythropathy (er"-ih-throp'-uh-thē) – disease of the red blood cells

erythropenia (ē-rith"-rō-pē'-nē-uh) – deficiency in the number of red blood cells

erythropoiesis (ē-rith"-rō-poy-ē'-sis) – the formation of red blood cells

erythropoietin (ē-rith"-rō-poy'-eh-tin) – hormone secreted by the kidney that stimulates production of erythrocytes

f

fibrin (fī'-brin) – threads of protein that form the basis of a blood clot

g

giardiasis (jī"-ar-dī'-uh-sis) – a diarrheal illness caused by the organism Giardia intestinalis (also known as Giardia lamblia)

gonorrhea (gah"-nō-rē'-uh) – one of the most common infectious bacterial diseases caused by the bacterium Neisseria gonorrhoeae; transmitted most frequently through sexual intercourse

granulocytosis (gran"-yoo-lō-sī-tō'-sis) – occurs when there is an abnormal increase in granulocytes in the blood, which may result from infection or inflammation of any type

h

helper cells – T cells that aid B cells in recognizing antigens and stimulating antibody production; also called T4 cells

hematogenous (hem"-uh-tahj'-eh-nus) – produced by or derived from the blood; disseminated by circulation or through the bloodstream

hemocytoblasts (stem cells) (hē"-mō-sī'-tō-blasts, stem selz) – immature cells

hemoglobin test (hē"-mō-glō'-bin tehst) – measures the total amount of hemoglobin in a sample of peripheral blood

hemolysis (hē-mol'-ih-sis) – the destruction of red blood cells

hemolytic anemia (hē"-mō-lit'-ik uh-nē'-mē-uh) – occurs when red cells are reduced due to excessive destruction

hemophilia (hē"-mō-fil'-ē-uh) – condition of excessive bleeding caused by a congenital lack of one of the protein substances (factor VIII) necessary for blood clotting

hepatitis A (hep"-uh-tī'-tis ā) – inflammation of the liver caused by the hepatitis A virus

herpes labialis (her'-pēz lā"-bē-al'-ihs) – infection caused by the herpes simplex virus; results in painful blisters (called *cold sores* or *fever blisters*) on the skin of the lips, mouth, gums, or skin around the mouth

human immunodeficiency virus (HIV) (hyoo'-mun ih"-myoo-nō-dē-fish'-en-sē dih-zēz') – the virus (retrovirus) that causes AIDS

humoral immunity (hyoo'-mur-ul ih-myoo'-nih-tē) – an immune response in which B cells change into plasma cells and secrete antibodies

hypercapnia (hī"-per-kap'-nē-uh) – an increased amount of carbon dioxide in the blood

hyperlipemia (hī"-per-lih-pē'-mē-uh) – an excessive quantity of fat in the blood

hypersplenism (hī"-per-splen'-izm) – a syndrome characterized by enlargement of the spleen

iatrogenic (ī"-at-rō-jen'-ik) – any adverse mental or physical condition induced in a patient by the effects of treatment by a physician or surgeon

immunoglobulins (ih"-myoo-nō-glob'-yoo-linz) – specific types of gamma globulin that are capable of acting as antibodies; examples are IgG (found in high concentration in the plasma) and IgA (found in breast milk, saliva, tears, and respiratory mucus); other immunoglobulins are AgM, IgD, and IgE

interferons (in"-ter-fēr'-ahnz) – antiviral proteins secreted by T cells; they also stimulate macrophages to consume bacteria

interleukins (in"-ter-loo'-kinz) – proteins that stimulate the growth of T-cell lymphocytes and activate immune responses

killer cells – T cells that envelop foreign cells, tumor cells, and bacteria; also called T8 cells

leukemia (loo-kē'-mē-uh) – disease of the bone marrow in which there is an excessive increase in cancerous white blood cells; four types are acute myelogenous (myelocytic), acute lymphocytic, chronic myelogenous (myelocytic), and chronic lymphocytic

leukocytopenia (loo"-kō-sī"-tō-pē'-nē-uh) – an abnormal decrease in leukocytes

listeriosis (lis-tēr"-ē-ō'-sis) – serious infection caused by eating food contaminated with the bacterium Listeria monocytogenes

lymphadenitis (lim-fad"-eh-nī'-tis) – inflammation of one or more lymph nodes

lymphadenopathy (lim-fad"-eh-nop'-uh-thē) – disease of the lymph nodes

lymphadenotomy (lim-fad"-eh-not'-uh-mē) – surgical incision into a lymph node

lymphangiogram (lim-fan"-jē-ō-gram) – test in which contrast medium is injected into lymph vessels in the foot, and x-rays are taken to show the path of lymph flow as it moves into the chest region; often used in the staging and diagnosis of lymphoma

lymphangiology (lim-fan"-jē-ol'-uh-jē) – the study of the lymphatic system

lymphocytopenia (lim"-fō-sī"-tō-pē'-nē-uh) – condition of fewer than normal lymphocytes in the blood

lymphogranuloma venereum (lim"-fō-gran"-yoo-lō'-muh veh-nēr'-ē-um) – a sexually transmitted disease caused by the bacteria Chlamydia trachomatis

lymphoid organs (lim'-foyd or'-gunz) – lymph nodes, spleen, and thymus gland

lymphopoiesis (lim"-fō-poy-ē'-sis) – the formation of lymphocytes or of lymphoid tissue

macrophages (mak'-rō-fā-jez) – cells in the spleen, liver, and bone marrow that destroy worn-out erythrocytes

mediastinal nodes (mē"-dē-uh-stī'-nul nōdz) – lymph nodes in the area between the lungs in the thoracic cavity

megakaryocytes (meg"-uh-kār'-ē-ō-sītz) – giant cells from which platelets, or thrombocytes, are formed in the red bone marrow

meningitis (men"-in-jī'-tis) – an infection that causes inflammation of the membranes covering the brain and spinal cord

mononucleosis (mahn"-ō-noo"-klē-ō'-sis) – an acute infectious disease that results in enlarged lymph nodes and increased numbers of lymphocytes and monocytes in the bloodstream; caused by the Epstein-Barr virus (EBV)

opportunistic infection (op"-ur-too-nis'-tik in-fek'-shun) – an infectious disease associated with AIDS; examples are candidiasis, herpes simplex, Pneumocystis carinii pneumonia, and toxoplasmosis

pernicious anemia (per-nish'-us uh-nē'-mē-uh) – develops when there is an insufficient number of mature erythrocytes; caused by an inability to absorb vitamin B12 into the body

phagocytosis (fag"-ō-sī-tō'-sis) – the process that occurs when phagocytes ingest and digest bacteria and particles

plasmapheresis (plaz"-muh-fer-ē'-sis) – the process of removing blood from the body and separating the cellular elements from the plasma by centrifuge

Pneumocystis carinii pneumonia (pneumocystis) (noo"-mō-sis'-tis kah-rin'-ē-ī noo-mō'-nē-uh) – a kind of pneumonia caused by the Pneumocystis carinii germ; the most common serious infection in persons with advanced HIV disease and AIDs

polycythemia vera (pahl"-ē-sih-thē'-mē-uh vē'-ruh) – refers to a general increase in the number of red blood cells

reticulocyte (reh-tik'-yoo-lō-sīt) – a developing red blood cell

retrovirus (reh'-trō-vī"-rus) – an RNA virus that makes copies of itself by using the host cell's DNA; this is in reverse (retro) fashion because the regular method is for DNA to copy itself onto RNA; a retrovirus like HIV carries an enzyme called reverse transcriptase that enables it to reproduce within the host cell

Reye's syndrome (rīz sin'-drōm) – a rare, sometimes fatal, disease of the brain that is accompanied by degeneration of the liver; occurs in children after acute viral infections such as chickenpox or an influenza-type illness; also associated with taking medications containing aspirin during the illness

Rh factor – antigen normally located on the surface of red blood cells of Rh-positive individuals

serodiagnosis (sē"-rō-dī"-ug-nō'-sis) – diagnosis made by observing the reactions of blood serum

shingles (shing'-gulz) – a painful illness caused by the varicella-zoster virus (the same virus that causes chickenpox)

sickle-cell anemia (sik'-ul sel uh-nē'-mē-uh) – a hereditary condition characterized by a crescent or sickle shape of erythrocytes caused by an abnormal type of hemoglobin in the red cell; occurs more frequently in people of African or African-American ancestry

sideropenia (sid"-er-ō-pē'-nē-uh) – a lack of iron in the blood

splenemia (splē-nē'-mē-uh) – condition in which the spleen is clogged with blood

suppressor cells (suh-pres'-er selz) – T-cell lymphocytes that inhibit the activity of B-cell lymphocytes

thalassemia (thal"-ah-sē'-mē-uh) – an inherited defect in the ability to produce hemoglobin; occurs most frequently in persons of Mediterranean background

thrombocyte (syn. platelet) (throm'-bō-sīt, plāt'-let) – clotting cell

thrombogenic (throm"-bō-jen'-ik) – formation of a blood clot

thrombolysis (throm-bahl'-ih-sis) – destruction of a blood clot

thromboplastin (throm"-bō-plas'-tin) – a protein released at the site of an injury when platelets clump; helps promote the formation of a fibrin clot

thymectomy (thī-mek'-tuh-mē) – surgical removal of the thymus gland

TruGene test (troo'-jēn test) – first FDA-approved test for analyzing genetic weaknesses in a patient's strain of HIV; assists physicians in choosing AIDS drugs that are likely to work best against the virus in that patient

Wegener's granulomatosis (veg'-nerz gran"-yoo-lo"-muh-tō'-sis) – an uncommon disease characterized by inflammation of the blood vessels (vasculitis)

Western blot (wes'-turn blaht) – a test used to detect the presence of HIV in serum

zidovudine (AVD) (zih-dō'-vuh-dēn) – a drug used to treat AIDS; originally called AZT

Transcription Tips

Transcribing dictation dealing with hematology and infectious diseases can be challenging. However, if you are familiar with diseases of red and white blood cells, infectious disease terminology, lab and diagnostic tests, infection-causing microorganisms, and potential biological and chemical weapons, your task will be easier.

diseases of red blood cells – anemia and its types—aplastic, pancytopenia, hemolytic, pernicious, and sickle-cell

diseases of white blood cells – leukemia (acute myelogenous, acute lymphocytic, chronic myelogenous, and chronic lymphocytic) and granulocytosis

Terms Relating to Infectious Diseases

carrier – an apparently well person in whom pathogenic microorganisms live and multiply without apparent ill effect and who can disseminate disease to others

communicable disease – an illness caused by a specific infectious agent or its toxic products that is transmitted directly or indirectly from an infected person or animal to a susceptible host

contamination – the presence of pathogenic microorganisms on a body or inanimate objects

endemic – a disease or infectious agent that is continuously present in a community, or the usual amount of the disease

epidemic – a temporary and significant increase in the incidence of a disease above what is normally expected in a given time

infection – the entry and multiplication of an infectious agent in the body of humans or animals

infectious agent – a parasite capable of producing infection

nosocomial infection – an infection or infectious disease that is contracted within the hospital or other institution

pathogens – microorganisms capable of producing disease under favorable conditions

parasites – microorganisms living on or in the bodies of other living organisms

saprophytes – microorganisms living on dead or decaying organic matter

sepsis – a pathologic state resulting from the presence of microorganisms or their poisonous products in the bloodstream

sporadic – the occasional occurrence of a disease at a low level of incidence

toxins – poisonous materials produced by bacteria

Diagnostic and Laboratory Tests

antiglobulin test (Coombs test) – test performed to demonstrate whether the patient's erythrocytes are coated with antibody; used to determine the presence of antibodies in infants of Rh-negative women

antinuclear antibodies (ANA) – blood test to identify antigen-antibody reactions

bleeding time – test that is performed by puncturing either the earlobe or the forearm to determine the time required for blood to stop flowing

blood typing – blood test to determine an individual's blood type and Rh factor

bone marrow aspiration – test for aplastic anemia, leukemia, certain cancers, and polycythemia; performed by removing bone marrow

coagulation time – test conducted to determine the time required for venous blood to clot in a test tube; normally less than 15 minutes

complete blood count (CBC) – blood test that yields a hematocrit, hemoglobin, red and white blood cell count, and differential

erythrocyte sedimentation rate (ESR) – blood test to determine the rate at which RBCs settle in a long, narrow tube; the distance the RBCs settle in 1 hour is the rate

hematocrit (Hct) – blood test performed on whole blood to determine the percentage of red blood cells in the total blood volume

hemoglobin (Hb, Hgb) – blood test to determine the amount of iron-containing pigment of the RBCs

partial thromboplastin time (PTT) – test performed on blood plasma to determine how long it takes for fibrin clots to form

platelet count – test performed on whole blood to determine the number of thrombocytes present

prothrombin time (PT) – test performed on blood plasma to determine the time needed for oxalated plasma to clot

red blood cell morphology – test performed to determine the shape or form of individual red cells; useful in diagnosing sickle-cell anemia

red blood count (RBC) – test performed on whole blood to determine the number of erythrocytes present

Western blot – test used to detect the presence of HIV in serum

white blood cell differential – blood test used to determine the number of different types of leukocytes (immature and mature forms)

white blood count (WBC) – blood test to determine the number of leukocytes present; an increase in the WBCs indicates infection and/or inflammation; a decrease in WBCs indicates aplastic anemia, pernicious anemia, or malaria

Microorganisms That Cause Infection

Microorganism	Species	Microorganism	Species
Clostridium	C. botulinum		N. meningitidis
	C. histolyticum	Proteus	P. vulgaris
	C. novyi	Pseudomonas	P. aeruginosa
	C. perfringens	Salmonella	S. typhosa
	C. septicum	Staphylococcus	S. aureus
	C. sporogenes		S. epidermidis
	C. tetani	Streptococcus	S. pneumoniae
Escherichia	E. coli	Viruses	
Mycobacterium	M. tuberculosis		
Neisseria	N. catarrhalis		
	N. gonorrhoeae		

Potential Biological Weapons

anthrax – a bacterium that is contracted through the skin, by inhalation, or by eating infected meat; produces a toxin that can be fatal

botulism – a rare but serious paralytic illness caused by a nerve toxin produced by the bacterium Clostridium botulinum

Ebola – a filovirus that is usually fatal; causes fever, chills, headaches, muscle aches, loss of appetite, vomiting, bloody diarrhea, abdominal pain, sore throat, and chest; blood fails to clot and patients bleed from every orifice

plague – highly infectious disease caused by the bacterium Yersinia pestis; transmitted by flea bites or by eating contaminated animal tissue; types are bubonic, pneumonic, and septicemic (most deadly)

ricin – poison derived from castor bean plants; can be turned into an aerosol and released; can be inhaled or ingested from poisoned food or contaminated water supply

smallpox – highly contagious viral disease that spreads and kills very quickly

tularemia – acute, plague-like infectious disease; transmitted by insect bites, eating undercooked meat from an infected animal, or drinking contaminated water

viral hemorrhagic fevers (VHFs) – a severe, multisystem syndrome caused by several families of viruses; affects multiple organ body systems; overall vascular system is damaged and body's regulatory ability is damaged

Potential Chemical Weapons

chlorine – greenish-yellow, odorous gas that has a choking smell and is very poisonous; destroys cells that line the respiratory tract

hydrogen cyanide – colorless gas or pale blue liquid that blocks oxygen from reaching the blood; irritates and burns the skin and eyes; high exposure can cause sudden death

mustard gas – yellow to brown gas that smells like garlic; potentially deadly agent that attacks the skin and eyes; causes severe blisters and, if inhaled, can damage lungs and other organs; may cause death by respiratory failure

phosgene – colorless gas that causes the lungs to fill with water, resulting in choking and suffocation

sarin – highly toxic nerve gas that affects the signaling mechanism by which nerve cells communicate; causes death by suffocation

VX – a nerve agent that works like sarin but is more toxic; one milligram on the skin will kill a person

Supportive Web Sites

www.aidsinfonet.org/
Click on "Index of Fact Sheets" or "Internet Bookmarks on AIDS" for helpful links.

www.cdc.gov/
Under "Contents," click on "Health Topics A-Z," then on links of interest.

http://familydoctor.org/
Under "Common Conditions," select topic of interest.

http://methodisthealth.com/
Under "Choose a Health Topic," choose "Infectious diseases" or another topic of interest.

http://my.webmd.com/
From the home page, do a search for "HIV Vaccine Glossary"; click on "HIV Vaccine Glossary"; this will lead to a site with an extensive list of terms.
Click on "Diseases and Conditions"; under the "All conditions" link, select "HIV/AIDS" for helpful sites.
Under "Medical Info," click on "Medical Library"; under "Health Guide A-Z," select "Health Topics," then click on a letter ("H" for information on HIV, for example).

www.nlm.nih.gov/
Under "Health Information," select "MEDLINEplus," then search for "hematology" and for "infectious diseases" for links of interest.
Also on the "MEDLINEplus" page, you can select "Health Topics" for links to other topics.

www.who.int/
Click on "Health Topics" and select links of interest.

Index of Hematology/Infectious Diseases Reports

(see table of contents for audio information)

Exercise #	Patient Name	Report/Procedure
✓ TE#1 6/12	Puckett, Marjorie	H&P (HIV)
✓ TE#2 13	Puckett, Marjorie	DS—pneumonia, HIV
✓ TE#3 14	Seymour, Matthew	Death Summary (Leukemia)
✓ TE#4 15	Utter, Matthew	H&P—AIDS
✓ TE#5 16	Flowers, Betty	DS—thrombocytopenic purpura
✓ TE#6 17	Ryder, Claude	DS—sickle cell/thalassemia

CHAPTER 13

NEUROLOGY/ NEUROSURGERY

Introduction

Neurology, neurosurgery, and *neuroradiology* are the medical specialties concerned with diagnosis and treatment of disorders of the brain, spinal cord, and peripheral nerves. The nervous system, which comprises the complicated communication network of the body, is the mechanism for the exchange of messages between the brain and more than 10 billion nerve cells. This interaction is what makes a human body into an intelligent, functioning individual.

Anatomically and functionally, the *nervous system* is divided into the brain, spinal cord, and nerves. The *brain* (encephalon) and the *spinal cord* (medulla spinalis) make up the *central nervous system (CNS).* The *peripheral nervous system (PNS)* is composed of a series of nerves that extend from the central nervous system to all portions of the body; the PNS coordinates all other body systems so that they work together as a unit.

Neurologists diagnose and treat diseases affecting the brain, spinal cord, peripheral nerves, and muscles. Disordered thought processes or emotions are treated by psychiatrists, although the two specialties overlap, particularly in relation to dementia or psychosomatic symptoms.

Contemporary neurologists interact closely with related specialists. Neurosurgeons treat tumors and subarachnoid hemorrhages; neuroradiologists image structural diseases of the brain and spinal cord; neurophysiologists investigate seizures using electroencephalography and diseases of nerve and muscle using nerve conduction studies and electromyography.

Headaches, strokes, epilepsy, Parkinson's disease, multiple sclerosis, and *sleep disorders* are common disorders treated by the neurologist. Neurological disorders may be caused by organic injury, congenital defects, or diseases such as infections. Diagnosis in neurology is founded on clinical principles, attending closely to the patient's history and to careful physical examination.

The related specialty of neurosurgery treats the surgical aspects of nervous system disease and disorder. Diskectomy, spinal fusion, and craniotomy for tumor or trauma are the procedures most commonly performed by neurosurgeons.

Neuroradiology is a developing area of expertise that uses various procedures to diagnose neurological abnormalities. Interventional radiologists also treat abnormalities. X-ray, ultrasound, nuclear studies, and magnetic resonance imaging are utilized to diagnose neurological disorders. As technology advances, other subspecialties will inevitably arise.

Critical Thinking Exercise

You are speaking to a medical transcription class, and a student asks what purpose a medical record serves.

What is your response?

Neurology/Neurosurgery Abbreviations

ACH	acetylcholine
AD	Alzheimer's disease
AJ	ankle jerk
ALS	amyotrophic lateral sclerosis
ANS	autonomic nervous system
APLD	automated percutaneous lumbar diskectomy
AVMs	arteriovenous malformations

BAER	brainstem auditory evoked response
BPV	benign positional vertigo
C	cervical
CAE	carotid artery endarterectomy
CAT	computerized axial tomography
CBS	chronic brain syndrome
CMG	cystometrogram
CNS	central nervous system
Co	cobalt
CP	cerebral palsy
CPAP	continuous positive airway pressure
CSF	cerebrospinal fluid
CVA	cerebrovascular accident
CVP	central venous pressure
DBS	deep brain stimulation
DCS	dorsal cord stimulation
DICOM	Digital Imaging and Communications in Medicine (teleradiology)
DT	delirium tremens
DTP	distal tingling on percussion
DTR	deep tendon reflexes
DV2	distribution
ECF	extended care facility
EEG	electroencephalogram
EMG	electromyogram
ENG	electronystagmograph
EST	electric shock therapy
FDA	frontodextra anterior
FS	frozen section
GBM	glioblastoma multiforme
GBS	Guillain-Barré syndrome
GCS	Glasgow Coma Scale
GSW	gunshot wound
GTCS	generalized tonic-clonic seizure; grand mal seizure
HA	headache
HDS	herniated disk syndrome
HNP	herniated nucleus pulposus
ICP	intracranial pressure
IFV	isolated fourth ventricle
IGS	image-guided surgery
IMV	intermittent mandatory ventilation
IVC	intraventricular catheter
KJ	knee jerk
L	lumbar
LGB	Landry-Guillain-Barré (syndrome)
LOA	left occiput anterior
LOP	left occiput posterior
LP	lumbar puncture
MD	muscular dystrophy
MEG	magnetoencephalography
MMSE	mini mental status exam
MR	mental retardation
MRA	magnetic resonance arteriogram
MRI	magnetic resonance imaging
MS	multiple sclerosis
MSI	magnetic source imaging
MSLT	mean (or multiple) sleep latency test
MVA	motor vehicle accident
MVV	maximal voluntary ventilation
NCV	nerve conduction velocity
NF	neurofibroma
NIHSS	National Institute of Health Stroke Scale
N.S.	neurosurgery
OBS	organic brain syndrome
OKN	opticokinetic nystagmus
PDD	primary degenerative dementia
PEG	pneumoencephalography
PET	positron emission tomography
PMS	petit mal seizure
PNS	peripheral nervous system
PSG	polysomnogram
RA	rheumatoid arthritis
RAS	reticular activating system
RIND	reversible, ischemic neurological deficit
RNA	ribonucleic acid
ROA	right occiput anterior
ROM	range of motion
ROP	right occiput posterior
SAH	subarachnoid hemorrhage
SBX	stereotactic brain biopsy
SSEP	somatosensory evoked potential

T	thoracic	**TNS**	transcutaneous nerve stimulation
TEE	transesophageal echocardiogram	**TPA**	tissue plasminogen activator
TENS	transcutaneous electrical nerve stimulation	**TS**	trauma score
TIA	transient ischemic attack	**W/S**	wake sleep check

Anatomic Illustrations

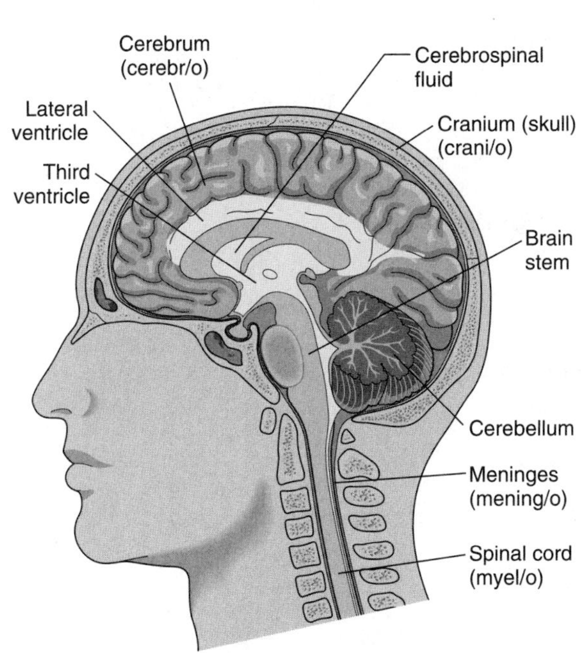

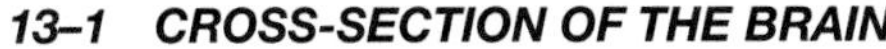

13–1 CROSS-SECTION OF THE BRAIN

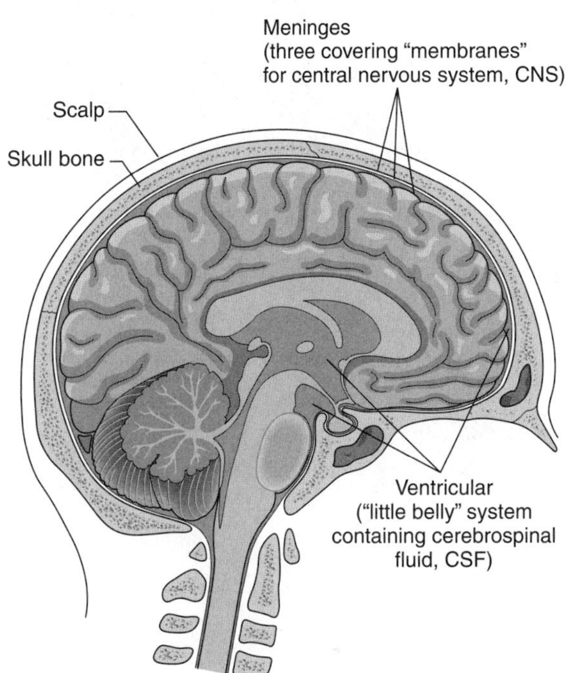

13–2 THE MENINGES AND VENTRICLES

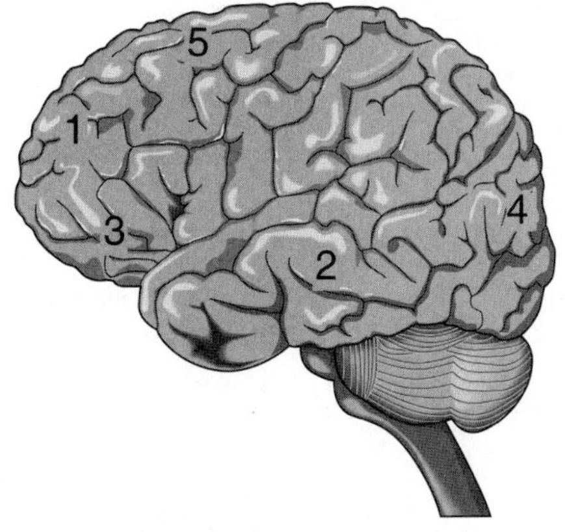

1. thinking area
2. hearing area
3. saying area
4. seeing area
5. writing area

13–3 SOME FUNCTIONAL AREAS OF THE BRAIN

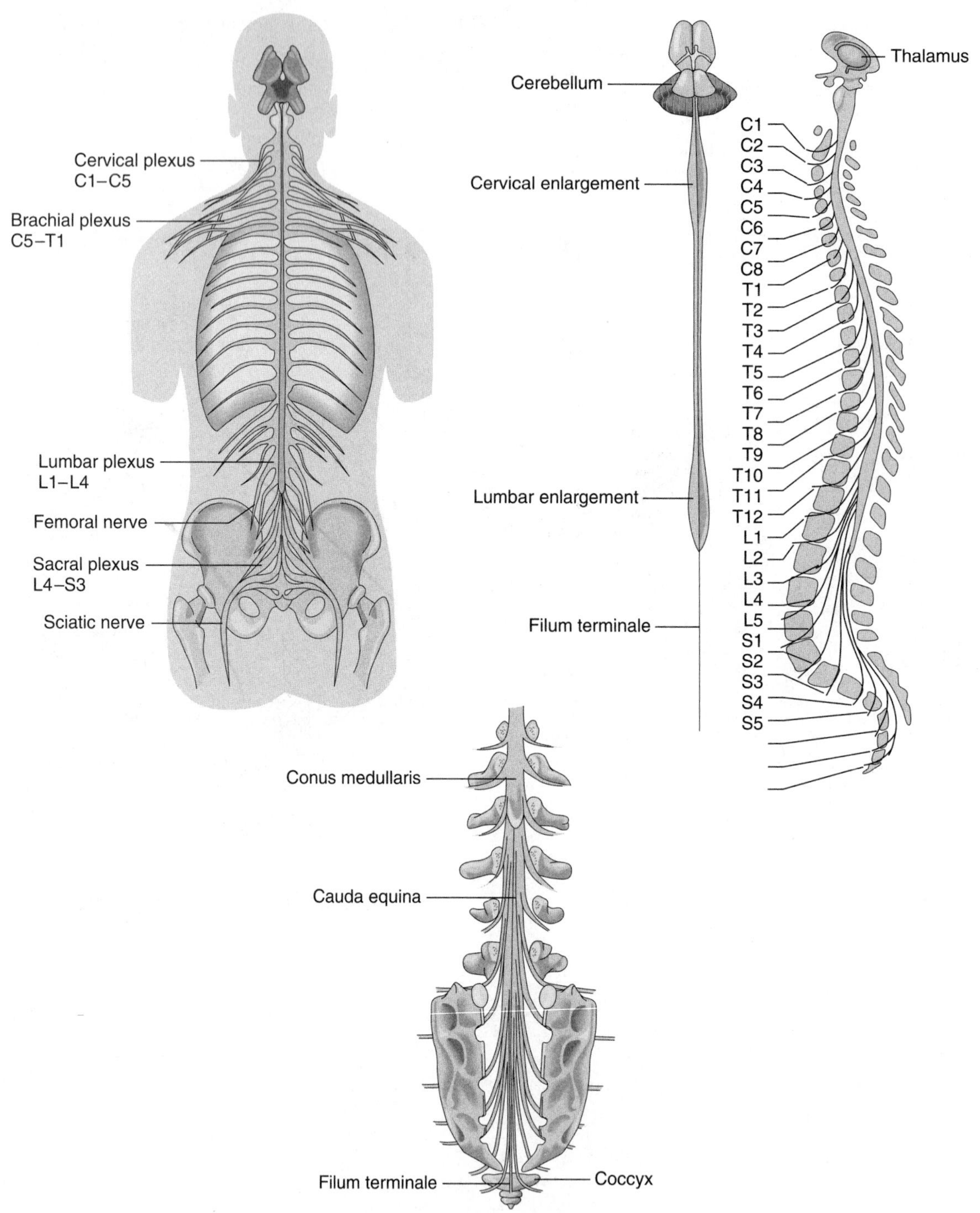
Cervical plexus
C1–C5
Brachial plexus
C5–T1
Lumbar plexus
L1–L4
Femoral nerve
Sacral plexus
L4–S3
Sciatic nerve
Cerebellum
Cervical enlargement
Lumbar enlargement
Filum terminale
Thalamus
C1
C2
C3
C4
C5
C6
C7
C8
T1
T2
T3
T4
T5
T6
T7
T8
T9
T10
T11
T12
L1
L2
L3
L4
L5
S1
S2
S3
S4
S5
Conus medullaris
Cauda equina
Filum terminale
Coccyx

13–4 SPINAL CORD (MYEL/O) AND NERVES

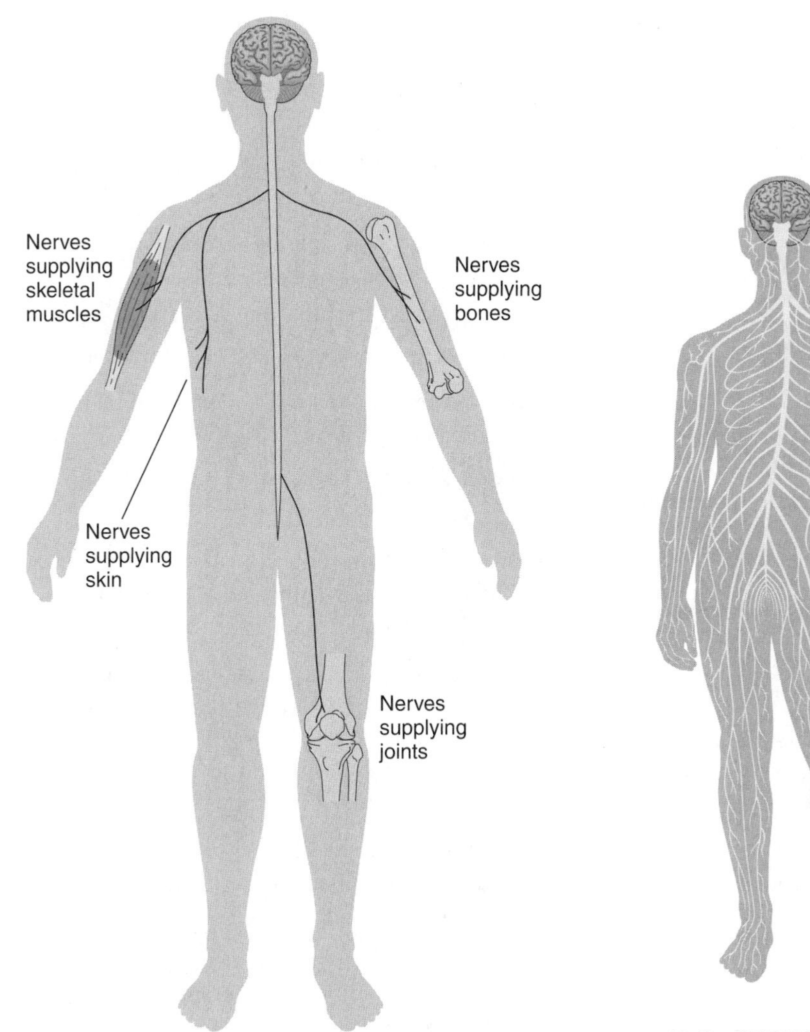

13–5 THE SOMATIC NERVOUS SYSTEM (SNS)

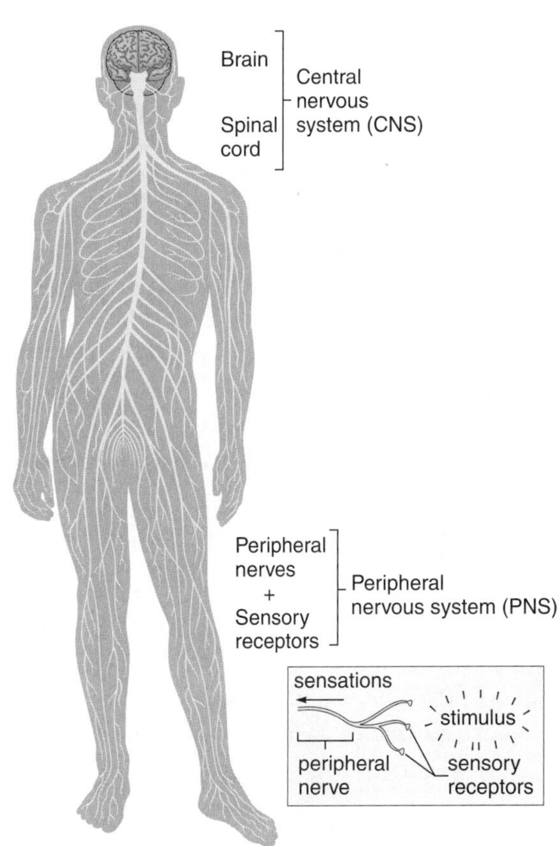

13–6 STRUCTURAL ORGANIZATION OF THE NERVOUS SYSTEM

Neurology/Neurosurgery Terminology

agrammatism (ā-gram'-uh-tizm") – inability to speak grammatically because of brain injury or disease

akinesia (ā"-kih-nē'-zē-uh) – absence or poverty of movements; the temporary paralysis of a muscle by the injection of procaine

Alzheimer's disease (syn. dementia) (altz'-hī-merz dih-zēz', dē-men'-shē-uh) – mental deterioration of unknown etiology characterized by advanced cortical atrophy and secondary ventricular dilatation

amyelia (ā"-mī-ē'-lē-uh) – congenital absence of spinal cord

amygdalotomy (uh-mig"-duh-lot'-uh-mē) – incision into the corpus amygdaloideum, a small mass of subcortical gray matter within the tip of the temporal lobe, anterior to the inferior horn of the lateral ventricle of the brain

amyotrophic lateral sclerosis (ALS) (ā"-mī-ō-trō'-fik lat'-er-ul skleh-rō'-sis) – degeneration involving the principal pyramidal tracts of the brain and spinal cord and the anterior horn cells in the spinal cord; results in loss of motor function; death usually occurs because of pharyngeal muscle failure

anencephalia (an"-en-seh-fā'-lē-uh) – congenital absence of the cranial vault with cerebral hemispheres completely missing or reduced to small masses attached to the base of the skull

anisocoria (an"-ih-sō-kōr'-ē-uh) – unequal pupils

aphasia (ā-fā'-zē-uh) – loss of the power of speech due to a central lesion

apoptosis (ā"-pō-tō'-sis) – "cell suicide"; condition in which cells shrivel rather than swell, with only minimal damage to surrounding cells

arteriovenous malformation (ar-tē"-rē-ō-vē'-nus mal-fōr-mā'-shun) – an abnormal connection of veins to arteries

astereognosis (ā-stār"-ē-ahg-nō'-sis) – loss of power to recognize objects or to appreciate their form by touching or feeling them

aura (aw'-ruh) – a subjective sensation or motor phenomenon that precedes and marks the onset of a paroxysmal attack such as a seizure or migraine headache

b

Biernacki's sign (bī-er-naht'-skēz sīn) – analgesia of the ulnar nerve in paralytic dementia and tabes dorsalis

Brantigan cage (bran'-tih-gun kāj) – internal fixation device used after lumbar spinal fusion

Brown-Sequard's syndrome (brown'-sah-karz' sin'-drōm) – a syndrome due to damage of one-half of the spinal cord

Brudzinski's sign (brood-zin'-skēz sīn) – a physical sign that suggests the presence of meningitis

c

cauda equina (kaw'-duh ē'-kwih-nuh) – "horse's tail"; the group of peripheral nerves that exit the spinal column below the end of the spinal cord

cephalalgia (sef"-ul-al'-jē-uh) – pain in the head; headache

cerebellum (sār"-eh-bel'-um) – the second largest portion of the brain; it is concerned with the coordination of movements and balance

cerebral dysrhythmia (sir'-ē-brul dis-rith'-mē-uh) – irregularity in the electrical impulses given off by the brain

cerebromeningitis (sir"-ē-brō-men"-in-jī'-tis) – inflammation of the brain and meninges

cerebrum (sir'-ē-brum) – the largest and uppermost portion of the brain; divided into two cerebral hemispheres

Charcot-Marie-Tooth disease (shar-kō'-mah-rē'-tooth dih-zēz') – progressive neuropathic (peroneal) muscular atrophy

cisterna (sis-ter'-nuh) – a closed space serving as a reservoir for lymph or other body fluid, especially one of the enlarged subarachnoid spaces containing cerebrospinal fluid

clonic (klah'-nik) – spasm in which rigidity and relaxation alternate in rapid succession

conus medullaris (kō'-nus med'-yoo-lār"-is) – medullary cone; the cone-shaped lower end of the spinal cord at the level of the upper lumbar vertebrae; the end of the spinal cord

cordectomy (kor-dek'-tuh-mē) – ablative destruction of a portion of the spinal cord

craniocele (krā'-nē-ō-sēl") – a protrusion of any part of the cranial contents through a defect in the skull

cranioclast (krā'-nē-ō-klast") – an instrument for performing craniotomy

craniotomy (krā"-nē-ot'-uh-mē) – any operation on the cranium

cryptococcosis (krip"-tō-kok-ō'-sis) – an infection that may involve the skin, lungs, or other parts but has a predilection to the brain and meninges

d

decerebrate (dē-sār'-eh-brāt) – to eliminate cerebral function by transecting the brain stem between the anterior colliculi and the vestibular nuclei or by ligating the common carotid arteries and the basilar artery at the center of the pons

demyelinate (dē-mī'-eh-lin-āt) – to destroy or remove the myelin sheath of a nerve or nerves

diastematomyelia (dī"-uh-stem"-ah-tō-mī-ē'-lē-uh) – a congenital defect, often associated with spina bifida, in which the spinal cord is split into halves by a bony spicule of fibrous band, each half being surrounded by a dural sac

diencephalon (dī"-en-sef'-uh-lahn) – the inner brain, thalamus and hypothalamus

diplegia (dī-plē'-jē-uh) – paralysis affecting like parts on both sides of the body; bilateral paralysis

dura mater (doo'-ruh mā'-tur) – the outermost, toughest, and most fibrous of the three membranes (meninges) covering the brain and spinal cord

dysautonomia (dis"-aw-tō-nō'-mē-uh) – a disorder of the autonomic nervous system (ANS) function

dystonia (dis-tō'-nē-uh) – a neurological muscle disorder characterized by involuntary muscle spasms

e

electromyography (ē-lek"-trō-mī-og'-ruh-fē) – the recording and study of the intrinsic electrical properties of skeletal muscle

encephalitis (en"-sef-uh-lī'-tis) – inflammation of the brain

encephalocele (en-sef'-uh-lō-sēl") – a herniation of a part of the brain through any opening in the skull

encephalomalacia (en-sef"-uh-lō-muh-lā'-shē-uh) – softening of the brain

encephalomyeloradiculitis (en-sef"-uh-lō-mī"-eh-lō-rah-dik"-yoo-lī'-tis) – inflammation of the brain, spinal cord, and spinal nerve roots

encephalopathy (en-sef"-uh-lop'-uh-thē) – any degenerative disease of the brain

epencephalon (ep"-en-sef'-uh-lahn) – cerebellum; metencephalon

ependymitis (ē-pen"-dih-mī'-tis) – inflammation of the ependyma, which is the lining membrane of the ventricles of the brain and of the central canal of the spinal cord

epileptologist (ep"-ih-lep-tahl'-uh-jist) – a practitioner who specializes in epilepsy and the treatment of epilepsy

f

fasciculation (fuh-sik"-yoo-lā'-shun) – a small, local contraction of muscles representing a spontaneous discharge of a number of fibers innervated by a single motor nerve filament

fiducials (fih-doo'-shuls) – fixed and accepted bases of reference or comparison

g

Gamma knife (gam'-uh nīf) – a stereotactic radiosurgical device that allows treatment of deep-seated brain tumors; the most commonly used method of radiosurgery

glioblastoma multiforme (glē"-ō-blas-tō'-muh mul'-tih-form) – a rapidly growing, malignant primary brain tumor, usually of the cerebral hemispheres, arising from cells called astrocytes; now called astrocytoma, grade 4, or malignant astrocytoma

glioma (glē-ō'-muh) – a tumor arising from supportive cells found in the brain and spinal cord

grand mal (gran mahl) – epilepsy in which a sudden loss of consciousness is immediately followed by generalized convulsions

Guillain-Barré syndrome (gē-yayn'-bar-rā' sin'-drōm) – a rare disease of the nervous system involving peripheral nerves, nerve roots, and spinal cord

h

hemangioblastoma (hē-man"-jē-ō-blas-tō'-muh) – a capillary hemangioma of the brain, consisting of proliferated blood vessel cells or angioblasts

hemianopia (hem"-ē-an-ō'-pē-uh) – loss of one-half of the visual field

hemilaminectomy (hem"-ē-lam"-ih-nek'-tuh-mē) – removal of the vertebral laminae on one side only

hemiparesis (hem"-ē-pah'-rē-sis) – muscular weakness affecting one side of the body

hypersomnia (hī"-per-sahm'-nē-uh) – excessive sleep with uncontrollable drowsiness

hypopnea (hī"-pō-nē'-uh) – abnormal decrease in the rate and depth of the respiratory movements

hypothalamus (hī"-pō-thal'-uh-mus) – the portion of the diencephalon that forms the floor and part of the lateral wall of the third ventricle

k

kernicterus (ker-nik'-ter-us) – a condition with severe neurological symptoms associated with high levels of bilirubin in the blood, as seen in liver failure

Kernig's sign (ker'-nigz sīn) – a symptom of meningitis evidenced by reflex contraction and pain in the hamstring muscles when the patient attempts to extend the leg after flexing the thigh upon the abdomen

kinesioneurosis (kih-nē"-sē-ō-noo-rō'-sis) – a functional nervous disorder characterized by motor disturbances such as spasms or tics

kyphoplasty (kī'-fō-plas"-tē) – procedure performed in conjunction with a vertebroplasty, whereby the collapsed vertebra is restored in height with a balloon before the plastic is injected

l

L-dopa (el-dō'-puh) – a drug used to supply dopamine, a neurotransmitter, in the treatment of Parkinson's disease

lateropulsion (lat"-er-ō-pul'-shun) – an involuntary tendency to go to one side while walking

leptomeninges (lep"-tō-meh-nin'-jēz) – the pia-arachnoid, a combined delicate web-like membrane that ultimately covers the brain; also called the pia mater

leptomeningitis (lep"-tō-men"-in-jī'-tis) – inflammation of the pia and arachnoid of the brain or spinal cord

linear accelerator (lin'-ē-ur ak-sel'-er-ā-tur) – equipment used in stereotactic radiosurgery to deliver a concentrated dose of radiation to a predetermined target, using x-rays

m

macrocrania (mak"-rō-krā'-nē-uh) – abnormal increase in the size of the skull, the facial area being disproportionately small in comparison

Magendie's foramen (mah-jen'-dēz fōr-a'-men) – an opening in the lower portion of the roof of the fourth ventricle through which the cerebrospinal fluid communicates with the subarachnoid space

magnetoencephalography (MEG) (mag-nē"-tō-en-sef'-uh-lah'-gruh-fē) – the recording of magnetic signals proportional to electroencephalographic waves emanating from electrical activity in the brain

medulla oblongata (meh-doo'-luh ahb-long-gah'-tuh) – the end of the brainstem that transitions into the spinal cord

meninges (meh-nin'-jēz) – the covering membranes of the brain and spinal cord

meningioma (me-nin"-jē-ō'-mah) – a hard, slow-growing, usually vascular tumor that arises from the meninges or covering membranes of the brain

meningoencephalitis (me-ning"-gō-en-sef"-uh-lī'-tis) – inflammation of the brain and meninges

meningomyelocele (me-ning"-gō-mī'-eh-lō-sēl") – protrusion of a part of the meninges and substance of the spinal cord through a defect in the vertebral column

MicroLYSIS (mī"-krō-lī'-sis) – ultrasound-enhanced drug delivery system that delivers thrombolytic drugs directly into the area of a brain clot

millijoule (mJ) (mil'-ih-jool) – a measurement used in YAG laser and argon laser applications (1/1000th of a joule)

myelomalacia (mī"-eh-lō-muh-lā'-shē-uh) – morbid softening of the spinal cord

n

narcolepsy (nar'-kō-lep"-sē) – a condition marked by an uncontrollable desire for sleep or by sudden attacks of sleep occurring at intervals

neurectomy (noo-rek'-tuh-mē) – excision of a nerve

neurilemma (noo"-rih-lem'-uh) – the delicate membranous sheath, or covering, of a peripheral nerve fiber

neurodegeneration (noo'-rō-dē-jen"-er-ā'-shun) – pertaining to the deterioration of nervous tissue

neurofibromatosis (noo"-rō-fī"-brō-muh-tō'-sis) – an inherited condition characterized by developmental changes in the nervous system, muscles, bones, and skin and marked superficially by the formation of multiple pedunculated soft tumors (neurofibromas) distributed over the entire body associated with areas of pigmentation

neurogenetics (noo"-rō-jeh-net'-iks) – pertaining to the development of nervous tissue

neuromatous (noo-rahm'-uh-tus) – affected with or of the nature of a tumor or new growth largely made up of nerve cells and nerve fibers

neuro-ophthalmologist (noo"-rō-of"-thuhl-mahl"-uh-jist) – a physician who diagnoses and treats patients suffering from optic nerve disorders, problems with eye and lid movement (double vision, lid spasm or droop), and unexplained visual loss

neuro-otologist (noo"-rō-ō-tahl'-uh-jist) – a physician who works with problems that cause vertigo and balance dysfunction, including labyrinthitis, benign positional vertigo, and Meniere's disease

nuclear imaging (PET and SPECT) (noo'-klē-ur im'-uh-jing) – imaging techniques that employ small amounts of radioactive isotopes (radionuclides) to measure cellular and/or tissue metabolism

nystagmus (nis-tag'-mus) – involuntary, rapid horizontal, vertical, rotatory, or mixed movement of the eyeball

o

obstructive sleep apnea (ahb-struk'-tiv slēp ap'-nē-uh) – a condition characterized by a particular snoring pattern, which is interrupted by pauses and then gasps, that causes periodic stopping of breathing during sleep

oligodendroglia (ol"-ih-gō-den-drahg'-lē-uh) – a glial cell of ectodermal origin that forms part of the support structure of the central nervous system

p

pacchionian (pak"-ē-ō'-nē-un) – smooth granular structures found in the meninges of the brain

pallidotomy (pah"-lih-dah'-tuh-mē) – production of lesions in the globus pallidus for the purpose of treating extrapyramidal disorders

paramyotonia (pār"-uh-mī"-ō-tō'-nē-uh) – a disease marked by tonic spasms due to disorder of muscular tonicity, especially a hereditary and congenital affection

paresthesia (pār"-es-thē'-zē-uh) – morbid or perverted sensation

parieto-occipital (puh-rī"-eh-tō-ok-sip'-ih-tul) – pertaining to the parietal and occipital bones or lobes

petit mal (peh-tē' mahl') – "absence seizures" that usually last for only a few seconds

pia mater (pē'-uh mā'-tur) – the innermost of the three membranes (meninges) covering the brain and spinal cord; one cell thick

pleocytosis (plē"-ō-sī-tō'-sis) – presence of a greater-than-normal number of cells in the cerebrospinal fluid

pneumocephalus (noo"-mō-sef'-uh-lus) – air within the skull

polyneuropathy (pahl"-ē-noo-rahp'-uh-thē) – a disease that involves multiple nerves

polysomnogram (pahl"-ē-sahm'-nuh-gram) – test conducted to evaluate sleep apnea syndrome

postictal (pōst-ik'-tul) – period of time during which the patient has neurological symptoms after a seizure

precuneus (prē-kyoo'-nē-us) – a small, square-shaped convolution on the medial surface of the parietal lobe of the cerebrum

proprioception (prō"-prē-ō-sep'-shun) – the sensory system mechanism concerned with movement of the body, its balance, posture, and coordination

quadriplegia (kwah"-drih-plē'-jē-uh) – paralysis of all four limbs

radiculitis (rah-dik"-yoo-lī'-tis) – inflammation of the root of a spinal nerve, especially of the portion of the root lying between the spinal cord and the intervertebral canal

radiculopathy (rah-dik"-yoo-lop'-uh-thē) – disease of the nerve roots

satellitosis (sat"-eh-lī-tō'-sis) – accumulation of neuroglial cells around neurons; seen whenever neurons are damaged

Schilder's disease (shil'-derz dih-zēz') – a rare, progressive demyelinating disorder that usually begins in childhood

schwannoma (shwon-nō'-muh) – a neoplasm of a peripheral nerve sheath

sella turcica (sel'-uh tur'-sih-kuh) – a bony shelf in approximately the central portion of the base of the skull that houses the pituitary gland

stereognosis (stār"-ē-ahg-nō'-sis) – the faculty of perceiving and understanding the form and nature of objects by the sense of touch

stereotactic (OR stereotaxic) radiosurgery (steh"-rē-ō-tak'-tik [steh"-rē-ō-taks'-ik] rā"-dē-ō-sur'-jur-ē) – the very precise delivery of radiation to a brain tumor without harm to the surrounding normal brain. To achieve this precision, special tools are used to pinpoint the location of the brain tumor; among them are the stereotactic frame, the CT or MRI scan, a computerized system for calculating the radiation dose to the brain tumor, and a precise system for delivering the radiation to the brain tumor

Sturge-Weber syndrome (encephalotrigeminal angiomatosis) (sturj-web'-er [en-sef"-uh-lō'-trī-jem'-ih-nul] an"-je-ō-muh-tō'-sis) – a congenital disorder characterized by a vascular facial birthmark and neurological abnormalities

subarachnoid (sub"-uh-rak'-noyd) – a potential situated or occurring between the arachnoid and the pia mater

synkinesis (sin"-kih-nē'-sis) – an associated movement; an unintentional movement accompanying a volitional movement

syringobulbia (sih-ring"-gō-bul'-bē-uh) – the presence of cavities in the medulla oblongata

syringomyelia (sih-ring"-gō-mī-ē'-lē-uh) – the presence of abnormal cavities filled with liquid in the spinal cord

teratoma (tar"-uh-tō'-muh) – a true neoplasm made up of a number of different types of tissue, none of which is native to the area in which it occurs

tetraplegia (teh"-truh-plē'-jē-uh) – quadriplegia

thalamus (thal'-uh-mus) – a structure within the diencephalon that serves as the main relay center for sensory impulses

tic douloureux (tihk doo-loo-roo') – trigeminal neuralgia; a disorder of the fifth cranial nerve

transverse myelitis (tranz-vurss' mī"-ē-lī'-tis) – a neurological disorder caused by inflammation across both sides of one level, or segment, of the spinal cord

trigeminal neuralgia (trī-jem'-ih-nul noor-al'-jē-uh) – facial pain

trismus (trihz'-mus) – motor disturbance of the trigeminal nerve, especially spasm of the masticatory muscles with difficulty in opening the mouth (lockjaw); a characteristic early symptom of tetanus

vagotonia (vā"-gō-tō'-nē-uh) – hyperexcitability of the vagus nerve; a condition in which the vagus nerve dominates in the general functioning of the body organs

ventriculocisternostomy (ven-trik"-yoo-lō-sis"-ter-nahss'-tuh-mē) – surgical establishment of a communication between the third ventricle of the brain and the cisterna magna for flow of cerebrospinal fluid in hydrocephalus

wallerian degeneration (wah-ler'-ē-un dē"-jen-er-ā'-shun) – fatty degeneration of a nerve fiber that has been severed from its nutritive centers

Transcription Tips

You will find it easier to transcribe neurology/neurosurgery dictation if you are familiar with the names and locations of the major organs and parts of the nervous system; combining forms, prefixes, and suffixes; and specialized terminology used in the field of neurology/neurosurgery. Familiarity with some of the communication disorders will also help.

The nervous system consists of:

- Three anatomic divisions:
  1. the central nervous system
  2. the autonomic nervous system
  3. the peripheral nervous system
- Four physiologic divisions:
  1. the sensory (afferent) system
  2. the motor (efferent) system, including the pyramidal and extrapyramidal divisions
  3. the autonomic nervous system, including the sympathetic and parasympathetic divisions
  4. the reticular activating system

Roots and/or Combining Forms

Root	Meaning	Root	Meaning
causo	burning	meningo, meningio	membranes, meninges
cerebello	cerebellum	myo	muscle
cerebro	cerebrum	myelo	spinal cord
comato	deep sleep	neuro	nerve
duro	duramater	ponto	pons
encephalo	brain	radiculo	nerve root
esthesio	feeling	syncopo	to cut off, cut short
glio	glue	taxo	order, coordination
kineso, kinesio	movement	thalamo	thalamus
lepto	thin, slender	theco	sheath
lexo	word, phrase	vago	vagus nerve

Glossary of Selected Nervous System Terms

amnesia – loss of memory

analgesia – inability to feel pain

anesthesia – loss of feeling

ataxia – lack of muscular coordination

autonomic nervous system – that part of the nervous system that cannot be controlled, governing the heart, smooth muscle, and glands

central nervous system – the system concerned with the brain and spinal cord

cerebral hemorrhage – one type of stroke

cerebrospinal fluid – the protective fluid contained within the brain and spinal cord

chorda – a tendinous or cord-like structure

coma – unconsciousness from which a patient cannot be awakened

cord – a stringlike structure; the portion of the central nervous system contained in the spinal canal

epilepsy – a deviation of the brain waves that may result in convulsions or motor sensory disturbances

foramen magnum – a passageway through the occipital bone for the spinal cord

frontal lobe – the foremost lobe of each cerebral hemisphere

hemiplegia – paralysis of one side of the body

hemisphere – either half of the brain

inertia – inactivity

Glossary of Selected Nervous System Terms

inversion – a turning inward

motor neuron – a nerve cell concerned with movement

neuron – nerve cell

occipital lobe – the posterior lobe of the cerebral hemisphere

palsy – paralysis

paraplegic – paralysis of the lower half of the body

parietal lobe – the lobe of the cerebral hemisphere located beneath the parietal bone

sensory neuron – any neuron concerned with sensory function

spinal cord – the nervous tissue within the vertebral canal

temporal lobe – the lobe of the cerebral hemisphere located behind the temporal bone

The 12 Cranial Nerves

abducens
acoustic
facial
glossopharyngeal
hypoglossal
oculomotor
olfactory
optic
spinal accessory
trigeminal
trochlear
vagus

Common Communication Disorders

anomia
aphasia
- Broca aphasia
- global aphasia
- Wernicke aphasia

apraxia
dysarthria
perseveration

Supportive Web Sites

www.hopkinsmedicine.org/
Search for "radiosurgery," then click on sites of interest for valuable information.

www.neurosurgery.org/
Click on "What is Neurosurgery" or "Patient Resources" and select links of interest; click on "Quick Find" and choose an area.

www.ninds.nih.gov/
Click on "Disorder Quick Links" or "Browse all Disorders" for helpful links to other information.

www.nlm.nih.gov/
Click on "Health Information," then "MEDLINEplus," then search for "neurology" or "neurosurgery"; select links of interest.

www.radionics.com
Click on available links or on "Quick Links" to find other links of interest.

Index of Neurology/Neurosurgery Reports

(see table of contents for audio information)

Exercise #	Patient Name	Report/Procedure
TE#1 6/19	Carlos, Juan	Placement of right internal pulse generator
TE#2	Edwards, Julie	Application of stereotactic CRW frame
TE#3 6/28	Diamond, Rhonda	Gamma knife stereotactic radiosurgery
TE#4 7/1	Purvis, Bo	Functional mapping of left thalamus (Vc)
TE#5	Farve, Brandon	Image-guided craniotomy for resection of dural AVM fistula
TE#6	Bordelon, Jeanelle	Bilateral bur holes for drainage of subdural hematomas
TE#7	Register, Brett	Right frontal craniotomy, clipping of aneurysms
TE#8	Weaver, Wanda Lynn	Left L5-S1 partial hemilaminectomy and disk excision
TE#9	Stephenson, Angela	Right pterional craniotomy, clipping of aneurysm

CHAPTER 14
PLASTIC SURGERY

Introduction

Simply stated, *plastic surgery* is the surgical method of repairing and/or reconstructing body structures that are defective or have been damaged by injury or disease. Some of these deformities may be present at birth; others are caused by burns, wounds, injury, disease, or the aging process. This method of surgery is employed to restore both function and appearance.

The word *plastic* is defined simply as "giving form or shape to a substance." As might be thought by many, neither the word *plastic* nor the substance bearing this name have any relationship to commercially prepared synthetic plastic materials and products. It is true, however, that medical-grade plastic materials may be used in some areas of reconstructive and cosmetic surgery.

The essence of plastic surgery is *tissue transplantation* and repositioning. *Tissues,* which include nerves, skin, bone, cartilage, tendon, mucous membrane, and fat, can be moved from sites near the damaged area or from remote parts of the body. In the new location, such tissue can substitute for damaged, deformed, or lost tissue and can protect exposed and functioning areas.

For optimum and lasting results, *grafts* are transferred from one part of the body to another part of the same individual. It is possible, though, for bone, cartilage, and corneas to be transplanted from one person to another.

Recent years have seen many advances in plastic surgery. Improved techniques have enabled surgeons to repair cleft lips so that the remaining scars are almost imperceptible. It is now common practice to transfer ultrathin sheets of good skin from one area to another by use of an instrument called the *dermatome.* New materials, such as the rubber-silicone compound *Silastic* and medical mesh grafts, are being used safely and successfully to round out facial contours and fill in depressions.

Plastic surgeons are frequently called upon to treat patients who have been burned. Burns are classified as first, second, third, or fourth degree depending on the depth of the burn. In many cases, grafting of tissue is required to restore function and appearance to the affected area(s).

The practice of plastic surgery is not confined to the head and neck, but is successfully performed on all parts of the body by general and specialty plastic surgeons. The general plastic surgeon may perform surgery on virtually any area of the body.

Critical Thinking Exercise

The attending physician calls the transcription department and asks if the transcriptionist is responsible for completion of the medical record—or could the intern or resident be held responsible for completion?

What is your response?

Plastic Surgery Abbreviations

ATL	antitension line
B-W	Braun-Wangensteen graft
CL	cleft lip
CP	cleft palate
CRIF	closed reduction & internal fixation
DIP	distal interphalangeal

FTSG	full-thickness skin graft
IP	interphalangeal
PIP	proximal interphalangeal
RSTL	relaxed skin tension lines
STSG	split-thickness skin graft
TBSA	total body surface area
TMJ	temporomandibular joint
TRAM	transverse rectus abdominis myocutaneous procedure

Anatomic Illustration

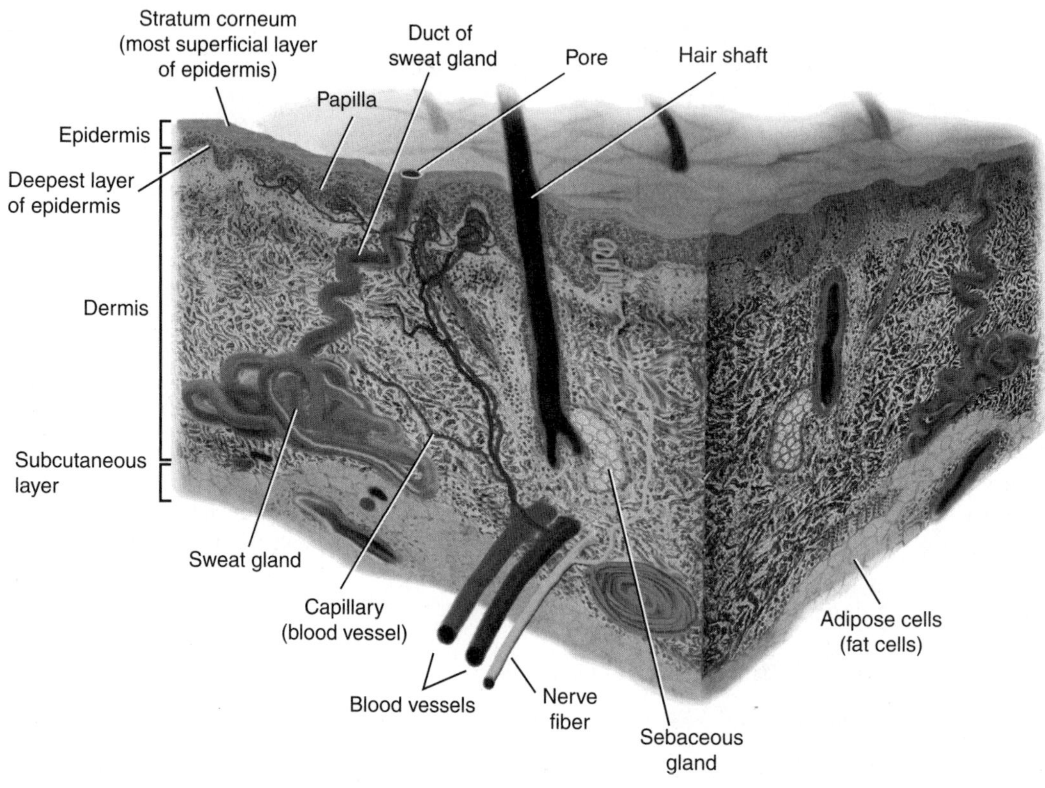

14–1 A CROSS-SECTION OF THE SKIN

Plastic Surgery Terminology

abdominoplasty (ab-dahm'-ih-nō-plas"-tē) – the surgery to remove excess skin and tighten the protuberant abdomen that results from multiple pregnancies

allograft (syn. homograft) (al'-ō-graft, hō'-mō-graft) – graft from one individual to another in the same species

autograft (aw'-tō-graft) – graft from one place to another on the same individual

autologous (aw-tol'-uh-gus) – in transplantation, refers to a graft in which the donor and recipient areas are in the same individual

blepharochalasis (blef"-uh-rō-kal'-uh-sis) – relaxation of the skin of the eyelid due to atrophy of the intercellular tissue

blepharoplasty (blef'-uh-rō-plas"-tē) – surgery on the eyelids to correct blepharochalasis

blepharoptosis (blef"-uh-rō-tō'-sis) – drooping of an upper eyelid due to paralysis

Botox (bō-tahks) – injection that temporarily relaxes facial muscles to eliminate wrinkles

brachioplasty (brā'-kē-ō-plas"-tē) – surgery to correct "batwing arms"; surgery to tighten or remove hanging skin of the inner arms

canthus (kan'-thus) – the angle at either end of the fissure between the eyelids; the points at which the upper and lower eyelids meet

cheilectomy (kī-lek'-tuh-mē) – excision of a lip

cheiloplasty (kī'-lō-plas"-tē) – surgical repair of a defect of the lip

cicatrix (sik'-uh-triks OR sik-ā'-triks) – the normal, nonraised scar left by a healed wound

cleft lip, cleft palate (kleft lip, kleft pal'-at) – congenital abnormalities affecting the upper lip and the hard and soft palate

craniofacial reconstruction (krā"-nē-ō-fā'-shul rē-kun-struk'-shun) – surgery for head and face deformities; most times a plastic surgeon and neurosurgeon work together in these procedures

dermabrasion (der"-muh-brā-zhun) – surgical removal of the frozen epidermis and as much of the dermis as necessary by mechanical means

dermatome (der'-muh-tōm) – instrument for incising the skin or for cutting thin slices for transplantation of skin

electrodermatome (ē-lek'-trō-der'-muh-tōm) – an electrical dermatome for cutting off even layers of large areas of skin in a short time; used in skin grafting, shaving scars, and the like

eschar (es'-kar) – a thick, coagulated crust or slough that develops following a thermal burn or chemical or physical cauterization of the skin

escharotomy (es-kar-ot'-uh-mē) – a surgical incision in a burn eschar to lessen constriction

escutcheon (es-kuh'-chun) – the pattern of distribution of the pubic hair

exsanguinate (eks-sang'-gwih-nāt) – to deprive of blood; bloodless

facioplasty (fā'-shē-ō-plas"-tē) – plastic surgery of the face

genioplasty (jē'-nē-ō-plas"-tē) – plastic surgery of the chin

hypermastia (hī"-per-mas'-tē-uh) – hypertrophy of the mammary gland

hypomastia (hī-pō-mas'-tē-uh) – abnormal smallness of the mammary glands

inframammary incisions (in"-fruh-mam'-uh-rē in-sih'-zhuns) – incisions made below the mammary gland

keloid (kē'-loyd) – a mass of raised, hyperplastic, fibrous connective scar tissue

keloplasty (kē'-lō-plas"-tē) – operative removal of a scar or keloid

laserbrasion surgery (lā'-zur-brā'-zhun sur'-jer-ē) – procedure that uses light beams to vaporize the top layers of the skin, to minimize the appearance of wrinkles, scars, or birthmarks

lipectomy (lip-ek'-tuh-mē) – the excision of a mass of subcutaneous adipose tissue, as from the abdominal wall

liposuction (lī-pō"-suk'-shun) – surgery to reduce excess fatty deposits

mammaplasty (OR mammoplasty) (mam'-uh-plas"-tē, mam'-ō-plas"-tē) – plastic reconstruction of the breast, as may be done to augment or reduce its size

mastopexy (mass'-tō-pek-sē) – mammaplasty performed to correct a pendulous breast

mastoplasty (mass'-tō-plas"-tē) – mammaplasty

mentoplasty (men"-tō-plas'-tē) – surgery done on the chin either to augment or reduce; results in better definition of the face

microdermabrasion (mī"-krō-der'-muh-brā'-zhun) – a mini-peeling of the skin surface, with minimal risk of dyspigmentation or scarring

myocutaneous (mī"-ō-kyoo-tā'-nē-us) – denoting a parcel comprising a muscle and its investments and vascular supply, the overlying skin, and the intervening tissues

orthognathic surgery (or"-thahg-nā'-thik sur'-jer-ē) – procedure performed in cooperation with a patient's dentist, orthodontist, or oral maxillofacial surgeon to correct problems with the "bite" or jaw alignment

otoplasty (ō'-tō-plas"-tē) – surgical correction of ear deformities and defects

palatoplasty (pal'-uh-tō-plas"-tē) – plastic reconstruction of the palate, including cleft palate operations

palatorrhaphy (pal"-uh-tōr-uh-fē) – surgical correction of a cleft palate

palpebral (pal'-pē-bruhl) – pertaining to an eyelid

Panas' operation (pan-ahz' op"-er-ā'-shun) – attachment of the upper eyelid to the occipitofrontalis muscle for correction of ptosis

pharyngoplasty (fah-ring'-gō-plas"-tē) – plastic operation on the pharynx

ptosis (tō-sis) – prolapse of an organ or a part

pyogenic (pī"-ō-jen'-ik) – producing pus

rhinocheiloplasty (rī"-nō-kī'-lō-plas"-tē) – plastic surgery of the nose and lip

rhinoplasty (rī'-nō-plas"-tē) – plastic surgical operation on the nose, whether reconstructive, restorative, or cosmetic

rhinotomy (rī-not'-uh-mē) – incision into the nose

rhytidoplasty (rit'-ih-dō-plas"-tē) – plastic surgery for the elimination of wrinkles from the skin

rhytidosis (rit"-ih-dō'-sis) – a wrinkling of the cornea

septorhinoplasty (syn. septoplasty) (sep"-tō-rī'-nō-plas"-tē, sep"-tō-plas"-tē) – a form of rhinoplasty performed to reconstruct the nasal passage or to relieve obstructions inside the nose to correct breathing problems

tantalum (tan'-tuh-lum) – a noncorrosive and malleable metal that has been used for plates or disks to replace cranial defects, for wire sutures, and for making prosthetic appliances

tarsorrhaphy (tahr-sōr'-uh-fē) – the operation of suturing together a portion of or the entire upper and lower eyelids for the purpose of shortening or closing entirely the palpebral fissure

temporomandibular joint (tem"-pō-rō-man-dib'-yoo-lur joynt) – the joint that connects the lower jaw to the skull

vermilion border (vur-mil'-yun bōr'-dur) – the red boundary of the lips that represents the highly vascular epithelial covering between the outer skin and moist oral mucosa of the mouth

xenograft (syn. heterograft) (zē'-nō-graft) – graft from one individual to another of a different species

xiphisternum (zif"-ih-ster'-num) – the xiphoid process

Transcription Tips

To be successful in transcribing plastic surgery dictation, you should be familiar with the accessory organs of the skin, in addition to the various layers of the skin. Recognizing terminology used in cosmetic surgery is also helpful.

Reconstructive surgery (plastic surgery) is performed to repair extravisceral defects and malformations, both congenital and acquired, and to restore function, as well as to prevent further loss of function.

Cosmetic surgery involves reconstruction of the cutaneous tissues around the neck and face and other parts of the body to restore function, correct defects, and remove the marks of time.

The following information provides data on selected confusing words, common cosmetic surgery procedures, types of grafts, and other typical surgery procedures.

Confusing Terms

allograft – transfer or transplants between two individuals of the same species

autograft – transfers or transplants from the same person

facioplasty – plastic surgery of the face

fascioplasty – plastic surgery on a fascia

isografts – grafts between identical twins

xenografts – grafts between two animals of different species

loupe – a pair of glasses worn by a surgeon in ocular surgery; "loupe magnification"

loop – instrument used to grasp and remove the lens; "lens loop"

mammaplasty (preferred) OR mammoplasty – plastic reconstruction of the breast

mammiplasty – plastic surgery on a nipple

skin graft (free graft) – a section of skin tissue that is separated from its blood supply and transferred as a free section of tissue to the recipient site

skin flap (pedicle graft) – a section of skin tissue used to cover or fill a defect

Common Cosmetic Plastic Surgery Procedures

abdominoplasty – surgery to remove excess skin and fat

blepharoplasty – surgery to repair baggy eyelids

chemical peeling – an approach to changing the condition of the skin; particularly suited for removing fine wrinkles from the face

dermabrasion – surgery that removes pockmarks, scars from acne, and certain other disfiguring marks

mammaplasty augmentation – surgery to increase breast size

mammaplasty reduction – surgery to reduce breast size

otoplasty – plastic surgery of the ear

rhinoplasty – reconstructive surgery of the nose

rhytidoplasty – facelift

suction lipectomy – body-contouring technique to aspirate fat by vacuum from the buttocks, flanks, abdomen, thighs, upper arms, knees, ankles, and chin

Types of Grafts

Most plastic surgery requires moving tissue from one part of the body to another. The moved tissue, or *graft,* is referred to as an *autograft;* skin, bone, cartilage, fat, fascia, muscle, or nerves may be taken.

Tissue transplanted from another person is called a *homograft (allograft).* The tissue can be obtained from living persons or taken from persons soon after death.

Heterografts (xenografts) consist of tissue from another species. Plastic surgery may be performed by means of free grafting—cutting tissue from one part of the body and moving it directly to another part.

Split-thickness grafts consist of the epidermis and varying thicknesses of the dermis. *Thin split-thickness grafts* have only a very thin layer of the dermis. *Intermediate* and *thick split-thickness grafts* have a thicker layer of dermis attached to the epidermis.

Full-thickness grafts are used primarily to cover small areas where matching skin color and texture are important, such as on the face.

Skin flaps are used when a large and deep defect is to be covered. "Sliding," "rotating," or "tubed" are a few of the terms used to identify various types of grafts that are never completely removed from the body at any one time, thereby maintaining a direct vascular supply.

Other Plastic Surgery Procedures

cleft palate repair – surgery to repair a congenital fissure in the roof of the mouth

ear reconstruction for microtia – microtia exists when there is a congenital absence of part or all of the external ear

hypospadias repair – hypospadias is a congenital anomaly where the urethra ends on the top surface of the penis or in the perineum

repair of acute burns – skin grafting is utilized to repair tissue that has been severely burned

repair of syndactyly – syndactyly exists when the digits of the hand or feet are webbed

tattooing – useful in plastic surgery for changing the color of grafted skin so that it more closely resembles the surrounding skin

Supportive Web Sites

www.facial-plastic-surgery.org/
Under "Patients," click on "Procedures" and links of interest such as "Glossary of Terms."

www.nlm.nih.gov/medlineplus/
Search on "plastic surgery" for links with detailed information; also click on "Encyclopedia" and search for specific topics.

www.plasticsurgery.org/
Read about "What's New in Plastic Surgery"; use the site's Search function to find topics of interest or click on "LEARN about Procedures" for detailed information on specific procedures.

Index of Plastic Surgery Reports

(see table of contents for audio information)

Exercise #	Patient Name	Report/Procedure
TE#1	Burton, Andrea	Abdominoplasty with rectus muscle plication
TE#2	Potvin, Michong	Carpal tunnel release
TE#3	Roe, Kenya	Augmentation mammaplasty
TE#4	Yokers, Celeste	Breast reduction
TE#5	Sossaman, Hank	Burn debridement and split-thickness skin graft of leg
TE#6	Zananelli, Thea	Mastectomy and breast reconstruction
TE#7	Raines, Mary	Excision of lip lesion
TE#8	Juan, Saleta	Repair of nasal/eyelid lacerations
TE#9	Childree, Kenneth	Burn scar release; skin graft; splint

CHAPTER 15

PEDIATRICS/ NEONATOLOGY

Introduction

Pediatrics is a specialized field of medicine that is concerned with disturbances of any system or function that might affect the health or orderly growth and development of the child. The pediatrician's commitment, extending beyond purely physical matters, is to secure for all children the opportunity to achieve their full native potential. In their role as understanding guardians of children's physical, mental, and emotional progress from conception to maturity, pediatricians are in the vanguard of social concern for children and their families. Generally pediatrics requires three years of residency training.

Neonatology is a subspecialized field of pediatrics that focuses on the human newborn. A *neonatologist* is an intensive-care physician who takes care of sick or premature infants. His or her knowledge of newborn physiology can assist in the management of congenital anomalies; surgical conditions of the neonate; failure to thrive; nutritional problems; genetic, neurologic, and biochemical diseases; and a host of conditions involving delayed maturity. Thus, neonatology is sharply limited in the age range it covers, but broad in its study of the interaction of normal physiology and disease processes. Training for neonatology requires three years of fellowship after successful completion of a pediatric residency.

Classifications of humans with which pediatricians and/or neonatologists work include *neonates* or *newborns, infants, children,* and *adolescents, youth,* or *teenagers.* A *neonate* (newborn) is a child from birth to 1 month of age. An *infant* is a child from 1 month to 24 months of age, and a *child* is a boy or girl from 2 to 13 years of age. Boys and girls aged 13 through 17 years are known as *adolescents, youths,* or *teenagers.*

Critical Thinking Exercise

A health care provider calls the transcription department and requests that a specific report be corrected from the electronic record that has already been signed electronically.

How would you respond to the caller?

Pediatrics/Neonatology Abbreviations

A&B	apnea and bradycardia
ABG	arterial blood gases
AC vent	assist control ventilation
ACAPI	anterior cerebral artery pulsatility index
ACHD	acyanotic congenital heart disease
AGA	appropriate for gestational age
alb	albumin
ALTE	acute life-threatening event
amp	ampicillin
ANC	absolute neutrophil count
AROM	artificial rupture of membranes
BAER	brain stem audioevoked response
BC	blood culture
Bili	bilirubin

BMV	bag and mask ventilation
BPD	bronchopulmonary dysplasia
BS	blood sugar, bowel sounds, or breath sounds
BW	birth weight
CAH	congenital adrenal hyperplasia
CCHD	cyanotic congenital heart disease
CDH	congenital diaphragmatic hernia
CHD	congenital heart disease
Claf	Claforan
CLD	chronic lung disease
clind	clindamycin
CMV	cytomegalovirus
coag	coagulase
CP	cerebral palsy
CPAP	continuous positive airway pressure
CPIP	chronic pulmonary insufficiency of prematurity
Cr	creatinine
CRP	C-reactive protein
CSF	cerebrospinal fluid
DA	dopamine
DB	date of birth
DIC	disseminated intravascular coagulation
DM	diabetes mellitus
DNA	deoxyribonucleic acid
DOL	day of life
EBM	expressed breast milk
Echo	echocardiogram
ECMO	extracorporeal membrane oxygenation
EEG	electroencephalogram
EKG or ECG	electrocardiogram/electrocardiography
Enf	Enfamil
ET	expiratory time
ETT	endotracheal tube
FAS	fetal alcohol syndrome
Fe	iron
FEN	fluid/electrolytes/nutrition
FiO_2	fraction of inspired oxygen
FOC	frontal occipital circumference
GENT	gentamycin
GER	gastroesophageal reflux
glc	glucose
glu	gluconate
H. flu.	Haemophilus influenza
HBsAg	hepatitis B surface antigen
HBV	hepatitis B vaccine
HC	head circumference
Hct	hematocrit
HCTZ	hydrochlorothiazide
Hgb	hemoglobin
H/H or H&H	hemoglobin/hematocrit
HIE	hypoxic-ischemic encephalopathy
HMD	hyaline membrane disease
HSV	herpes simplex virus
HUS	head ultrasound
ICH	intracranial hemorrhage
IDM	infant of diabetic mother
I/E or I:E	inspiratory to expiratory time ratio
Ig	immunoglobulin
IMV	intermittent mandatory ventilation
IT	inspiratory time
I/T	immature total neutrophil ratio
ITP	idiopathic thrombocytopenic purpura
IUGR	intrauterine growth retardation
IVH	intraventricular hemorrhage
L	liter
LBW	low birth weight
LGA	large for gestational age
LP	lumbar puncture
L/S or L:S	lecithin/sphingomyelin ratio (test of fetal lung maturity)
M	murmur
MAP	mean arterial pressure
MAS	meconium aspiration syndrome
MawP	mean airway pressure
MCA	multiple congenital anomalies
mec	meconium
Mg	magnesium
$MgSO_4$	magnesium sulfate
MSF	meconium-stained fluid
N. cat.	Neisseria catarrhalis
N. gon.	Neisseria gonorrhoeae

N. men.	Neisseria meningitidis
NB	newborn
NCPAP	nasal continuous positive airway pressure
NEC	necrotizing enterocolitis
Neo	neonatal
NG	nasogastric
NICU	neonatal intensive care unit
NS	normal saline
NSVD	normal spontaneous vaginal delivery
N&V	nausea and vomiting
O&B	Ortolani and Barlow
OCT	oxytocin challenge test
OG	oral gastric or orogastric (feeding)
OI	oxygenation index
OM	otitis media
$PaCO_2$	arterial carbon dioxide tension
PaO_2	arterial oxygen tension
PBLC	preterm (premature) birth live child
PCN	penicillin
PDA	patent ductus arteriosus
PEEP	positive end-expiratory pressure
PFC	persistent fetal circulation
PFTs	pulmonary function tests
PHH	posthemorrhagic hydrocephalus
PIE	pulmonary interstitial emphysema
PIP	post (or peak) inspiratory pressure
PKU	phenylketonuria
plts	platelets
PPHN	persistent pulmonary hypertension of the newborn
PPV	positive-pressure ventilation
PROM	prolonged or premature rupture of membranes
PS	pulmonary stenosis
PUBS	percutaneous umbilical blood sampling
PVL	periventricular leukomalasia
RDS	respiratory distress syndrome
REM	rapid eye movement
ROP	retinopathy of prematurity
RRR	regular rate and rhythm
S. aureus	Staphylococcus aureus
S. epi	Staphylococcus epidermidis
SaO_2	arterial oxygen saturation
SEH	subependymal hemorrhage
SGA	small for gestational age
SIDS	sudden infant death syndrome
Sim	Similac
SIMV	synchronized intermittent mechanical ventilation
SROM	spontaneous rupture of membrane
SSC	Similac special care formula (followed by number = calorie count)
Strep	Streptococcus
SZ	seizure
T_3	triiodothyronine
T_4	levothyroxine
TAPVR	total anomalous pulmonary venous return
TBLC	term birth live child
Theo	theophylline
TOF	tetralogy of Fallot
TOGV	transposition of the great vessels
Toxo	toxoplasmosis
TPN	total parenteral nutrition
TRIG	triglycerides
TSH	thyroid-stimulating hormone
TTNB	transient tachypnea of the newborn
TV	tidal volume
UAC	umbilical artery catheter
UC	urine culture
U/S	ultrasound
UVC	umbilical venous catheter
Vanc	vancomycin
VBG	venous blood gas
VCUG	voiding cystourethrogram
VIT	vitamin
VLBW	very low birth weight
VSD	ventricular septal defect
VSS	vital signs stable

Pediatrics/Neonatology Terminology

a

amniocentesis (am"-nē-ō-sen-tē'-sis) – surgical transabdominal puncture of the amniotic sac using a needle and syringe in order to remove amniotic fluid

amnioscopy (am"-nē-ahss'-kuh-pē) – direct visual observation of the fetus, color, and amount of amniotic fluid by use of a specially designed endoscope inserted into the amniotic cavity via the abdominal wall

anencephaly (an"-en-sef'-uh-lē) – congenital absence of the cranial vault, with cerebral hemispheres completely missing or reduced to small masses attached to the base of the skull

Apgar score (ap'-gar skōr) – a system of scoring the physical condition of infants one minute after birth; the heart rate, respiration, muscle tone, response to stimuli, and color are each rated 0, 1, or 2

asphyxia (as-fik'-sē-uh) – condition resulting from an insufficient intake of oxygen

atresia (ah-trē'-zē-uh) – congenital absence or closure of a normal body opening or tubular structure

c

caput succedaneum (kap'-it suk"-sē-dā'-nē-um) – swelling occurring in and under the fetal scalp during labor

cephalhematoma (sef"-ul-hē"-muh-tō'-muh) – a tumor or swelling filled with blood beneath the pericranium

chorioamnionitis (kō"-rē-ō-am"-nē-ō-nī'-tis) – inflammation of the fetal membranes caused by bacterial infection

cleft lip or palate (kleft lihp, kleft pal'-ut) – birth defect characterized by a split through the lip, the roof of the mouth, or soft tissue in the back of the mouth resulting from failure of these structures to close normally during early fetal development

craniotabes (krā"-nē-ō-tā'-bēz) – in infancy, abnormal softening of the skull bones

d

Down syndrome (down sin'-drōm) – a variable combination of birth defects that include mental retardation and characteristic facial features

e

equinovarus (ē-kwī"-nō-vār'-us) – clubfoot; defect characterized by certain ankle and foot abnormalities, where the foot is twisted inward and downward

f

fontanelle (alt. sp. fontanel) (fahn"-tuh-nehl') – an unossified space or soft spot lying between the cranial bones of the skull of a fetus

g

gastroschisis (gas-trahs'-kih-sis) – a congenital fissure that remains open in the wall of the abdomen

h

hyaline membrane disease (hī'-uh-lin mem'-brān dih-zēz') – a disorder affecting newborn infants (particularly premature) characterized by the development of a hyaline-like membrane lining the terminal respiratory passages

hyperbilirubinemia (hī"per-bil"-ih-roo"-bih-nē'-mē-uh) – an excessive amount of bilirubin in the blood

hyperinsulinemia (hī"-per-in"-soo-lih-nē'-mē-uh) – the presence of an excessive amount of insulin in the blood

hypomagnesemia (hī"-pō-mag"-neh-sē'-mē-uh) – decreased magnesium in the blood; results in increased neuromuscular irritability

hypotonia (hī"-pō-tō'-nē-uh) – the condition of diminished tone of the skeletal muscles

hypoxia (hī-pok'-sē-uh) – deficiency of oxygen

i

intussusception (in"-tuh-suh-sep'-shun) – the slipping of one part of an intestine into another part just below it

k

Klinefelter's syndrome (klīn'-fel-terz sin'-drōm) – caused by an extra X chromosome; affects only males

l

lactobezoar (lak"-tō-bē'-zōr) – a solid mass of milk products in the stomach or intestines of an infant

m

meconium (mē-kō'-nē-um) – first feces of a newborn infant

mucopolysaccharidosis (myoo"-kō-pahl"-ē-sak"-uh-rī-dō'-sis) – a genetic disorder caused by the lack of an enzyme essential for breaking down sugar molecules and used in building connective tissues in the body

myelomeningocele (mī"-eh-lō-meh-ning'-gō-sēl) – spina bifida with portion of cord and membranes protruding

myringotomy (mih"-ring-got'-uh-mē) – surgery for otitis media in which the surgeon makes a small incision in the eardrum

n

neonatal necrotizing enterocolitis (nē"-ō-nā'-tul nek'-rō-tī"-zing en"-ter-ō-kō-lī'-tis) – a severe disease of the GI tract of the newborn, particularly the premature

neonatal septicemia (nē"-ō-nā'-tul sep"-tih-sē'-mē-uh) – bacterial infection documented by a positive blood culture in the first four weeks of life

Ohtahara syndrome (ō-tah-hah'-rah sin'-drōm) – a neurological disorder characterized by seizures, usually within the first three months of life

omphalocele (om'-fah-lō-sēl") – a congenital hernia of the navel

patent ductus arteriosus (PDA) (pā'-tent duk'-tus ar-tēr"-ē-ō'-sus) – persistence of a communication between the main pulmonary artery and the aorta after birth

perinatology (pār"-ih-nā-tahl'-uh-jē) – study of the fetus and infant from 20–29 weeks of gestation to 1–4 weeks after birth

polyhydramnios (pahl"-ē-hī-dram'-nē-ōs) – an excess of amniotic fluid in the bag of waters in pregnancy

progeria (prō-jē'-rē-uh) – a form of infantilism that causes a child to age prematurely

renal agenesis (rē'-nul ā-jen'-eh-sis) – absence of one or both kidneys

respiratory distress syndrome (RDS) (reh'-spih-ruh-tōr"-ē dih-strehs' sin'-drōm) – hyaline membrane disease

spina bifida (spī'-nuh bihf'-ih-duh) – a neural tube birth defect characterized by a malformation of vertebrae, involving malformation and protrusion of the spinal cord and spinal nerve roots

tachypnea (tak"-ip-nē'-uh) – abnormal rapidity of respiration

tetralogy of Fallot (teh-trahl'-uh-jē uv fal-ō') – a combination of congenital cardiac defects characterized by pulmonary stenosis, interventricular septal defect, dextroposition of the aorta so that it overrides the interventricular septum and receives venous as well as arterial blood, and right ventricular hypertrophy

trisomy (trī'-sō-mē) – condition that occurs when an individual or cell has an extra chromosome

truncus arteriosus (trun'-kus ar-tē"-rē-ō'-sus) – birth defect in which a large, single arterial vessel is present at the top of the heart, from which the aortic arch and the pulmonary and coronary arteries originate

tympanostomy (tim"-puh-nahs'-tuh-mē) – surgery for otitis media in which a tube is inserted into the eardrum to allow continuous drainage of fluid from the middle ear

vesicoureteral reflux disease (veh"-sih-kō-yoo-rē'-ter-ul rē'-fluks dih-zēz') – condition in which urine stored in the bladder can "backwash" up the ureters to the kidney

Transcription Tips

Transcription in pediatrics/neonatology can be challenging. However, knowledge of related terminology, similar words, major congenital abnormalities, newborn reflexes, respiratory problems, and neonatal infections will make the task much easier.

The neurological exam report on a newborn and young infant may include terms such as blinking reflex due to loud noise, blinking reflex due to bright light, palmar grasp reflex, rooting reflex, trunk incurving, vertical suspension position, stepping response, tonic neck reflex, mass reflexes, and Perez reflex.

Confusing Terms

dilatation – condition of being stretched beyond the normal dimensions

dilation – act of being dilated or stretched

feces – the excrement discharged from the intestines

facies – pertaining to the anterior or ventral aspect of the head from forehead to chin

hyperglycemia – abnormally increased content of sugar in the blood

hyperglycinemia – hereditary disorder involving excessive glycine in the blood

hypoglycemia – abnormally low content of sugar in the blood

keratosis – horny growth

ketosis – a condition characterized by an abnormally elevated concentration of ketone bodies in the body tissues and fluids

nephritis – inflammation of a kidney

neuritis – inflammation of a nerve

palate – the partition separating the nasal and oral cavities

palliate – to reduce the severity of

Selected Major Congenital and Chromosomal Anomalies Identifiable in the Neonate

Body System/Tissue	Defect
central nervous	hydrocephalus meningocele myelomeningocele spina bifida occulta
skeletal muscle	dislocation of hip talipes equinovarus (clubfoot)
genitourinary	exstrophy of the bladder hypospadias
gastrointestinal tract	cleft lip and palate esophageal atresia with or without tracheo-esophageal fistula imperforate anus intestinal stenosis or atresia omphalocele
abdominal wall	diaphragmatic eventration or paralysis diaphragmatic hernia heart disease Hirschsprung's disease tracheoesophageal fistula

Genetic Disorders

Aicardi syndrome – rare disorder characterized by partial or complete absence of the structure that links the two hemispheres of the brain, infantile spasms, mental retardation, and an ocular abnormality of the retina of the eye

Angelman syndrome – a neurological disorder characterized by severe congenital mental retardation, unusual facial appearance, and muscular abnormalities

cleidocranial dysplasia – genetic disorder of bone development

cloacal exstrophy – very rare and complicated birth defect involving eversion of the gastrointestinal tract

Genetic Disorders

clubfoot – one of the most common birth defects; refers to certain ankle and foot abnormalities usually present at birth; the foot is twisted inward and downward

Coffin Lowry syndrome – rare genetic disorder characterized by craniofacial and skeletal abnormalities, mental retardation, short stature, and hypotonia

craniosynostosis – a deformity of the infant skull that results when the skull sutures between various skull bones fuse prematurely

Crouzon syndrome – one of large group of birth defects in which there is abnormal fusion of the bones of the skull and face

Fragile X syndrome – most common genetically inherited form of mental retardation

Friedreich's ataxia – inherited disease, with sclerosis of the dorsal and lateral columns of the spinal cord, that causes progressive damage to the nervous system

hereditary spherocytosis – disorder of the red blood cell membrane characterized by spherocytosis, abnormal fragility of erythrocytes, jaundice, and splenomegaly

Hermansky-Pudlak syndrome (HPS) – a genetic disorder characterized by a rare form of albinism that is associated with low visual acuity, bruising and prolonged bleeding, and lung fibrosis

holoprosencephaly – disorder caused by failure of the forebrain of the embryo to divide to form bilateral cerebral hemispheres; results in a deficit in midline facial development

Hurler syndrome – a rare genetic disease characterized by a missing enzyme essential for breaking down sugar molecules and used in building connective tissues in the body; a type of mucopolysaccharidosis (MPS)

hypospadias – relatively common birth defect in males; characterized by the urethra opening on the underside of the penis or on the perineum

Klippel-Feil syndrome – rare disorder characterized by the congenital fusion of any two of the seven cervical vertebrae, resulting in shortness of the neck

Kostmann's syndrome – inherited disorder of the bone marrow

leukodystrophy (leukodystrophies) – a group of genetic disorders characterized by imperfect development or maintenance of the myelin sheath covering nerve fibers in the brain

Menkes disease – genetic neurodegenerative disorder of copper metabolism

myotonia congenital – genetic neuromuscular disorder characterized by slow relaxation of the muscles

Refsum's disease (syndrome) – one of a group of genetic disorders called *leukodystrophies* that affect growth of the myelin sheath

Rothmund-Thomson syndrome (RS) – hereditary disease characterized by progressive degeneration, scarring, and abnormal pigmentation of the skin together with stunting of growth, baldness, cataracts, depressed nasal bridge, and malformations of the teeth, nails, and bone

Sandhoff's disease – rare, genetic lipid-storage disorder that causes progressive deterioration of the central nervous system

Sturge-Weber syndrome – congenital disorder characterized by a vascular birthmark and neurological abnormalities

Tay-Sachs disease – a fatal, inherited disease of the central nervous system; death occurs by age 5

Treacher Collins syndrome – a genetic birth defect that may affect the size and shape of the ears, eyelids, cheek bones, and upper and lower jaws

Reflexes of the Newborn

auditory blink reflex – eyes quickly close if the examiner loudly claps his or her hands above 3 cm from the infant's head

Babinski's reflex – extension of the great toe and flaring of the outer toes when the sole of the foot is stimulated

crossed extensor reflex – when one leg is extended and the knee is held straight, while the sole of the foot is stimulated, the opposite leg will flex

Landau sign – when the baby is suspended horizontally, with the head depressed against the trunk and the neck flexed, the legs will flex and be drawn up to the trunk

Moro reflex – response to sudden loud noise; the body stiffens and the arms go up and out, then forward and toward each other

neck righting – when the head is turned to one side, the shoulder and trunk, followed by the pelvis, will turn to that side

optical blink reflex – when light is suddenly shined into the open eyes, the eyes will close quickly with a quick dorsal flexion of the head

palmar grasp – pressure on palm of hand will elicit grasp

plantar grasp – pressure on sole of foot behind toes causes flexion of toes

positive-supporting reflex – when held in an erect position, baby will stiffen the lower extremities and support his or her weight

pupillary reflexes – ipsilateral constriction to light

rooting – when the corner of the mouth is touched and an object is moved toward the cheek, an infant will turn the head toward the object and open the mouth

tonic neck reflex – sudden jolt will cause head to turn to one side with the leg and arm on that side extended, while the extremities on the other side flex

Respiratory Problems of the Neonate

- aspiration syndromes
  - meconium aspiration syndrome
- chronic lung disease of the neonate
- persistent pulmonary hypertension
- pneumonias
  - intrauterine (congenital) pneumonia
  - neonatal pneumonia
- pneumothorax and pneumomediastinum
- pulmonary hypoplasia
- pulmonary interstitial emphysema
- retained lung fluid syndromes

Respiratory Problems That Can Be Corrected Surgically

- choanal atresia
- congenital cystic adenomatoid malformation
- congenital lobar emphysema
- micrognathia and glossoptosis

Other Neonatal Conditions

- ABO incompatibility
- hemolytic disease (erythroblastosis fetalis)
- hepatitis B
- hyperbilirubinemia
- jaundice
- jaundice secondary to enclosed hemorrhage
- kernicterus (bilirubin encephalopathy)
- Rhesus incompatibility
- varicella-zoster virus

Infections of the Neonate

conjunctivitis
enteritis
meningitis
omphalitis
osteomyelitis
otitis media
peritonitis
septicemia
tetanus
tuberculosis
urinary tract infection

Nonbacterial Infections

AIDS
herpes simplex
TORCH syndrome (T = toxoplasmosis, O = other viruses and congenital syphilis, R = rubella, C = cytomegalovirus, and H = herpes simplex)

Supportive Web Sites

www.my.webmd.com/
Click on "Medical Library," "Health Guide A-Z," and "Health Topics"; search for "pediatrics" or click on individual letters A–Z for other links of interest.

www.nlm.nih.gov/medlineplus/
Search for "pediatrics," "neonatology," "genetic disorders," "birth defects," and other topics for links of interest; also click on "Encyclopedia" and search for specific topics.

www.oncolink.com/
Click on "Types of Cancer," then on "Pediatric Cancers" for links of interest.

www.tchin.org/
Click on "Resources," then "Resource Room," then on links of interest.
Under "Dictionaries," click on "Glossary of Childhood Onset Heart Disease" for a list of words and definitions.

Index of Pediatrics/Neonatology Reports

(see table of contents for audio information)

Exercise #	Patient Name	Report/Procedure
TE#1	Richardson, Tony	H&P
TE#2	Howard, BABY BOY #2	DS
TE#3	Gavan, Kenneth	DS
TE#4	Younce, BABY BOY	Death Summary
TE#5	McCall, BABY BOY	DS
TE#6	Carthage, BABY BOY #2	H&P
TE#7	Bakutis, Jennifer	DS

CHAPTER 16

OTORHINOLARYNGOLOGY

ACTH AD
AP ANTER
ASIS ANT
AV ARTER
BA BARIU
BPD BIPA
CAT COM
CGY CENT
CURIE
CPB CON

Introduction

The three medical specialties of *otology, rhinology,* and *laryngology* refer to the structure, function, and diseases of the ears, nose, and throat respectively and are usually practiced together.

An *otologist* is a physician who is concerned with the medical and surgical diagnoses of the diseases of the ear, which is composed of three basic parts—the *external* (or outer) ear, the *middle* ear, and the *internal* (or inner) ear. The outer ear is composed of the *pinna* and the *external auditory canal.* The middle ear consists of the *tympanic membrane,* the *malleus,* the *incus,* the *stapes,* and the *oval window.* The inner ear is made up of the *cochlea,* the auditory liquids and receptors in the organ of *corti,* and the auditory nerve fibers.

A *rhinologist* is a doctor who treats the nose and its diseases. The three basic parts of the nose are the *external nose,* the *internal nose,* and the *sinuses,* which are the openings that appear in the interior of the nose and occur in pairs, one for each side of the face. They are known as the *maxillary, frontal, ethmoid,* and *sphenoid* sinuses. *Sinusitis* is an inflammation of the sinuses.

A physician who studies the throat and the tracheobronchial tree is called a *laryngologist.* What lay people call the throat is referred to by medical people as the *pharynx* and is composed of three natural divisions—the *nasopharynx,* the *oropharynx,* and the *laryngopharynx* (hypopharynx). Acute *pharyngitis* is an inflammation of the throat. Chronic pharyngitis can be classified as hypertrophic, atropic, or chronic grandular.

Physicians who are concerned with the medical and surgical diagnoses of diseases of all three divisions—ears, nose, and throat—are known as *otorhinolaryngologists.*

Critical Thinking Exercise

The hospital you are working for is being reviewed for accreditation by the Joint Commission on Accreditation of Healthcare Organizations (JCAHO) in six months. Because yours is a very busy department, sometimes the date of the report and the date of transcription differ by days, weeks, or even months. Hospital officials have asked you to change the date of transcription to match the date of the report so that the record will look good to the evaluators.

What is your response? Explain your answer.

Otorhinolaryngology Abbreviations

AC	air conduction
AD	right ear
AS	left ear
AU	both ears
BC	bone conduction
BOM	bilateral otitis media
db, dB	decibel
EENT	eyes, ears, nose, throat
EES	erythromycin ethylsuccinate
ENG	electronystagmography
ENT	ears, nose, throat
ETF	eustachian tubal function

FESS	functional endoscopic sinus surgery
HD	hearing distance
IAC	internal auditory canal
IRT	infrared tympanic thermometry
mp	mouthpiece
NSR	nasal septal reconstruction
OM	otitis media
oto	otology
PE tube	polyethylene tube
PND	postnasal drip
PORP	partial ossicular replacement prosthesis
SAL	sensory acuity level
SD	septal defect
SISI	short increment sensitivity index
SMR	submucous resection
SOM	serous otitis media
Staph	Staphylococcus
Strep	Streptococcus
T&A	tonsillectomy and adenoidectomy
TM	tympanic membrane
TMJ	temporomandibular joint
TORP	total ossicular replacement prosthesis
URI	upper respiratory infection
ZMC	zygomaticomalar

Anatomic Illustrations

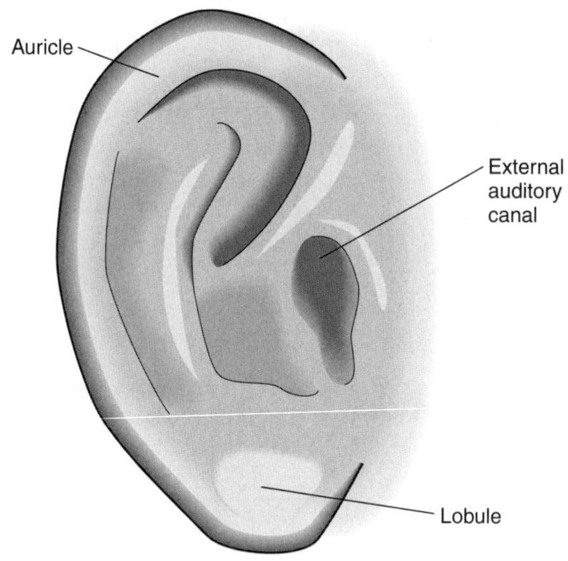

16–1 EXTERNAL VIEW OF THE EAR

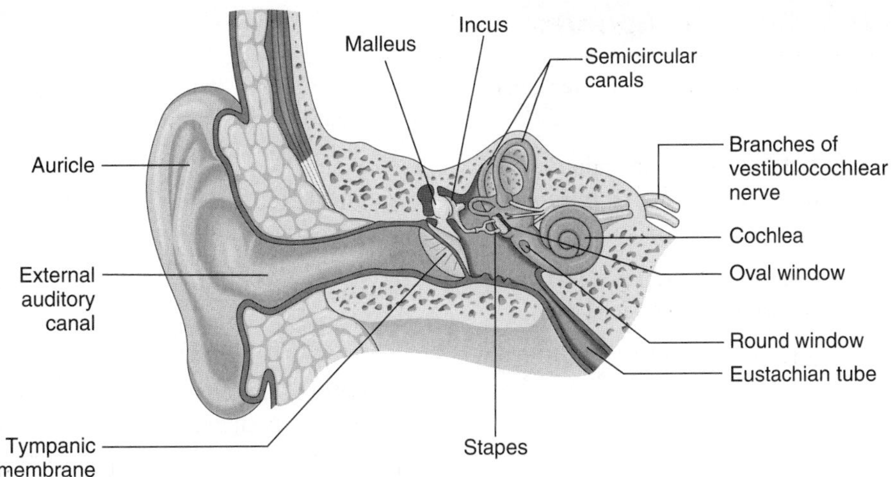

16–2 STRUCTURES OF THE EAR

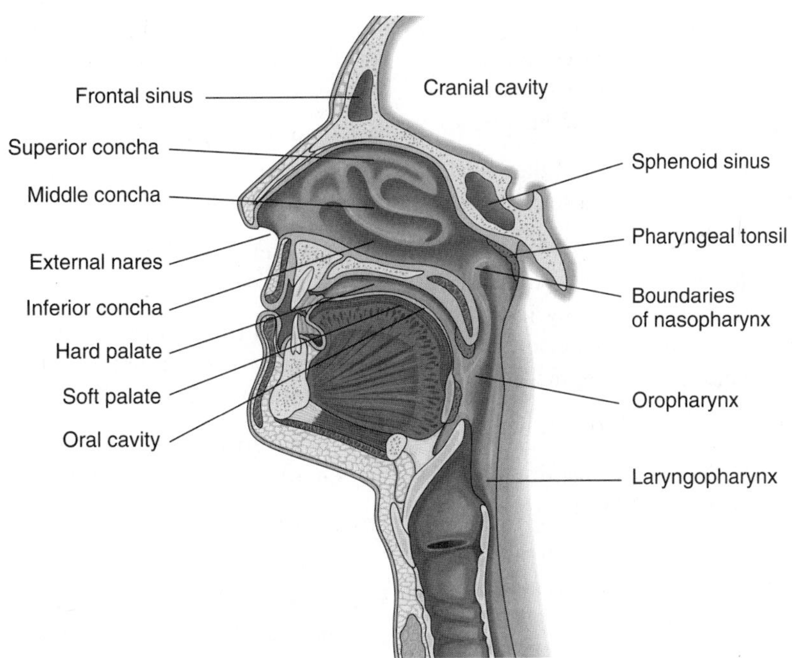

16–3 SAGITTAL SECTION OF THE FACE AND NECK, SHOWING THE NOSE, NASAL CAVITY, AND PHARYNX

Otorhinolaryngology Terminology

a

adenoidectomy (ad"-eh-noyd-ek'-tuh-mē) – removal of adenoids

antrostomy (an-trahs'-tuh-mē) – the operation of making an opening into an antrum for purposes of drainage

attic (at'-ik) – a cavity situated on the tegmental wall of the tympanic cavity, just above the facial canal

c

Caldwell-Luc procedure (kald'-wel-look' prō-sēd'-jur) – sinus operation

cerumen (seh-roo'-men) – earwax

cheiloschisis (kī-lahs'-kih-sis) – harelip

cheilosis (kī-lō'-sis) – a condition marked by fissuring and dry scaling of the vermilion surface of the lips and angles of the mouth

chorda tympani nerve (kōr'-duh tim'-puh-nī nurv) – a nerve originating from the facial nerve and distributed to the submandibular, sublingual, and lingual glands and the anterior two-thirds of the tongue

Chvostek's sign (vahs'-teks sīn) – a spasm of the facial muscles resulting from tapping the muscles or the branches of the facial nerve

Coakley's operation (kōk'-lēz op-er-ā'-shun) – an operation for disease of the frontal sinus by incising through the cheek, removing the anterior wall, and curetting away the mucous membrane

cochlea (kōk'-lē-uh) – the essential organ of hearing

concha (kahng'-kuh) – a structure or part that resembles a shell in shape; also called the turbinate

corniculum laryngis (kōr-nik'-yoo-lum lār"-in'-jis) – a conical nodule of elastic cartilage surmounting the apex of each arytenoid cartilage

coryza (kō-rī'-zuh) – head cold

cricoid (krī'-koyd) – the cricoid cartilage; a ring-like cartilage forming the lower and back part of the larynx

cricoidectomy (krī"-koy-dek'-tuh-mē) – complete removal of the cricoid cartilage

d

decibel (deh'-sih-bul) – a unit used to express the ratio of two powers; one decibel is equal to approximately the smallest difference in acoustic power that the human ear can detect

desensitization (dē-sen"-sih-tih-zā'-shun) – a condition in which the organism does not react immunologically to a specific antigen

e

endolymphatic (en"-dō-lim-fat'-ik) – pertaining to the endolymph, the fluid contained in the membranous labyrinth of the ear

epiglottis (ep"-ih-glah'-tis) – the lid-like cartilaginous structure overhanging the entrance to the larynx; prevents food from entering the larynx and trachea while swallowing

epistaxis (ep"-ih-stak'-sis) – nosebleed

epitympanum (ep"-ē-tim'-puh-num) – the upper portion of the tympanic cavity above the tympanic membrane; contains the head of the malleus and the body of the incus

ethmoidectomy (eth"-moy-dek'-tuh-mē) – removal of ethmoid cells that open into the nasal cavity

eustachian tube (auditory tube) (yoo-stā'-shun OR yoo-stā'-kē-un toob) (aw'-dih-tōr"-ē toob) – a canal connecting the nasopharynx and the middle ear cavity

external auditory canal (eks'-tur"-nul aw'-dih-tōr-ē kuh-nal') – the canal that leads from the pinna to the tympanic membrane

extirpate (eks'-tur-pāt) – to completely remove an organ or a tissue

f

fenestration (fen"-eh-strā'-shun) – the surgical creation of a new opening in the labyrinth of the ear for the restoration of hearing in cases of otosclerosis

follicular tonsillitis (fō-lik'-yoo-lur tahn"-sih-lī'-tis) – an acute inflammation of the tonsils and their crypts

fronto-occipital (frun"-tō-ok-sip'-ih-tul) – pertaining to the forehead and the occiput

frontoparietal (frun"-tō-pah-rī'-eh-tul) – pertaining to the frontal and parietal bones

frontotemporal (frun"-tō-tem'-pō-rul) – pertaining to the frontal and temporal bones

g

geniohyoid (jē"-nē-ō-hī'-oyd) – pertaining to the chin and hyoid bone

genyantralgia (jen"-ē-an-tral'-jē-uh) – pain in the maxillary sinus

glossoepiglottic (glahs"-ō-ep-ih-glah'-tik) – pertaining to the tongue and epiglottis

glossopharyngeal (glah"-sō-făr-in'-jē-ul) – pertaining to the tongue and the pharynx

glossotomy (glah-sot'-uh-mē) – incision into the tongue

h

hemilaryngectomy (hem"-ē-lăr"-in-jek'-tuh-mē) – excision of one-half of the larynx

hyoid bone (hī'-oyd bōn) – a horseshoe-shaped bone situated at the base of the tongue, just above the thyroid cartilage

hypopharynx (hī"-pō-făr'-inks) – the division of the pharynx that lies below the upper edge of the epiglottis and opens into the larynx and esophagus

i

in situ (in sit'-yoo, in sī'-tyoo) – in the natural or normal place

incudostapedial (ing"-kyoo-dō-stah-pē'-dē-ul) – pertaining to the incus and stapes

incus (ing'-kus) – the middle of the three bones of the ear; with the stapes and malleus, conducts vibrations from the tympanic membrane to the inner ear; also called the *anvil*

k

Kiesselbach's area (kē'-sul-bahks ā'-rē-uh) – the nose

l

labyrinth (lab'-ih-rinth) – a system of intercommunicating cavities or canals, especially that constituting the internal ear

laryngitis (lăr"-in-jī'-tis) – an inflammation of the mucous membrane lining the larynx accompanied by edema of the vocal cords

laryngocentesis (lah-ring"-gō-sen-tē'-sis) – surgical puncture of the larynx

laryngopharyngectomy (lah-ring"-gō-făr"-in-jek'-tuh-mē) – excision of the larynx and pharynx

laryngoscopy (lăr"-ing-gahs'-kuh-pē) – examination of the interior of the larynx, especially that performed with the laryngoscope

lymphoepithelioma (lim"-fō-ep"-ih-thē"-lē-ō'-muh) – a poorly differentiated radiosensitive squamous cell carcinoma involving lymphoid tissue of the region of the tonsils and nasopharynx

m

malleus (mal'-ē-us) – the largest of the auditory bones and the one attached to the membrana tympani; also called the *hammer* because of its shape

membrana tympani (mem-brā'-nuh tim'-puh-nī) – eardrum

Meniere's disease (men"-ē-ārz' dih-zēz') – deafness, tinnitus, and vertigo resulting from nonsuppurative disease of the labyrinth

myasthenia gravis (mī"-as-thē'-nē-uh gra'-vis) – a syndrome of fatigue and exhaustion of the muscular system marked by progressive paralysis of muscles without sensory disturbance or atrophy; may affect any muscle of the body, but especially those of the face, lips, tongue, throat, and neck

myringotomy (mir"-in-got'-uh-mē) – surgical incision of the eardrum in an area that tends to heal readily, to avoid spontaneous rupture at a site that rarely closes

n

nasolacrimal (nā"-zō-lak'-rih-mul) – pertaining to the nose and lacrimal apparatus

o

occipitomastoid (ok-sip"-ih-tō-mas'-toyd) – pertaining to the occipital bone and the mastoid process

olfactory center (ol-fak'-tuh-rē sen'-tur) – the center of smell

oropharynx (ō"-rō-făr'-inks) – division of the pharynx that lies between the soft palate and the upper edge of the epiglottis

ossicle (ahss'-ih-kul) – a small bone

otalgia (ō-tal'-jē-uh) – earache; pain in the ear

otitis media (ō-tī'-tis mē'-dē-uh) – inflammation of the middle ear

otorhinolaryngology (ō"-tō-rī"-nō-lăr"-ing-gahl'-uh-jē) – the branch of medicine dealing with diseases of the ear, nose, and throat; also called *otolaryngology*

otorrhagia (ō"-tō-rā'-jē-uh) – bleeding from the ear

otorrhea (ō"-tō-rē'-uh) – purulent drainage from the ear

otosclerosis (ō"-tō-skleh-rō'-sis) – a progressive condition in which the normal bone of the inner ear is replaced by abnormal osseous tissue

p

palatoglossal (pal"-uh-tō-glahs'-ul) – pertaining to the palate and tongue

palatopharyngeal (pal"-uh-tō-fah-rin'-jē-ul) – pertaining to the palate and pharynx

pansinusitis (pan"-sī-nuh-sī'-tis) – inflammation of all the sinuses

paracentesis tympani (păr"-uh-sen-tē'-sis tim'-puh-nī) – incision of the tympanic membrane for drainage or irrigation

parotid (puh-rot'-id) – situated or occurring near the ear, as the parotid gland

parotitis (păr"-ō-tī'-tis) – inflammation of the parotid gland

perilymphatic (păr"-ē-lim-fat'-ik) – pertaining to the perilymph, or around a lymphatic vessel

peritonsillar abscess (pār"-ī-tahn'-sih-lur ab'-sehss) – abscess near or around a tonsil; infection extends from the tonsil to form an abscess in surrounding tissue

pharyngoplegia (făr"-ing-gō-plē'-jē-uh) – paralysis of the muscles of the pharynx

piriform sinus (pĕr'-ih-form sī'-nus) – pear-shaped sinus

preauricular (prē"-aw-rik'-yoo-lur) – situated in front of the auricle of the ear

presbycusis (prez"-bī-kyoo'-sis) – a progressive, bilateral hearing loss occurring with age

pseudocholesteatoma (soo"-dō-kō"-les-tē-uh-tō'-muh) – a mass of cornified epithelial cells resembling cholesteatoma in the tympanic cavity in chronic middle ear inflammation

r

rhinitis (rī-nī'-tis) – an inflammatory condition of the mucous membranes of the nose and accessory sinuses

rhinorrhea (rī"-nō-rē'-uh) – "runny nose"

Rosenmuller's fossa (rō'-zen-mil"-erz fah'-suh) – a slit-like depression in the pharyngeal wall behind the opening of the eustachian tube

S

Scarpa's membrane (skar'-puhz mem'-brān) – secondary tympanic membrane

secretory otitis media (sē-krē'-tōr-ē [OR sē'-kreh-tōr-ē] ō-tī'-tis mē'-dē-uh) – thick, cloudy, viscous exudate in the middle ear containing cells and mucous strands

septoplasty (sep'-tō-plas"-tē) – plastic surgery on the nasal septum to correct defects or deformities

septorhinoplasty (sep"-tō-rī'-nō-plas"-tē) – a combined operation to repair defects or deformities of the nasal septum and of the external nasal pyramid

serous otitis media (sē'-rus ō-tī'-tis mē'-dē-uh) – thin, clear, amber fluid in the middle ear

Silastic tube (sī-las'-tik toob) – trademark for polymeric silicone substance having the properties of rubber; used in surgical prostheses

sphenopalatine (sfē"-nō-pal'-uh-tīn) – pertaining to or in relation with the sphenoid and palatine bones

stapedectomy (stā"-pē-dek'-tuh-mē) – complete removal of the stapes

stapes (stā'-pēz) – the innermost of the auditory ossicles, shaped somewhat like a stirrup; also called the *stirrup*

staphyledema (staf"-il-ē-dē'-muh) – an enlargement or swollen part of the uvula

Stensen's duct, foramen (sten'-senz dukt, fō-rā'-men) – the duct that drains the parotid gland and empties into the oral cavity opposite the second superior molar

t

temporomandibular (tem"-pō-rō-man-dib'-yoo-lur) – pertaining to the temporal bone and the mandible

thyromegaly (thī"-rō-meg'-uh-lē) – enlargement of the thyroid gland; goiter

tinnitus (tih-nī'-tus) – a noise in the ears, as ringing, buzzing, roaring, clicking, and the like

tympanic membrane (tim-pan'-ik mem'-brān) – eardrum; the membrane separating the external from the middle ear

tympanitis (tim"-puh-nī'-tis) – inflammation of the eardrum

tympanoeustachian (tim"-puh-nō-yoo-stā'-kē-un [OR -yoo-stā'-shun]) – pertaining to the tympanic cavity and auditory tube

tympanomandibular (tim"-puh-nō-man-dib'-yoo-lur) – pertaining to the middle ear and the mandible

tympanomastoiditis (tim'-puh-nō-mas"-toy-dī'-tis) – inflammation of the middle ear and the pneumatic cells of the mastoid process

tympanoplasty (tim'-puh-nō-plas"-tē) – surgical reconstruction of the hearing mechanism of the middle ear

tympanotomy tube (tim"-puh-naht'-uh-mē toob) – tube inserted in the membrane tympani

tympanum (tim'-puh-num) – middle ear

u

uvula (yoo'-vyoo-luh) – the soft, fleshy mass hanging from the soft palate

V

vallecula (vah-lek'-yoo-luh) – the depression between the epiglottis and the root of the tongue on either side

vomer (vō'-mer) – the unpaired flat bone that forms the inferior and posterior part of the nasal septum

Z

zygomaticomaxillary (zī"-gō-mat"-ih-kō-mak'-sih-lăr"-ē) – pertaining to the zygoma and maxilla

Transcription Tips

When transcribing dictation in otorhinolaryngology (ENT), you should be familiar with the equipment, examination techniques, and mechanical testing employed when evaluating the ears, nose, and throat areas, particularly in an office setting. An in-depth knowledge of ENT terminology and combining forms and/or roots will also be beneficial.

The nose is more than a passageway for movement of air into the lungs; it also preconditions the air by warming it, humidifying it, and cleaning it. The pharynx, commonly referred to as the throat, separates into the trachea and esophagus immediately above the larynx.

Equipment

audiophone – instrument that conducts sound to the auditory nerve through teeth or bone

esophagoscope – instrument used to examine the esophagus

myringoscope – instrument used to examine the eardrum

nasal speculum – instrument used to examine the nose

otoscope – instrument used to examine the ear

Thermoscan instant thermometer – device used to take the temperature in the ear

Tests and/or Procedures

audiogram – a record produced when hearing is measured

Bekesy, Doerfler-Stewart, Lombard, Rinne, Weber – hearing tests

laryngoscopy – visual examination of the larynx

Roots and/or Combining Forms

Root	Meaning	Root	Meaning
acouso	hearing	neuro, neur	nerve
adeno, aden	gland	oligo	few, deficient
aero, aer	air, gas	oro	mouth
audio	hearing, the sense of hearing	ossiculo	ossicle
		osteo, oste	bone
auro, auriculo	ear	oto, ot	ear
cephalo, cephal	head	patho	disease
cheilo, cheil	lip	pharyngo	pharynx
chordo	cord	phono, phon	sound
cochleo	cochlea	py, pyo	pus
erythro	red	rhino, rhin	nose
eu	normal	salpingo	eustachian tube, auditory tube
glosso, gloss	tongue		
laryngo	larynx	stapedo	stapes
leuco, leuko	white	steno	narrowed
mastoido	mastoid process	tracheo	trachea
micro, micr	small	tropho	nourishment
myringo	eardrum, tympanic membrane	tympano	eardrum, middle ear
		vaso	vessel
naso	nose	veno	vein

Confusing Terms

aural – pertaining to the ear
oral – pertaining to the mouth

canker – an ulceration, primarily of the mouth and lips
chancre – the primary lesion of syphilis

facial – pertaining to the face
fascial – pertaining to the fascia

malleolus – a bone of the ankle
malleus – a bone of the ear

mucous (adj) – pertaining to or resembling mucus
mucus (n) – secretion of the mucous membrane

nuchal – the back, nape, or scruff of the neck
knuckle – dorsal aspect of any phalangeal joint

Supportive Web Sites

http://medmark.org/
Click on "Otorhinolaryngology," then scroll down to the section entitled "For Consumers" and select links of interest.

www.cancer.gov
Click on "Cancer Information," "Types of Cancer," then links of interest.

www.my.webmd.com
Under "Medical Info," click on "Diseases and Conditions"; select related links as desired.

www.nlm.nih.gov
Click on "Health Information," then "MEDLINEplus" and "Health Topics"; select "Ear, Nose, & Throat" under "Diseases and Conditions" for links of interest.

Index of Otorhinolaryngology Reports

(see table of contents for audio information)

Exercise #	*Patient Name*	*Report/Procedure*
TE#1	Almond, Duane	Bilateral myringotomy
TE#2	Edwards, Betty Jean	Tonsillectomy and adenoidectomy
TE#3	Riveria, Esmelda	Cochlear implantation
TE#4	Riveria, Esmelda	Repositioning of cochlear implant
TE#5	Weams, Suzette	Microlaryngoscopy
TE#6	Schneider, Carolyn	Tympanoplasty
TE#7	Yougo, Herman	Flexible bronchoscopy
TE#8	Weible, Katherine	Bilateral FESS
TE#9	Toufo, Ernest	Bilateral endoscopic polypectomy

CHAPTER 17
OPHTHALMOLOGY

Introduction

The specialized field of medicine that deals with medical and surgical disorders of the eyes, as well as the treatment thereof, is known as *ophthalmology.* Physicians specializing in this field are called ophthalmologists and must have an MD degree, of course, plus three to five years of specialized training in a hospital.

Various anatomical structures within the eye cooperate to make sight possible. When light enters the eye, it passes through the cornea, pupil, lens, and vitreous body, thereby stimulating sensory receptors on the retina or innermost layer of the eye.

External structures of the eye are the *eyelids; conjunctiva; orbit; lacrimal gland, sac, canaliculi,* and *nasolacrimal duct; orbit;* and *muscles. Internal structures* are the *eyeball* and its various parts and the *nerve fibers* that connect the eyeball to the brain. The *sclera* and the *cornea* compose the outer layer of the eyeball. The *iris, ciliary body,* and *choroid* make up the middle layer. The inner layer is composed of the *retina.* The *lens* is located behind the iris and is suspended by ligaments.

Ophthalmologists treat eye diseases such as *glaucoma, tumors,* and *infections.* The most frequently performed surgical procedure on the eye for people 65 years of age and older is for removal of cataracts. A relatively new procedure performed by ophthalmologists is *LASIK.* This procedure can improve vision for patients with nearsightedness, farsightedness, or astigmatism.

In addition to performing surgical procedures, ophthalmologists prescribe glasses to correct visual problems such as *nearsightedness, farsightedness, astigmatism,* and other visual defects.

A distinction should be made between the *ophthalmologist,* the *optometrist,* and the *optician.* Whereas the ophthalmologist, or oculist as one is sometimes called, prescribes glasses and treats diseases of the eyes, the optometrist is skilled in measuring a patient's vision and prescribing glasses. This physician may also prescribe eye exercises to improve vision or correct visual defects.

When given the prescription by an optometrist or oculist, the optician makes and sells the proper glasses. An optometrist is usually also an optician, whereas the ophthalmologist is not.

Critical Thinking Exercise

You are under a quality assurance program and are expected to produce 98% accuracy. Your score has fallen from 98% to 97.6% according to the latest review, but you disagree with the way the quality specialist has scored your documents.

How would you handle this situation?

Ophthalmology Abbreviations

AC	anterior chamber
ALP	argon laser photocoagulation
ALT	argon laser trabeculoplasty
ARC	anomalous retinal correspondence
AV	arteriovenous
BDR	background diabetic retinopathy
BLP	bare light perception
BRVO	branch retinal vein occlusion

CACG	chronic angle closure glaucoma
CME	cystoid macular edema
CNM	choroidal neovascular membrane
COAG	chronic open angle glaucoma
CRAO	chronic (or central) retinal artery occlusion
CRVO	central retinal vein occlusion
D	diopter
DME	diabetic macular edema
DVA	distance visual acuity
ECCE	extracapsular cataract extraction
EM	emmetropia
EOG	electro-oculogram
EOM	extraocular movement; extraocular muscles
ERG	electroretinogram
ERM	epiretinal membrane
ET	esotropia
GPC	giant papillary conjunctivitis
HT	hypermetropia, hypertropia
ICCE	intracapsular cataract cryoextraction
IOL	intraocular lens
IOP	intraocular pressure
L&A, l/a	light and accommodation
LASER	light amplification by stimulated emission of radiation
LTP	laser trabeculoplasty
MY	myopia
NLP	no light perception
NPC	near point of convergence
NRC	normal retinal correspondence
NVA	near visual acuity
NVG	neovascular glaucoma
OD, RE	oculus dexter (right eye)
OS, LE	oculus sinister (left eye)
OU	oculus uterque (each eye OR both eyes)
PD	prism diopter
PDR	proliferative diabetic retinopathy
PERLA	pupils equal, react to light and accommodation
PERRLA	pupils equal, round, and react to light and accommodation
PI	peripheral iridectomy
PK	penetrating keratoplasty
PPLV	pars plana lensectomy-vitrectomy
PPV	pars plana vitrectomy
PRH	preretinal hemorrhage
PRK	photorefractive keratectomy
PRP	panretinal photocoagulation
PVD	posterior vitreous detachment
RB	retinoblastoma
RD	retinal detachment
REM	rapid eye movement
RP	retinitis
RPE	retinal pigment epithelion
RPED	retinal pigment epithelial detachment
SMD	senile macular degeneration
SOAG	secondary open angle glaucoma
SRF	subretinal fluid
SRNVM	subretinal neovascular membrane
ST	esotropia
TOD	tension of right eye
TOS	tension of left eye
TRD	traction retinal detachment
VA	visual acuity
VC	acuity of color vision
VH	vitreous hemorrhage
VF	visual field
VOU	vision of each eye
XT	exotropia
+	plus or convex
–	minus or concave

Anatomic Illustrations

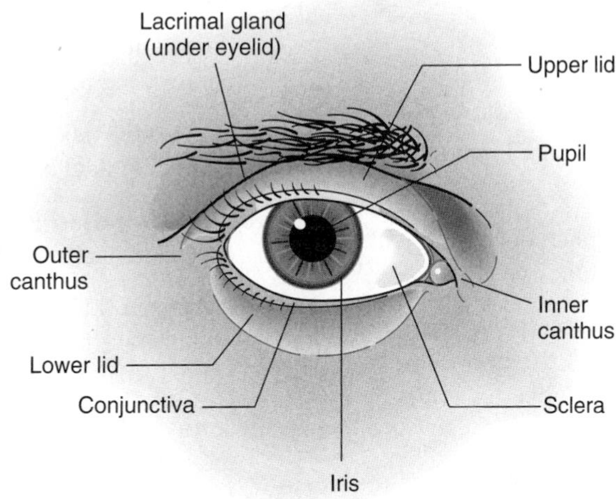

17–1 EXTERNAL VIEW OF THE EYE

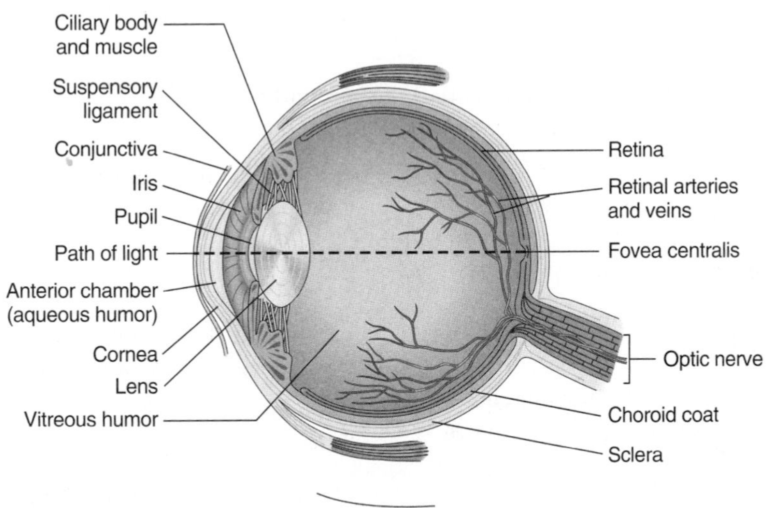

17–2 LATERAL VIEW OF THE EYEBALL INTERIOR

Ophthalmology Terminology

a

amaurosis (am"-aw-rō'-sis) – blindness, especially blindness occurring without apparent lesion of the eye, as from disease of the optic nerve, spine, or brain

amaurosis centralis (am"-aw-rō'-sis sen-tral'-is) – blindness due to disease of the central nervous system

amblyopia (am"-blē-ō'-pē-uh) – dimness of vision without detectable organic lesion of the eye

ametropia (am"-eh-trō'-pē-uh) – discrepancy between the size and refractive powers of the eye, such that images are not brought to a proper focus on the retina

anisocoria (an"-ih-sō-kōr'-ē-uh) – inequality of the pupils in diameter

aphakia (ā-fā'-kē-uh) – absence of the lens of the eye; may occur congenitally or from trauma but is most commonly caused by extraction of a cataract

aqueous humor (ā'-kwē-us hyoo'-mur) – clear fluid of the eyeball between the cornea and the lens

Argyll-Robertson pupil (ar-gī l' rob'-ert-sun pyoo'-pul) – a pupil that is miotic and that responds to accommodation effort, but not to light

asthenopia (as"-thē-nō'-pē-uh) – weakness or easy fatigue of the visual organs, attended by pain in the eyes, headache, dimness of vision, etc.

astigmatism (ah-stig'-muh-tizm) – abnormal curvature of the lens or cornea of the eye

b

Bitot's spots (bē'-tōz spahtz) – superficial, foamy gray, triangular spots on the conjunctiva, consisting of keratinized epithelium

blepharitis (blef"-uh-rī'-tis) – inflammation of the eyelids

blepharoplegia (blef"-uh-rō-plē'-jē-uh) – paralysis of an eyelid

blepharorrhaphy (blef"-uh-rōr'-uh-fē) – the operation of suturing the eyelids together

c

canthotomy (kan-thaht'-uh-mē) – surgical division of the outer canthus

canthus (kan'-thus) – either angle at the ends of the eyelid

cataract (kat'-uh-rakt) – an opacity of the lens of the eye

cataract, cerulean (kat'-uh-rakt, seh-roo'-lē-en) – blue cataract

cataract, intumescent (kat'-uh-rakt, in-too-mess'-ent) – a cataract in which the lens is swollen and opaque

chorioretinal (kō"-rē-ō-ret'-ih-nul) – pertaining to the choroid and retina

choroideremia (kō"-roy-der-ē'-mē-uh) – hereditary primary choroidal degeneration

choroiditis (kō"-royd-ī'-tis) – inflammation of the choroid and ciliary processes

chromatopsia (krō"-muh-top'-sē-uh) – a visual defect in which colorless objects appear to be tinged with color

ciliectomy (sil"-ē-ek'-tuh-mē) – excision of a portion of the ciliary margin of the eyelid and the roots of the lashes

cilium (sil'-ē-um) – eyelash

conjunctiva (kahn"-junk-tī'-vuh) – the delicate membrane lining the eyelids and the front of the eyeballs

conjunctivitis (kun-junk"-tih-vī'-tis) – inflammation of the conjunctiva

corectopia (kōr-ek-tō'-pē-uh) – abnormal situation of the pupil

corneal abscission (kōr'-nē-ul ab-sish'-un) – excision of the prominence of the cornea in staphyloma

corneoiritis (kōr"-nē-ō-ī-rī'-tis) – inflammation of the cornea and iris

corneosclera (kōr"-nē-ō-skleh'-ruh) – the cornea and sclera regarded as forming one organ

cyclectomy (sī-klek'-tuh-mē) – excision of a portion of the ciliary border

cyclochoroiditis (sī"-klō-kō"-royd-ī'-tis) – inflammation of the choroid and ciliary body

cyclodiathermy (sī"-klō-dī'-uh-ther"-mē) – destruction of a portion of the ciliary body by diathermy; employed as therapy in cases of glaucoma

d

dacryoadenitis (dak"-rē-ō-ad"-eh-nī'-tis) – inflammation of a lacrimal gland

dacryocystoptosis (dak"-rē-ō-sis"-top-tō'-sis) – prolapse or downward displacement of the lacrimal sac

dacryops (dak'-rē-ahps) – a watery state of the eye

diopsimeter (dī"-ahp-sim'-eh-tur) – a device for measuring the field of vision

diplopia (di-plō'-pē-uh) – the perception of two images of a single object

discission (dis-sizh'-un) – the surgical rupturing of the capsule so that the aqueous humor may gain access to the lens of the eye

dysmegalopsia (dis"-meg-uh-lop'-sē-uh) – a disturbance of the visual appreciation of the size of objects in which they appear larger than they are

dysopia (dis-ō'-pē-uh) – defective vision

e

embryotoxon (em"-brē-ō-tok'-sun) – a ring-like opacity of the margin of the cornea

emmetropia (em-eh-trō'-pē-uh) – the normal condition of the eye as far as refraction is concerned

endophthalmitis (en"-dahf-thal-mī'-tis) – inflammation involving the ocular cavities and their adjacent structures

enophthalmos (en-ahf-thal'-mohs) – a backward displacement of the eyeball into the orbit

enucleation (ē-noo"-klē-ā"-shun) – excision of the eyeball

epiphora (ē-pif'-ur-uh) – an abnormal overflow of tears down the cheek, mainly due to stricture of the lacrimal passages

episcleritis (ep"-ih-skleh-rī'-tis) – inflammation of the tissues overlying the sclera

erysiphake (er-is'-ih-fāk) – an instrument for removing the lens in cataract by suction

euchromatopsy (yoo-krō'-muh-top"-sē) – normal color vision

evisceration (ē-viss"-er-ā'-shun) – removal of the contents of the eyeball, with the sclera being left intact

exophthalmometer (ek"-sahf-thal-mahm'-eh-tur) – an instrument for measuring the amount of exophthalmos

exophthalmos (ek"-sahf-thal'-mohs) – abnormal protrusion of the eyeball

g

glaucoma (glaw-kō'-muh) – a group of eye diseases characterized by an increase in intraocular pressure; causes pathological changes in the optic disk and typical defects in the field of vision

goniotomy (gahn"-ē-aht'-uh-mē) – Barkan's operation for a type of glaucoma characterized by an open angle and normal depth of the anterior chamber

h

hemeralopia (hem"-er-uh-lō'-pē-uh) – day blindness; defective vision in a bright light

hemianopia (hem"-ē-ah-nō'-pē-uh) – defective vision or blindness in half of the visual field

heterochromia (het"-er-ō-krō'-mē-uh) – diversity of color in a part or parts that should normally be of one color

homokeratoplasty (hō"-mō-kār'-uh-tō-plas"-tē) – corneal grafting with tissue derived from another individual of the same species

hordeolum (hōr-dē'-ō-lum) – a stye

hyperopia (hī"-per-ō'-pē-uh) – farsightedness

hyphema (hī-fē'-muh) – hemorrhage within the anterior chamber of the eye

hypoxic (hī-pok'-sik) – pertaining to or characterized by hypoxia, low oxygen content or tension

i

iridectomize (ir"-ih-dek'-tuh-mīz) – to remove part of the iris by excision

iridectomy (ir"-ih-dek'-tuh-mē) – surgical excision of part of the iris

iridencleisis (ir"-ih-den-klī'-sis) – the surgical creation of a permanent drain by incarceration of a slip of the iris within a corneal or limbal incision to act as a wick through which the aqueous humor is filtered from the anterior chamber to the subconjunctival tissues; done to reduce intraocular pressure

iridesis (ī-rih'-dē-sis) – the operation of repositioning the pupil by bringing a sector of the iris through a corneal or limbal incision and fixing the sector with a suture

iridocorneosclerectomy (ir"-ih-dō-kōr"-nē-ō-skleh-rek'-tuh-mē) – surgical incision of a portion of the iris, cornea, and sclera for glaucoma

iridocyclectomy (ir"-ih-dō-sī-klek'-tuh-mē) – surgical removal of a portion of the iris and of the ciliary body

iridokeratitis (ir"-ih-dō-kār"-uh-tī'-tis) – inflammation of the iris and cornea

iridomesodialysis (ir"-ih-dō-mē"-sō-dī-al'-ih-sis) – surgical loosening of adhesions around the inner edge of the iris

iridotomy (ir"-ih-daht'-uh-mē) – incision of the iris, as in creating an artificial pupil

Ishihara's test (ish"-ih-hah"-rahz tehst) – a test for color vision made by the use of a series of plates composed of round dots of various sizes and colors

isopia (ī-sō'-pē-uh) – equality of vision in the two eyes

keratectasia (kār"-uh-tek-tā'-zē-uh) – protrusion of a thinned, scarred cornea

keratoconjunctivitis (kār"-uh-tō-kun-junk"-tih-vī'-tis) – inflammation of the cornea and iris

keratometry (kār"-uh-tom'-eh-trē) – the measurement of the cornea made by an instrument called a keratometer, which measures the curve of the cornea

kerectomy (keh-rek'-tuh-mē) – surgical removal of a part of the cornea

lenticulo-optic (len-tik"-yoo-lō-ahp'-tik) – pertaining to the lenticular nucleus and the optic thalamus

leukokoria (loo"-kō-kō'-rē-uh) – a condition characterized by appearance of a whitish reflex or mass in the pupillary area behind the lens

levator palpebrae muscle (leh-va'-tōr pal'-pē-brē mus'-ul) – a muscle that raises the upper eyelid

megalophthalmos (meg"-uh-lahf-thal'-mohs) – abnormally large size of the eyes

metamorphopsia (met"-uh-mōr-fahp'-sē-uh) – a disturbance of vision in which objects are seen as distorted in shape

microphthalmia (mī"-krawf-thal'-mē-uh) – abnormal smallness of the eyes

myopia (mī-ō'-pē-uh) – nearsightedness

nyctalopia (nik"-tuh-lō'-pē-uh) – night blindness

nystagmus (nih-stag'-mus) – an involuntary, rapid movement of the eyeball

ophthalmodynamometer (awf-thal"-mō-dī"-nuh-mahm'-eh-ter) – an instrument for measuring the retinal arterial pressure

ophthalmodynia (awf-thal"-mō-dī'-nē-uh) – pain in the eye

ophthalmoplegia (awf-thal"-mō-plē'-jē-uh) – inability to move the eye

ophthalmotropometer (awf-thal"-mō-trō-pahm'-eh-ter) – an instrument for measuring eye movements

perimetry (peh-rim'-eh-trē) – determination of the extent of the peripheral visual field by use of a perimeter

phacoemulsification (fa'-kō-ē-mul'-sih-fih-kā-shun) – the surgical process of using an ultrasonic device to disintegrate a cataract, which is then aspirated and removed; called the "no-stitch surgery"

photo-ophthalmia (fō"-tō-awf-thal'-mē-uh) – ophthalmia caused by intense light, such as electric light, rays of welding arc, or reflection from snow

photocoagulation (laser treatment) (fō"-tō-kō-ag"-yoo-lā'-shun) – condensation of protein material by the controlled use of light rays

phthisis bulbi (tī'-sis bul'-bē) – shrinkage and wasting of the eyeball

pinguecula (ping-gwek'-yoo-luh) – a yellowish spot of proliferation on the bulbar conjunctiva near the sclerocorneal junction, usually on the nasal side

proptosis (prahp-tō'-sis) – a forward displacement or bulging, especially of the eye

Purkinje-Sanson images (pur-kin'-jē-sah-saw' ih-muh-jez) – reflected images formed on the anterior surface of the cornea and the anterior and posterior surfaces of the crystalline lens

radial keratotomy (rā'-dē-ul kār"-uh-taht'-uh-mē) – surgical procedure where slit-like cuts are made in the cornea to flatten it for a correction of myopia (nearsightedness)

retinopathy (ret"-ih-nahp'-uh-thē) – any noninflammatory disease of the retina

retrobulbar (reh"-trō-bul'-bur) – behind the eyeball

Schiotz's tonometer (shē-uts'-ez tuh-nahm'-eh-tur) – an instrument that registers intraocular pressure by direct application to the cornea

sclerectoiridectomy (skleh-rek"-tō-ir"-ih-dek'-tuh-mē) – operation that excises a portion of the sclera and of the iris for glaucoma

sclerectomy (skleh-rek'-tuh-mē) – excision of the sclera by scissors, by punch, or by trephining

scleritis (skleh-rī'-tis) – inflammation of the sclera

scleronyxis (skleh"-rō-nik'-sis) – surgical puncture of the sclera

scotoma (skō-tō'-muh) – an area of depressed vision within the visual field, surrounded by an area of less depressed or of normal vision

sphincterectomy (sfingk"-ter-ek'-tuh-mē) – excision of any sphincter, such as the sphincter iridis

strabismus (struh-biz'-mus) – cross eye

stye (sty) (stī) – a localized inflammatory swelling of one of several sebaceous glands of the eyelid

synchysis (sin'-kih-sis) – a softening or fluid condition of the vitreous body of the eye

trichiasis (trih-kī'-uh-sis) – the condition of ingrowing eyelashes

ulectomy (yoo-lek'-tuh-mē) – excision of scar tissue (i.e., in secondary iridectomy)

uvea (yoo'-vē-uh) – the iris, ciliary body, and choroid considered together

Van Lint akinesia (van lihnt ā"-kih-nē'-sē-uh) – a type of seventh nerve block, by local anesthetic, to stop the patient from closing the lids during an operation

vitrectomy (vih-trek'-tuh-mē) – excision of the vitreous body

vitreous (vih'-trē-us) – glass-like or hyaline; often used alone to designate the vitreous body of the eye

vitreous humor (vih'-trē-us hyoo'-mur) – the fluid that fills the inner space of the eyeball between the lens and retina

Weiss' procedure (vīs' prō-cē-jur) – blepharoplasty

xanthelasma (zan"-theh-laz'-muh) – the commonest form of xanthoma, affecting the eyelids and characterized by soft yellowish spots or plaques

xerophthalmia (zē"-rawf-thal'-mē-uh) – dryness of the conjunctiva and cornea due to vitamin A deficiency

Transcription Tips

For greatest efficiency in transcribing ophthalmology dictation, you should be able to identify the major parts of the eye and their locations, external and internal examination procedures, abnormal conditions of the eye and associated structures, and typical surgical procedures.

External Examination Procedures
(examination of the eyes and adnexa without the aid of special apparatus)

color vision tests – tests done to determine the person's ability to perceive primary colors and shades of colors

refraction – a clinical measurement of the error of focus in an eye

Snellen chart – to determine visual acuity

visual fields – to determine function of retina, optic nerve, and optic pathways

Internal Examination Procedures
(examination of the eyes using special apparatus)

gonioscopy – direct visualization of the junction of the iris and cornea

ophthalmoscopic examination – the use of an ophthalmoscope to examine the interior of the eye

tonometry – the measurement of intraocular tension or pressure

Selected Operative Procedures

enucleation – removal of the entire eyeball

evisceration – removal of the eye contents but leaving the sclera and attached muscles intact

exenteration – removal of all orbital contents for certain malignancies

kerorefractive procedures – radial keratotomy and epikeratophakia

laser photocoagulation and cryotherapy treatments – laser treatment and cryocoagulation

surgeries

of the conjunctiva – pterygium excision, reformation of the cul-de-sac

of the cornea – keratoplasty (corneal transplant)

of the eyelids – canthotomy, plastic repair of entropion, plastic repair of blepharochalasis, blepharopigmentation, and eyebrow enhancement

for glaucoma – iridectomy, Elliot trephination, anterior and posterior lid sclerectomies, cyclodialysis, trabeculectomy, goniotomy, laser trabeculoplasty, argon laser iridotomy, cyclocryotherapy

of the lacrimal gland and apparatus – dacryocystorhinostomy

of the lens – cataract extraction (intracapsular method, extracapsular method, phacoemulsification)

for retinal detachment – episcleral technique, scleral resection

for strabismus – myectomy, tuck

vitrectomy – anterior vitrectomy, pars plana vitrectomy

Abnormalities of the Eyelids

ectropion – the margin of the lids

entropion – an inward turning of the lid margin

periorbital edema – soft swelling of both lids

ptosis – drooping of the upper lid

Selected Abnormal Eye Conditions

arcus senilis – a thin, grayish-white arc or circle not quite at the edge of the cornea

blepharitis – inflammation of the eyelid

chalazion – a beady nodule in an otherwise normal eyelid

corneal scar – a superficial grayish-white opacity on the cornea

dacryocystitis – inflammation of the tear sac(s)

pinguecula – a yellowish triangular nodule on the bulbar conjunctiva on either side of the iris

pterygium – a triangular thickening of the bulbar conjunctiva that grows slowly across the cornea

stye OR sty (acute hordeolum) – a painful, tender, red infection around a hair follicle of the eyelashes

xanthelasma – slightly raised, yellowish, well-circumscribed place in the skin

Diagnostic and/or Laboratory Tests

color vision tests – given to judge one's ability to identify differences in color

exophthalmometry – use of the exophthalmometer to measure the forward protrusion of the eye to evaluate an increase or decrease in exophthalmos

gonioscopy – use of a gonioscope to examine the anterior chamber of the eye for evaluation of ocular motility and rotation

keratometry – use of a keratometer to measure the cornea

ocular ultrasonography – uses high-frequency sound waves delivered through a small probe placed on the eye to measure intraocular lenses, detect orbital and periorbital lesions, length of the eye, and curvature of the cornea

ophthalmoscopy – use of the ophthalmoscope to examine the interior of the eyes to identify changes in the blood vessels in the eye and to diagnose systemic diseases

tonometry – use of a tonometer to measure intraocular pressure of the eye to screen for glaucoma

visual acuity – standard vision test to measure acuteness or sharpness of vision. The Snellen eye chart, from which the patient reads letters of various sizes from 20 feet, may be used.

Supportive Web Sites

http://medmark.org/
Click on "ophthalmology"; scroll to the section "For Consumers" and click on links of interest.

www.cancer.gov
Click on "Cancer Information" and "Types of Cancer"; under "Cancers by Body Location/System," click on "eye," then links of interest.

www.my.webmd.com
Search for a particular eye condition or disease about which you desire more information.

www.nlm.nih.gov
Click on "Health Information," then "MEDLINEplus"; search for "ophthalmology" and links of interest.

Index Of Ophthalmology Reports

(see table of contents for audio information)

Exercise #	Patient Name	Report/Procedure
TE#1	Rhian, Gretchen	Cataract extraction
TE#2	Israel, Jonathan	Trabeculectomy
TE#3	Luigi, Sandra	Penetrating keratoplasty
TE#4	Ramirez, Jesus	Viscocanulotomy
TE#5	Tennison, David	Vitrectomy
TE#6	Davis, Terry	Keratoplasty
TE#7	Schwartz, Clarence	Retinal detachment
TE#8	Sanchez, Teresa	Blepharoplasty/levator repair
TE#9	Rogers, Missy	Phacoemulsification
TE#10	Townsend, Anderson	Pseudophakic keratoplasty
TE#11	Yelverton, Paige	Oculinum injection

CHAPTER 18

PSYCHIATRY

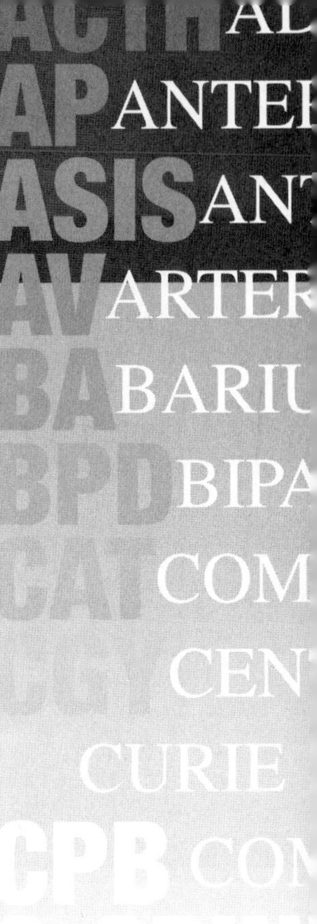

Introduction

The branch of medicine that deals with functional nervous disorders or mental disease is known as *psychiatry.* A *psychiatrist* treats both conscious and unconscious processes of the *psyche*—the human faculty for thought, judgment, and emotion.

Psychiatrists who analyze the thinking and actions of patients suffering from psychiatric illnesses perform the study, treatment, and prevention of mental illness. Mental illness can result from a variety of causes. Generally psychological and social factors contribute significantly; however, some mental illnesses stem from chemical bases.

Patients with psychiatric problems are treated by *physical means, drugs,* or *psychotherapy,* which makes use of reassurance, suggestion, hypnosis, or discussion of the patient's condition in an effort to help the patient understand the nature of the problem and meaning of the symptoms.

Therapeutic techniques used by psychiatrists are *drug therapy, psychotherapy,* and *electroconvulsive therapy.* Drug therapy is accomplished through the use of *neuroleptic* drugs, which modify the psychotic symptoms displayed by the patient. Antidepressants, antianxiety agents, and phenothiazines (major tranquilizers) are categories of neuroleptic drugs.

Psychiatrists treat patients with such disorders as anxiety, eating, mood, personality, sexual and gender identity, dementia and delirium, dissociative, schizophrenia, substance-related, and somatoform.

Psychiatrists complete four years of medical school and additional years of training in the techniques and procedures of *psychotherapy,* the treatment of mental disorders. Psychiatrists may also pursue additional training to become *child psychiatrists,* who work with children; or *forensic psychiatrists,* who work with legal officials to determine mental competence in criminal cases.

Psychologists differ from psychiatrists in the education they receive and the treatment methods they are allowed to use. A psychologist is a nonmedical professional who completes either a master's or doctor of philosophy degree in a field such as *clinical psychology, experimental psychology,* or *social psychology.* Whereas the psychiatrist can use drugs or electroconvulsive therapy in treatment, the psychologist cannot without permission from a physician.

Critical Thinking Exercise

Mr. Jacobson calls the medical transcription department and asks if his psychiatric electronic medical records are secure.

What would you tell him?

Psychiatry Abbreviations

AD	Alzheimer's disease (dementia)
ADHD	attention-deficit-hyperactivity disorder
CA	chronological age
CBS	chronic brain syndrome
CR	conditioned reflex
CS	conditioned stimulus
DOT	date of testing
DSM	Diagnostic and Statistical Manual of Mental Disorders
DT	delirium tremens

ECT	electroconvulsive therapy
EEG	electroencephalogram
ESP	extrasensory perception
EST	electric shock therapy
IMP	Inpatient Multidimensional Psychiatric (Scale)
MMPI	Minnesota Multiphasic Personality Inventory
MSRPP	Multidimensional Scale for Rating Psychiatric Patients
OBS	organic brain syndrome
ODD	oculodentrodigital (dysplasia)
OT	occupational therapy
PEG	pneumoencephalogram
PMA	Primary Mental Abilities Tests
SAD	seasonal affective (mood) disorder
SB	Stanford-Binet Test
TAT	Thematic Apperception Test
UCR	unconditioned reflex
WAIS	Wechsler Adult Intelligence Scale
WISC	Wechsler Intelligence Scale for Children

Psychiatry Terminology

a

acrophobia (ak"-rō-fō'-bē-uh) – morbid dread of high places

agoraphobia (ag"-uh-ruh-fō'-bē-uh) – fear of being in a large open space

ambivalence (am-bih'-vuh-lunts) – the simultaneous existence of conflicting attitudes, as of love and hate toward the same object

amentia (ā-men'-shē-uh) – feeblemindedness; a mental disorder characterized by marked mental confusion, sometimes so severe as to approach stupor

amok (uh-mahk') – a psychic disturbance marked by a period of depression followed by violent attempts to kill people

analysand (uh-nal'-ih-sand) – one who is being psychoanalyzed

anamnesis (an"-am-nē'-sis) – the collected data concerning a patient, his or her previous environment, and experiences, including any abnormal sensations, moods, or acts observed by the patient or by others and the dates of their appearance and duration, as well as any results of treatment

anorexia nervosa (an"-ō-rek'-sē-uh ner-vō'-suh) – a serious nervous condition in which the patient loses his or her appetite and systematically eats little food, so that he or she becomes greatly emaciated

antipsychotic (an"-tī-sī-kaht'-ik) – a neuropharmacolic agent that principally affects psychomotor activity and is generally without hypnotic effects, as a tranquilizer

Asperger's syndrome (autistic psychopathy) (uh-sper'-gerz sin'-drōm, aw-tis'-tik sī-kop'-uh-thē) – a pervasive developmental disorder characterized by severe and sustained impairment in social interaction, development of restricted and repetitive patterns of behavior, interests, and activities

ataractics (at"-uh-rak'-tikz) – tranquilizing agents widely used in psychiatric disorders such as agitation, aggressive outbursts, psychomotor overactivity, etc.; antianxiety agents

b

Bender-Gestalt test (ben'-der geh-stawlt' tehst) – a psychological test used for evaluating perceptual-motor coordination, for assessing personality dynamics, for assessing organic brain impairment, and for measuring neurological maturation

bradyphrasia (brād"-ē-frā'-zē-uh) – slowness of speech due to mental disorder

bradypsychia (brād"-ē-sī'-kē-uh) – slowness of mental reactions

c

carphology (kar-fahl'-uh-jē) – the involuntary picking at the bedclothes seen in severe fevers and in conditions of great exhaustion

catalepsy (kat'-uh-lep"-sē) – a morbid state in which there is a waxy rigidity of the limbs; if the limbs are placed in various positions, those positions will be maintained for a time

catatonia (kat-uh-to'-nē-uh) – stupor

chorea insaniens (kō-rē'-uh in-sā'-nē-enz) – chorea with symptoms of insanity, chiefly seen in pregnant women

coprophilia (kahp"-rō-fil'-ē-uh) – a psychopathologic interest in filth, especially in feces and in defecation

cyclothymia (sī"-klō-thih'-mē-uh) – a temperament characterized by cyclic alternations of mood between elation and depression

cyclothymic personality (sō"-klō-thī'-mik per"-suh-nahl'-ih-tē) – an individual manifesting mood swings from elation to depression

d

dereism (dē'-rē-izm) – mental activity in which fantasy runs on unhampered by logic and experience

dysboulia (dis-boo'-lē-uh) – abnormal weakness or disturbance of the will

dyslexia (dis-lek'-sē-uh) – an inability to read understandingly due to a central lesion

e

echopraxia (ek"-ō-prak'-sē-uh) – the spasmodic and involuntary imitation of the movements of another

ego-dystonic (ē"-gō-dis-tahn'-ik) – denoting any impulse, idea, or the like that is repugnant to and inconsistent with an individual's conception of himself or herself

electronarcosis (ē-lek"-trō-nar-kō'-sis) – anesthesia produced by passing an electric current through the brain by electrodes placed on the temples

enosimania (en"-ahss-ih-mā'-nē-uh) – obsessive belief of having committed an unpardonable offense

euphoria (yoo-fōr'-ē-uh) – in psychiatry, an abnormal or exaggerated sense of well-being, particularly common in the manic state

f

flagellation (flaj"-eh-lā'-shun) – whipping or being whipped to achieve erotic pleasure

g

grandiosity (gran"-dē-ahss'-ih-tē) – a condition characterized by delusions of grandeur

h

hebephrenic schizophrenia (hē'-bē-frē-nik skitz"-uh-frē'-nē-uh) – shallow inappropriate emotions, disorganized thinking, unpredictable childish behavior and mannerisms, indicative of gross personality disorganization

i

ideation (ī"-dē-ā'-shun) – the distinct mental presentation of objects

k

Korsakoff's psychosis (kōr'-suh-kawfs sī-kō'-sis) – a chronic brain syndrome associated with a prolonged use of alcohol

l

lability (lah-bil'-ih-tē) – in psychiatry, emotional instability; a tendency to show alternating states of gaiety and somberness

libido (lih-bē'-dō) – in psychoanalysis, the motive power of the sex life

m

malingering (mah-ling'-ger-ing) – the willful, deliberate, and fraudulent feigning or exaggeration of the symptoms of illness or injury done for the purpose of a consciously desired end

manic-depressive (man'-ik-dē-preh'-siv) – alternating between attacks of mania and depression

mesmerism (mez'-mer-izm) – hypnotism

metaphrenia (met"-uh-frē'-nē-uh) – the mental condition in which the interests are withdrawn from the family or group and directed to personal gain or aggrandizement

milieu therapy (mē-lyoo' thār'-uh-pē) – the utilization of a modified and controlled environment in the treatment of mental disease

mydriasis (mī-drī'-uh-sis) – extreme or morbid dilatation of the pupil; dilatation of the pupil as the effect of a drug

n

neurasthenia (noo"-rass-thē'-nē-uh) – a neurosis characterized by chronic weakness, easy fatigability, and sometimes exhaustion

neurosis (noo-rō'-sis) – disorder in which the dominant trait is anxiety

neurotic (noo-rot'-ik) – a nervous person in whom emotions predominate over reason; pertaining to or affected with a neurosis

nihilism (nī'-il-izm) – a form of delusion in which, to the patient, everything no longer exists

nympholepsy (nim'-fō-lep"-sē) – ecstasy; transport, especially of an erotic nature

o

obnubilation (ob-noo"-bih-lā'-shun) – a clouded state of the mind

oligophrenia (ol"-ih-gō-frē'-nē-uh) – defective mental development

p

panphobia (pan-fō'-bē-uh) – fear of everything; a vague morbid dread of some unknown evil

paresthetic (pār"-es-thet'-ik) – relating to or marked by paresthesia

petit mal epilepsy (peh-tē' mahl' ep'-ih-lep"-sē) – epilepsy in which there is sudden momentary loss of consciousness with only minor myoclonic jerks; seen especially in children

phagomania (fag"-ō-mā'-nē-uh) – an insatiable craving for food, or an obsessive preoccupation with the subject of eating

postictal (post-ik'-tul) – following a stroke or seizure, such as an acute epileptic attack

psychometry (sī-kahm'-eh-trē) – the measurement of intelligence; psychological testing

psychoneurosis (sī"-kō-noo-rō'-sis) – an emotional disorder due to unresolved conflicts, anxiety being its chief characteristic

psychosis (sī-kō'-sis) – a general term for any major mental disorder of organic and/or emotional origin characterized by derangement of the personality and loss of contact with reality

psychosomatic (sī"-kō-sō-mat'-ik) – pertaining to the mind-body relationship; having bodily symptoms of psychic, emotional, or mental origin

psychotogen (sī-kot'-uh-jen") – a drug that produces psychotic manifestations

psychotropic (sī"-kō-trō'-pik) – exerting an effect on the mind

r

recidivism (rē-sid'-ih-vizm) – the relapse or recurrence of a disease

Rorschach test (rōr'-shahk tehst) – a personality test that attempts to detect conscious or unconscious personality traits and conflicts by eliciting the individual's associations to a set of ink blots

rumination, obsessive (roo"-mih-nā'-shun, ahb-seh'-siv) – the constant preoccupation with certain thoughts, with inability to dismiss them from the mind

s

schizoid personality (skitz'-oyd) – an individual who is oversensitive, shy, seclusive, unsociable, eccentric, and autistic

schizophrenia (skitz"-uh-frē'-nē-uh) – severe mental disorder of psychotic depth marked by disturbances in behavior, mood, and ability to think

selenoplegia (seh-lē"-nō-plē'-jē-uh) – a morbid condition once believed to be due to the influence of the moon's rays

somatization (sō"-mah-tih-zā'-shun) – in psychiatry, the conversion of mental experiences or states into bodily symptoms

somnambulism (sahm-nam'-byoo-lizm) – a hypnotic state in which the subject has full possession of his or her senses but no subsequent recollection; sleep walking

t

tangentiality (tan-jen'-shē-al'-ih-tē) – a disturbance in the associative thought process in which the patient tends to digress readily from one topic under discussion to other topics that arise in the course of associations

w

workup (adj., noun) (wurk'-up) – the lab, x-ray, or other procedures involved in the diagnostic study of a patient with regard to the symptoms or complaints

Transcription Tips

To transcribe psychiatry dictation efficiently, you should know that the content of a psychosocial workup, or psychological assessment, differs in many ways from other types of medical reports. A psychiatrist, psychologist, or other allied health care professional dictates this report following a thorough examination of the patient. Generally the following sections are included: assessment procedures; a reason for referral and for admission; observation of behavior; test results, some of which are displayed in tabular form; suggested diagnoses; and summary and recommendations. Because the psychosocial workup must be very thorough, these reports can be quite lengthy.

You should also become familiar with roots and/or combining forms, terms that identify major psychiatric disorders and symptoms, therapeutic techniques, and selected psychiatric tests.

Because the psychiatrist, psychologist, or other allied health care professional may refer to some of the common phobias in dictation, knowledge of the scientific terms that describe the phobias is valuable.

Roots and/or Combining Forms

Root	Meaning	Root	Meaning
affect	emotion	mento	mind
anxio	uneasy, anxious, distressed	neuro	nerve
auto	self	philo	attraction to, love
hallucino	hallucination, to wander in the mind	phreno	mind
hypno	sleep	psycho	mind
iatro	treatment	schizo	split
		somato	body

Selected Psychiatric Disorders

anxiety disorders – phobic disorders, obsessive-compulsive disorder, post-traumatic stress disorder, generalized anxiety disorder

delirium, dementia, and Alzheimer's disease

dissociative disorders – dissociative identity disorder, dissociative amnesia, dissociative fugue

eating disorders – anorexia nervosa, bulimia nervosa

mood disorders – bipolar disorders (cyclothymia), depressive disorders (dysthymia, seasonal affective disorder)

personality disorders – antisocial, histrionic, narcissistic, paranoid, schizoid, schizotypal, borderline, avoidant, dependent, obsessive-compulsive, multiple

schizophrenia – paranoid, disorganized, catatonic, undifferentiated, residual; schizophreniform, schizoaffective, delusional disorders

sexual and gender identity disorders – exhibitionism, fetishism, pedophilia, sexual masochism, sexual sadism, transvestic fetishism, voyeurism

somatoform disorders – conversion disorder, hypochondriasis, somatization, body dysmorphic disorder

substance-related disorders – alcohol, amphetamines, cannabis (marijuana), cocaine, hallucinogens (LSD, mescaline), opioids (heroin, morphine, codeine, methadone), sedatives, anxiolytics, hypnotics, caffeine, nicotine, inhalants, phencyclidine (PCA)

Therapeutic Techniques

drug therapy – antianxiety agents, antidepressants, lithium, phenothiazines, antipsychotic agents

electroconvulsive therapy (ECT) – electric current application to the brain

psychotherapy – behavior, family, group, play, sex therapy; hypnosis; psychoanalysis, psychodynamic, cognitive therapy

Selected Psychiatric Tests

Abnormal Involuntary Movement Scale (AIMS)
Barranquilla Rapid Survey Intelligence (BARSIT)
Beck Depression Inventory (BDI)
Beery-Buktinica Developmental
Bender-Gestalt (BGT)
Bender Visual-Motor Gestalt (BVMGT)
Bryant-Schwan Design (BSDT)
Children's Apperception (CAT)
Del Rio Language Screening (DRLST)
dexamethasone suppression (DST)
Differential Aptitude (DAT)
Draw-A-Person Test
Edinburg Articulation (EAT)
Ego-Ideal and Conscience Development (EICDT)
Eidetic Parents (EPT)
Franck Drawing Completion (FDCT)
Freeman Anxiety Neurosis and Psychosomatic (FANPT)
Guilford-Zimmerman personality (GZ)
Halstead Aphasia (HAT)
Halstead-Reitan Neuropsychologic (HRNTB)

Selected Psychiatric Tests

Hamburg-Wechsler Intelligence (HAWIC)
Hamilton Anxiety Scale (Ham-A)
Hamilton Depression Scale (Ham-D)
House-Tree-Person (HTP, H-T-P)
Lincoln-Oseretsky Motor Performance (LOMPT)
Mertens Visual Perception (MVPT)
Millon Clinical Multiaxsial Inventory (MCMI)
Minnesota Multiphasic Personality Inventory (MMPI)
Minnesota Percepto-Diagnostic (MPDT)
Monotic Word Memory (MWMT)
Nalline
OISE Picture Reasoning (PRT)
Oliphant Auditory Discrimination Memory (OADMT)
Otis-Lennon Mental Ability (OLMAT)
Physiognomic Cue (PCT)
Porteus Maze (PMT)
Reitan-Indiana Aphasia Screening (RIAST)
Reitan-Klove Tactile Form Recognition
Rorschach Contest (RCT)
Slosson Intelligence (SIT)
Stanford-Binet Intelligence Scale
STYCAR Hearing (SHT)
STYCAR Language (SLT)
STYCAR Vision (SVT)
Suprathreshold Adaptation (STAT)
Symbol Digit Modalities (SDMT)
Tactile Finger Recognition (TFRT)
Test of Articulation Competence, Fisher-Logemann (FLTAC)
Test of Psycholinguistic Abilities, Illinois (ITPA)
tetrahydrocannabinol (THC)
Teutonomania
Teutonophobia
thaasophobia
"Thai sticks" (slang term, cannabis)
thalassomania
thanatomania
thanatos (death instinct)
Thematic Apperception Test (TAT, T.A.T.)
thematic paralogia
Wechsler Adult Intelligence Scale (WAIS)
Wepman Auditory Discrimination
Woodcock-Johnson Psychoeducational (WJPTB)
Yerkes-Bridges (YBT)

Supportive Web Sites

http://medmark.org/
Click on "psychiatry"; click on links of interest.

www.my.webmd.com
Click on "Diseases and Conditions"; scroll to "Mental Health" and click on links of interest.

www.nlm.nih.gov
Click on "Health Information," then "MEDLINEplus"; search for "psychiatry" and click on links of interest.

Index of Psychiatry Reports

(see table of contents for audio information)

Exercise #	*Patient Name*	*Report/Procedure*
TE#1	Adkins, Daniel	Consultation—Neuropsychological evaluation
TE#2	Bullard, Katrina	H&P (eating disorder)
TE#3	Randel, Justin	Discharge summary (drug dependent)
TE#4	DeVito, Leslie	Psychological assessment
TE#5	Pietrosewicz, Terry	Discharge summary
TE#6	Hearin, Viola	Discharge summary

CHAPTER 19

DENTISTRY/ ORAL SURGERY

Introduction

Physicians in the practice of *dentistry* are concerned with the *teeth, oral cavity, facial bones,* and *associated structures,* including the diagnosis and treatment of their diseases and the restoration of defective or missing tissue.

In addition to the general dentist, five clinical specialties exist in dentistry. Of these, hospital services commonly use four.

The *general dentist* has had four or more years of specialty training. He or she provides restorative and general dental care to patients in the hospital setting.

The *pedodontist* or *pediatric dentist* practices comprehensive preventive and therapeutic oral health care for children from birth through adolescence. A pedodontist undergoes two or more years of postdoctoral specialty training.

Periodontics is a specialty of dentistry that encompasses the prevention, diagnosis, and treatment of diseases of the supporting and surrounding tissues of the teeth or their substitutes. The specialist in periodontics will have graduated from a two- or three-year postdoctoral specialty program.

Oral and *maxillofacial surgery* is a special area of dentistry that includes the diagnosis, surgical and adjunctive treatment of diseases, injuries, and defects involving both the functional and aesthetic aspects of the hard and soft tissues of the oral and maxillofacial region. The oral and maxillofacial surgeon is the product of a four- to six-year postdoctoral program of specialty training. Although this is considered a dentistry-based specialty, significant numbers of surgeons are now being trained in a double MD/DDS degree program.

Critical Thinking Exercise

Now that you have completed your training as a medical transcriptionist and will begin work in the near future, you decide that your ultimate goal is to be a supervisor of MTs.

How can you determine what the qualifications are for this position? List resources that provide such information.

Dentistry/Oral Surgery Abbreviations

AB	axiobuccal
ABC	axiobuccocervical
ABG	axiobuccogingival
ABL	axiobuccolingual
AC	axiocervical
AD	axiodistal
ADC	axiodistocervical
ADG	axiodistogingival
ADI	axiodistoincisal
ADO	axiodisto-occlusal
AFH	anterior facial height
AG	axiogingival
AI	axioincisal
AL	axiolingual

ALA	axiolabial
ALAG	axiolabiogingival
ALAL	axiolabiolingual
ALC	axiolinguocervical
ALG	axiolinguogingival
ALO	axiolinguo-occlusal
AM	axiomesial
AMC	axiomesiocervical
AMD	axiomesiodistal
AMG	axiomesiogingival
AMI	axiomesioincisal
AMO	axiomesio-occlusal
AO	axio-occlusal
AP	axiopulpal
BA	buccoaxial
BAC	buccoaxiocervical
BAG	buccoaxiogingival
BC	buccocervical
BD	buccodistal
BG	buccogingival
BL	buccolingual
BM	buccomesial
BO	bucco-occlusal
BP	buccopulpal
BWX	bite-wing x-rays
CRN	crown
DB	distobuccal
DBO	distobucco-occlusal
DBP	distobuccopulpal
DC	distocervical
DG	distogingival
DL	distolingual
DLA	distolabial
DLAI	distolabioincisal
DLI	distolinguoincisal
DLO	distolinguo-occlusal
DLP	distolinguopulpal
DMF	decayed, missing, and filled
DO	disto-occlusal
DP	distopulpal
DPL	distopulpolingual
D5RL	dextrose 5% with lactated Ringers
F/	full upper denture
/F	full lower denture
FCC	fracture-compound comminuted
F/M	full mouth
FMX	full mouth x-rays
FSC	fracture-simple comminuted
Fx	fracture
GA	gingivoaxial
GBA	gingivobuccoaxial
GLA	gingivolinguoaxial
IP	incisoproximal
MB	mesiobuccal
MBO	mesiobucco-occlusal
MBP	mesiobuccopulpal
MG	mesiogingival
MID	mesioincisodistal
ML	mesiolingual
MLA	mesiolabial
MLAI	mesiolabioincisal
MLI	mesiolinguoincisal
MLO	mesiolinguo-occlusal
MLP	mesiolinguopulpal
MO	mesio-occlusal
MOD	mesio-occlusodistal restoration of tooth
MP	mesiopulpal
MPL	mesiopulpolingual
MPLA	mesiopulpolabial
OC	occlusocervical region of tooth
P/	partial upper denture
/P	partial lower denture
PFH	posterior facial height
PNS	posterior nasal spine
PRP	posterior ramal plane
PTM	pterygomaxillary fissure
RC	root canal
REC CRN	recement crown
SSC	stainless steel crown
TMJ	temporomandibular joint

Anatomic Illustrations

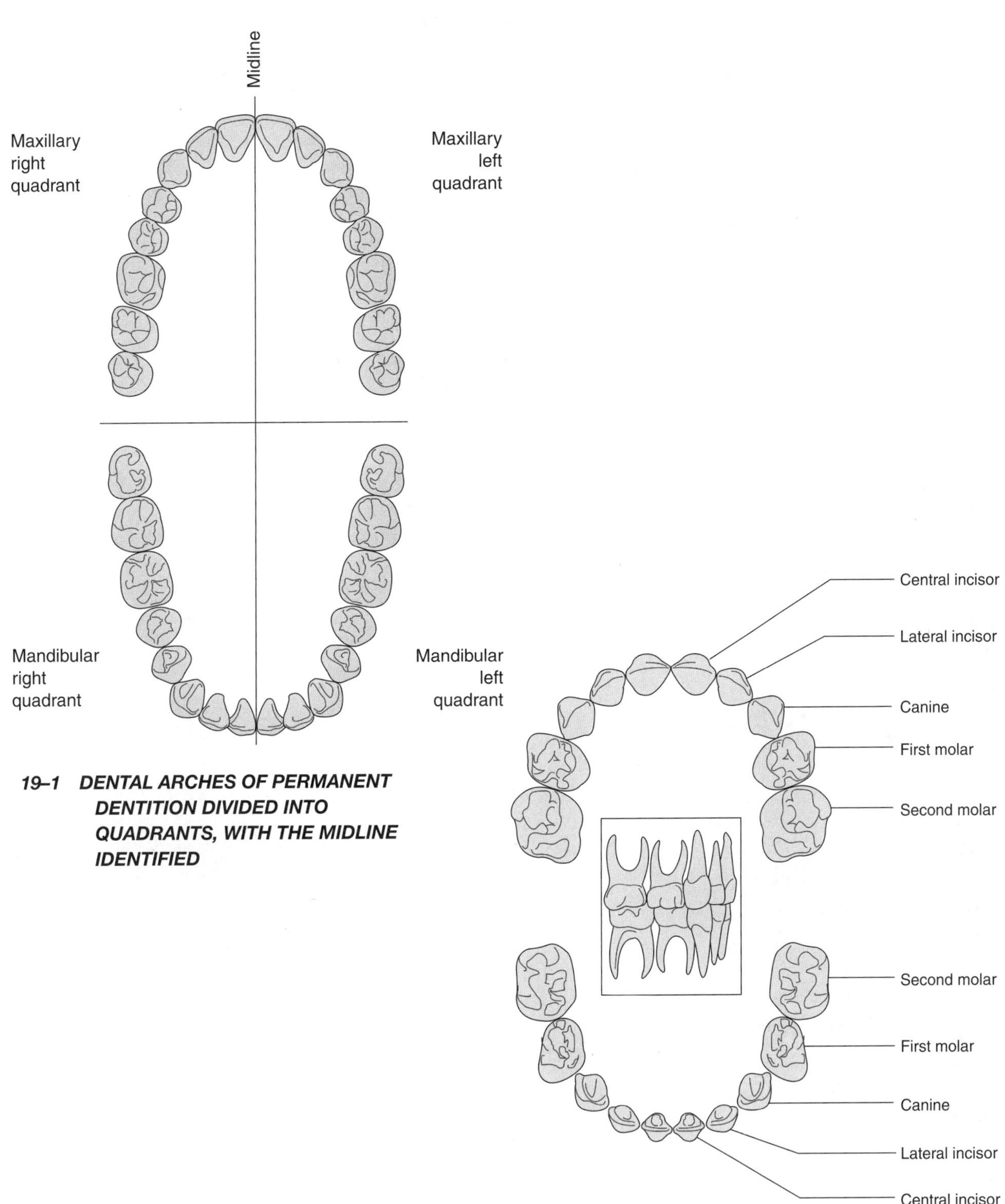

19–1 DENTAL ARCHES OF PERMANENT DENTITION DIVIDED INTO QUADRANTS, WITH THE MIDLINE IDENTIFIED

19–2 THE DECIDUOUS DENTITION, WITH EACH TOOTH IDENTIFIED BY NAME

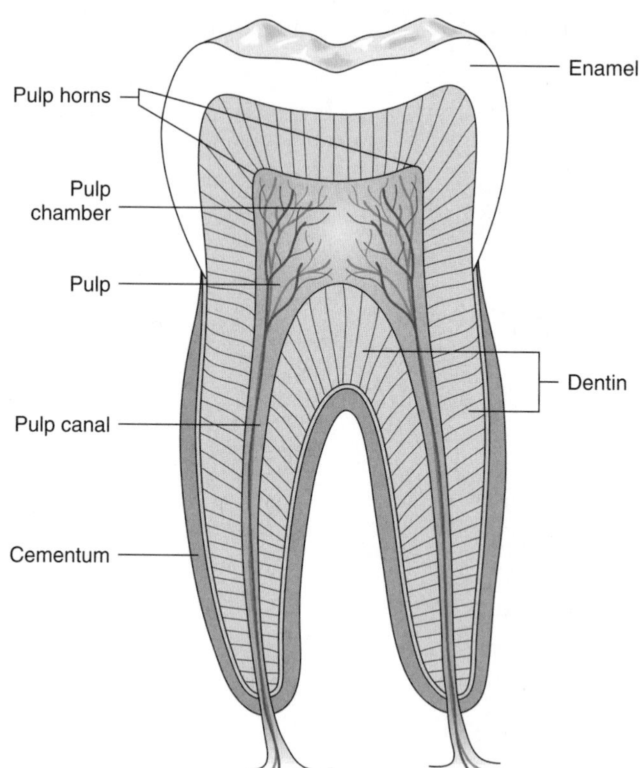

19–3 CROSS-SECTION OF THE TOOTH

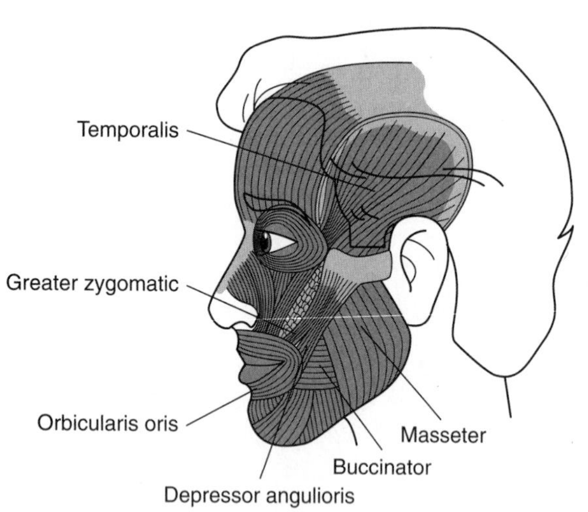

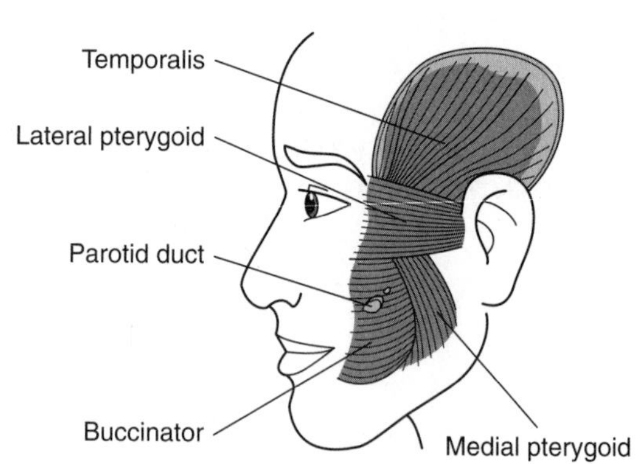

19–4 MUSCLES OF THE FACE

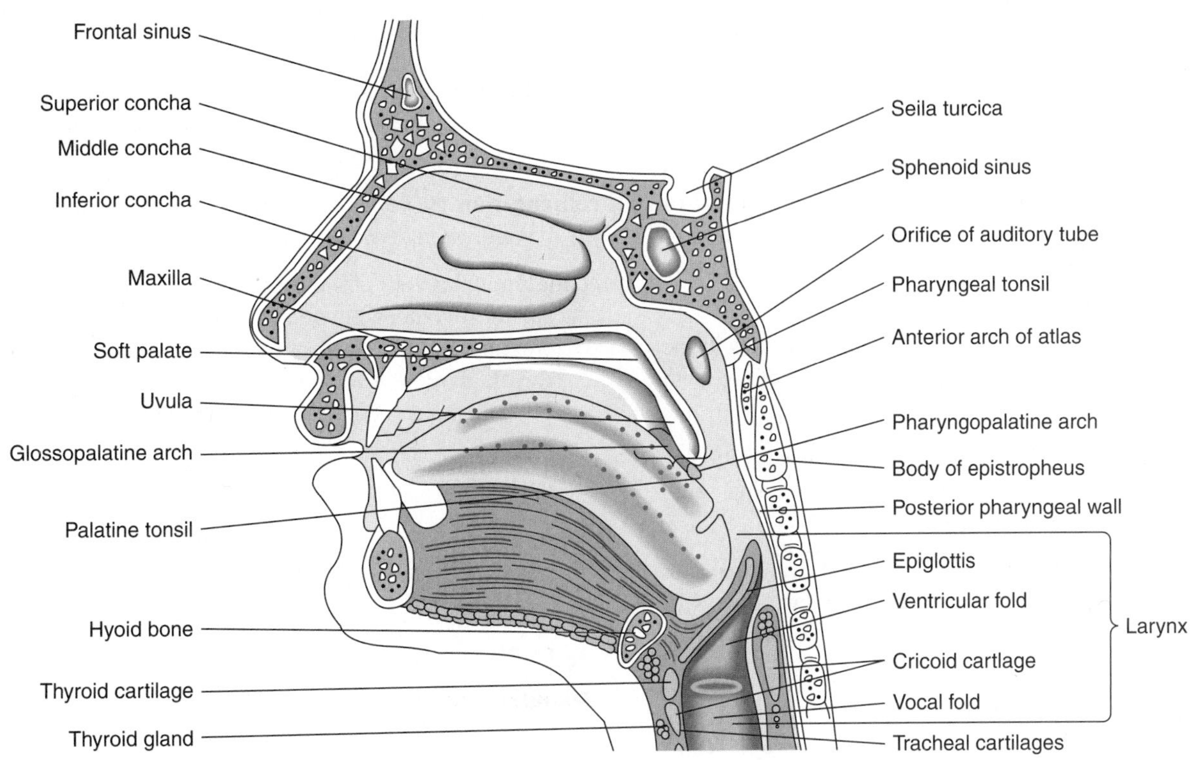
Frontal sinus
Superior concha
Middle concha
Inferior concha
Maxilla
Soft palate
Uvula
Glossopalatine arch
Palatine tonsil
Hyoid bone
Thyroid cartilage
Thyroid gland
Seila turcica
Sphenoid sinus
Orifice of auditory tube
Pharyngeal tonsil
Anterior arch of atlas
Pharyngopalatine arch
Body of epistropheus
Posterior pharyngeal wall
Epiglottis
Ventricular fold
Cricoid cartlage
Vocal fold
Larynx
Tracheal cartilages

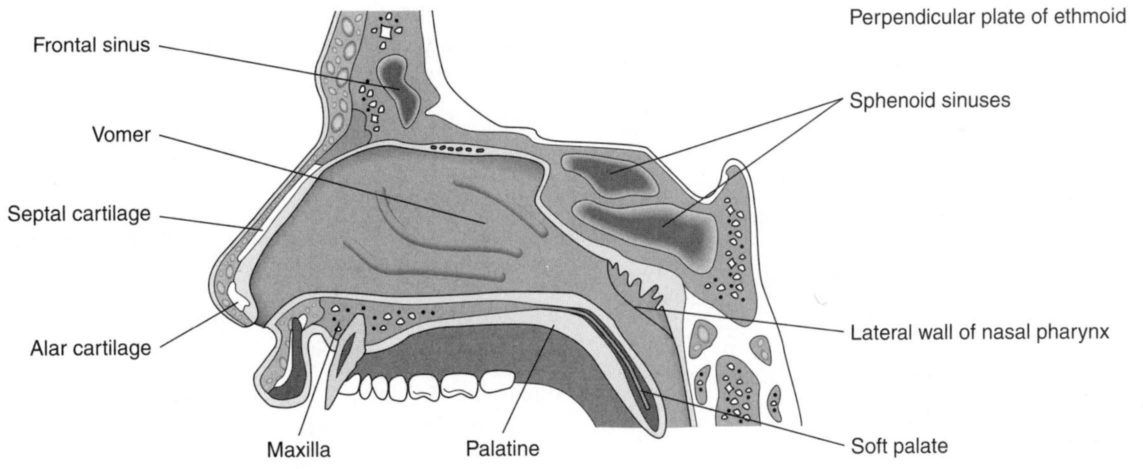
Frontal sinus
Vomer
Septal cartilage
Alar cartilage
Maxilla
Palatine
Perpendicular plate of ethmoid
Sphenoid sinuses
Lateral wall of nasal pharynx
Soft palate

19–5 STRUCTURES OF THE ORAL AND NASAL CAVITIES

Dentistry/Oral Surgery Terminology

a

alveolalgia (al"-vē-ō-lal'-jē-uh) – pain occurring in a dental alveolus

alveolectomy (al"-vē-ō-lek'-tuh-mē) – excision of a portion of alveolar bone to aid in the removal of teeth, in the restoration of the normal contour following the removal of teeth, and in the preparation of the mouth for dentures

alveoli (al-vē'-o-lē) – the bony cavities or sockets in the mandible and maxilla in which the roots of the teeth are attached

alveoloclasia (al-vē"-ō-lō-klā'-zē-uh) – disintegration or resorption of the inner wall of a tooth alveolus, causing looseness of the teeth

alveoloplasty (al-vē'-ō-lō-plas"-tē) – surgical alteration of the shape and order of the alveolar process in preparation for immediate or future denture construction

alveolus (pl. alveoli) (al-vē'-ō-lus, al-vē'-ō-lē) – a general term used in anatomical nomenclature to designate a small sac-like dilatation

amelodentinal (am"-eh-lō-den'-tih-nul) – pertaining to the enamel and dentin of a tooth

ankyloglossia (ang"-kih-lō-glos'-ē-uh) – tongue-tied

apertognathia (ah-per"-tog-nā'-thē-uh) – open-bite deformity

apoxemena (ā"-pok-sem'-eh-nuh) – the material removed from a periodontal pocket; treatment of periodontitis

apoxesis (ā"-pok-sē'-sis) – the removal of detritus from a periodontal pocket

arcus dentalis (ar'-kus den-tal'-is) – the curving structure formed by the crowns of the teeth in their normal position in the jaw

avulsed teeth (ah-vulst' tēth) – traumatic loss of teeth from their bony alveoli or sockets

b

bone rongeur (bōn raw-zhur') – an instrument for cutting tissue, particularly bone

brachygnathia (brak-ig-nā'-thē-uh) – "bird face"; retrognathic or small mandible, either congenital or associated with the interference of condylar growth because of trauma or infection

buccinator muscle (buk'-sih-nā"-tur mus'-ul) – muscle of chin that compresses the cheek and retracts the angle of the mouth

buccolingual (buk"-ō-ling'-gwul) – pertaining to the cheek and tongue; pertaining to the buccal and lingual surfaces of a posterior tooth

c

cementation (sē"-men-tā'-shun) – the attachment of restorative material to a natural tooth with cement

cephalometrics (sef"-uh-lō-met'-riks) – method of measuring distances between bony landmarks of the cranium and face from a reproducible cephalogram for the purpose of evaluating facial growth and development, including soft tissue profiles

cheilorrhaphy (kī-lōr'-ā-fē) – surgical repair of a deformed lip

concrescence (kahn-kres'-enz) – union of two completely formed teeth by fusion of the roots

condylectomy (kahn"-dih-lek'-tuh-mē) – surgical removal of a condyle or a portion thereof

d

Deknatel sutures (dek'-nuh-tel soo'-tyoorz) – synthetic nonresorbable surgical suture material

Denhardt mouth gag or Molt mouth prop (den'-hart mowth gag) – an adjustable metal mouth prop

dens-in-dente (denz-in-den'-tē) – developmental anomaly of a tooth that gives the impression of a "tooth within a tooth"

dentigerous cyst (den-tij'-er-us) – containing or bearing a tooth or teeth

dentition (den-tish'-un) – the teeth in the dental arch; ordinarily used to designate the natural teeth in position in their alveoli

dentoalveolar (den"-tō-al-vē'-ō-lur) – pertaining to a tooth and its alveolus

diastema (dī"-uh-stē'-muh) – a space between two adjacent teeth in the same dental arch

e

eminectomy (em"-ih-nek'-tuh-mē) – removal of the articular eminence of the temporomandibular joint

endodontics (en"-dō-dahn'-tiks) – the branch of dentistry concerned with the etiology, prevention, diagnosis, and treatment of diseases and injuries that affect the tooth pulp, root, and periapical tissue

endo-osseous implant (en"-dō-ahss'-ē-us) – a synthetic implantable device used to restore edentulous or partially edentulous jaw bones

exodontia (ek"-sō-dahn'-shē-uh) – exodontics or the removal of natural teeth

f

fluorosis (floo"-ō-rō'-sis) – a mottled discoloration of the enamel of the teeth resulting from ingestion of excessive amounts of fluoride during tooth development

g

gingivectomy (jin"-jih-vek'-tuh-mē) – surgical excision of all loose, infected, and diseased gum tissue from necks of teeth

gingivitis (jin"-jih-vī'-tis) – inflammation involving the gingival tissue only

glossopalatinus muscle (glahs"-ō-pal"-uh-tī'-nus mus'-ul) – muscle originating in the undersurface of the soft palate that elevates the tongue and constricts the throat

gutta-percha (gut"-uh-per'-chuh) – rubber-based compound used as a temporary filling material in dentistry or used as a permanent root canal filling in endodontics

h

hydroxyapatite (hī-drok"-sē-ap'-uh-tīt) – an inorganic crystalline compound found in the matrix of bone and the teeth, which gives rigidity to these structures

hypercementosis (hī"-per-sē"-men-tō'-sis) – excessive development of secondary cementum on the surfaces of tooth roots

i

incisolabial (in-sī"-zō-lā'-bē-ul) – denoting the incisal and labial surfaces of an anterior tooth

k

Kirschner wire (kersh'-ner wīr) – heavy, rigid wire, threaded at one end, used with a hand drill to pass through a fractured bone or a segment of a bone to which traction can be applied

l

laterognathia (lat"-er-ō-nā'-thē-uh) – horizontal deformity to one or the other side of the maxilla or mandible in relation to the rest of the face

LeFort fracture (leh-fōr' frak'-chur) – fracture of the maxilla; three types exist depending on the anatomical location

m

macrodontia (mak-rō-dahn'-shē-uh) – abnormal increase in the size of the teeth

malposed (mal-pōzd') – not in the normal position

mandible (man'-dih-bul) – the bone of the lower jaw

masseteric (mas"-eh-tār'-ik) – pertaining to the masseter muscle

masticating (mas'-tih-kā-ting) – chewing

maxilla (mak-sil'-uh) – upper jaw

maxillomandibular (mak-sil"-ō-man-dib'-yoo-lur) – pertaining to the maxilla and the mandible

mesial (mē'-zē-ul) – nearer the center line of the dental arch

micrognathia (mī"-krō-nā'-thē-uh) – unusual or undue smallness of the jaw

mucocele (myoo'-kō-sel) – dilatation of a cavity with accumulated mucous secretion; usually a minor salivary gland

mucoperiosteum (myoo"-kō-pār"-ē-ahss'-tē-um) – periosteum underlying mucous membranes, as in the oral cavity

mylohyoid muscle (mī"-lō-hī'-oyd mus'-ul) – the muscle that elevates the hyoid bone and supports the floor of the mouth

o

occlusal (ō-kloo'-zul) – pertaining to the masticating surface of a tooth

odontalgia (syn. dentalgia) (ō-dahn-tal'-jē-uh, den-tal'-jē-uh) – pain in a tooth

odontectomy (ō"-dahn-tek'-tuh-mē) – excision of an erupted tooth or of an unerupted or impacted tooth

odontogenic (ō-dahn"-tō-jen'-ik) – forming teeth; arising in tissues that give rise to the teeth

odontoma (ō-dahn-tō'-muh) – a tumor found only in the jaws, consisting of the constituent parts of teeth in aberrant forms

operculectomy (ō-per"-kyoo-lek'-tuh-mē) – surgical removal of the mucosal flap partially or completely covering an unerupted tooth

p

periapical (pār"-ē-ap'-ih-kul) – relating to tissues encompassing the apex of a tooth, including periodontal membrane and alveolar bone

pericementitis (pār"-ē-sē"-men-tī'-tis) – inflammation of the tissues adjacent to the tooth root

pericementoclasia (pār"-ē-sē-men"-tō-klā'-zē-uh) – disintegration of the periodontal ligament and alveolar bone without loss of overlying gingival tissue

prognathism (prahg'-nuh-thizm) – marked forward projection of the mandible or the maxilla beyond a normal distance from the cranial base

prosthodontics (prahss"-thō-dahn'-tiks) – the branch of dentistry concerned with the construction of artificial appliances designed to restore and maintain oral function by replacing missing teeth and sometimes other oral structures or parts of the face

pterygoid muscle (tār'-ih-goyd mus'-ul) – one of four muscles, in two sets (internal and external), running from the mandible to the pterygoid plate of the sphenoid bone

pulpitis (pul-pī'-tis) – inflammation of the dental pulp

retrognathic (reh"-trō-nāth'-ik) – pertaining to or characterized by retrognathia, underdevelopment of the maxilla and/or mandible

rhizodontropy (rī"-zō-dahn'-truh-pē) – the fixation of an artificial crown upon the natural root of a tooth

rhizodontrypy (rī"-zō-dahn'-trih-pē) – perforation of the root of a tooth to allow the escape of morbid material

sialodochoplasty (sī"-uh-lō-dō'-kuh-plas"-tē) – surgical procedure for the repair of a defect and/or restoration of a portion of a salivary gland duct

staphylorrhaphy (staf"-ih-lōr'-uh-fē) – surgical procedure performed on the soft palate

temporomandibular joint (tem"-pō-rō-man-dib'-yoo-lur – the encapsulated, double, synovial joints between the condyles of the mandible and the base of the skull

torus mandibularis (tōr'-us man-dib'-yoo-lah-rihs) – bone projections on the inside of the mandible

vermilion border (vur-mil'-yun bōr'-dur) – the exposed red portion of the upper or lower lip

vestibuloplasty (ves-tib'-yoo-lō-plas"-tē) – surgical modification of the gingival-mucous membrane relationships in the vestibule of the mouth, including deepening of the vestibular trough, repositioning of the frenum or muscle attachments, and broadening of the zone of attached gingiva after periodontal treatment

Z-plasty (ze'-plas"-tē) – a plastic operation for the relaxation of contractures in which a Z-shaped incision is made, the middle bar of the Z being over the contracted scar, and the triangular flaps rotated so that their apices cross the line of contracture

Transcription Tips

When transcribing dentistry/oral surgery dictation, you need to become familiar with the major functional parts of a tooth, its location, and function. Knowledge of the dentition process, dental abnormalities, and unhealthy conditions of the teeth and mouth will also aid in the transcription process.

Components of a Tooth

enamel – covers the outer surface of the tooth; formed prior to eruption of the tooth by special epithelial cells called ameloblasts

dentine – strong, bony substance that constitutes the main body of the tooth; its principal constituents are similar to those of bone

cementum – bony substance secreted by cells that line the tooth socket

pulp – substance that makes up the inside of the tooth; composed of connective tissue with an abundant supply of nerves, blood vessels, and lymphatics

Parts of a Tooth

crown – the portion that protrudes above the gum into the mouth

root – the portion in the bony socket of the jaw

neck – the collar between the crown and root where the tooth is surrounded by its gum

Dentition

Human beings and most other mammals develop two sets of teeth during a lifetime. The first teeth are called the *deciduous teeth* or milk teeth; humans have 20 of these. They erupt between the sixth month and second year of life and last until approximately the sixth to thirteenth year. After each deciduous tooth is lost, a permanent tooth replaces it; and an additional 8 to 12 molars appear posteriorly in the jaw, making the total number of permanent teeth 28 to 32 (32 if one grows four wisdom teeth).

Communication among dental practitioners is aided by use of a system of tooth designation. Currently three systems are in use, although no single system is internationally accepted. In the United States, the ***Universal System*** is popular. This system assigns a different number to each tooth, beginning with the upper right third permanent molar (see Figure 19–1).

Deciduous teeth are indicated by capital letters, beginning with "A" for the upper right second deciduous molar and ending with "T" for the lower right second deciduous molar.

The ***Palmer System*** divides the dentition into four quadrants with a horizontal line and a vertical line; it then assigns a number from 1 to 8 to the teeth in each quadrant, beginning with the central incisor. Deciduous teeth are designated by capital letters A–E.

The third system, from the *Federation Dentaire Internationale (FDI),* identifies teeth by assigning two numbers to each tooth.

Dental Abnormalities

The two most common dental abnormalities are *malocclusion* and *caries. Malocclusion* is usually the result of a hereditary abnormality that causes the teeth of one jaw to grow in an abnormal direction. *Caries* is the gradual decay and disintegration of the soft or bony tissue of a tooth.

Unhealthy Conditions of the Teeth and Mouth

Ludwig angina – diffuse purulent inflammation of the floor of the mouth, its facial spaces, muscles, and glands; must involve all three spaces: submandibular, sublingual, and submesial

periapical abscess – an abscess that develops around the root of a tooth

periodontal disease – a disease of the tissues that support the teeth (periodontium); affects the gingivae, bone, cementum, and periodontal membrane

periodontitis – inflammation or infection of the parotid gland or ducts; occurs in debilitated patients whose oral hygiene is poor, whose mouths have been permitted to become dry, or who have not chewed solid food regularly

stomatitis – an inflammation of the mouth that may be caused by drugs such as barbiturates, pathogenic organisms, mechanical trauma, irritants, or nutritional disorders

aphthous stomatitis – canker sores

catarrhae stomatitis – any mild inflammation of nonspecific origin affecting the mouth

Vincent angina (syn. trench mouth) – necrotizing ulcerative gingivitis

Supportive Web Sites

www.ada.org
Click on "oral health topics" for a list of numerous related sites and links.

www.hsls.pitt.edu
This is the URL for the University of Pittsburgh's Health Sciences Library System. This site yields numerous links relating to dentistry/oral surgery, depending on what you search for.

www.nlm.nih.gov
Click on "Health Information," then "MEDLINEplus"; search for "dentistry" or "oral surgery" and choose links of interest.

www.smiles4ever.com
Good site for information on removal of teeth and associated procedures/conditions.

Index Of Dentistry/Oral Surgery Reports

(see table of contents for audio information)

Exercise #	*Patient Name*	*Report/Procedure*
TE#1	Talburt, Gloria	Surgery—repair of condylar fracture
TE#2	Kindall, Wendy	Extractions and restorations
TE#3	Smiles, Patricia	Op. Rep.—Maxillary and mandibular bony exostoses
TE#4	Bush, Tommy	H&P and Op. Rep. for prognathism
TE#5	Yuen, Susan	Operation—bone staple
TE#6	Brown, Brett	Operation—sagittal split
TE#7	Penn, Oneida	Operation—alveoloplasty
TE#8	Blackledge, J.	Operation—maxillary osteotomy
TE#9	Mueller, Derrick	Operation—sliding osteotomy

CHAPTER 20

STUDENT EXERCISES

Introduction

This chapter will challenge your problem-solving abilities with situations you might encounter on the job as a medical transcriptionist. You can demonstrate your expertise in transcribing some "different" kinds of reports, in solving critical thinking exercises comprised of realistic on-the-job dilemmas, and in proofreading and correcting sample reports. Your expertise in using research skills will also be tested in completing exercises in this chapter.

Section I (eclectic transcription exercises) includes dictation for types of reports different from what you have heard in the other chapters. These exercises will acquaint you with types of medical reports or correspondence generated in a clinic, office, or emergency room setting. In a clinic and/or office setting, physicians dictate progress notes and/or follow-up reports on a patient to be transcribed onto a continuation form.

In this section you will have the opportunity to transcribe

- A white paper from ophthalmology (TE#1)
- "Histories" taken on three patients in an office setting prior to doing refractive surgery (from ophthalmology) (TE#2)
- Progress notes to be transcribed onto a continuation form (used in a clinic or office setting) (TE#3)
- Two letters (TE#4)
- An emergency room record (TE#5)

Section II (realistic on-the-job dilemmas) provides opportunities to demonstrate your critical thinking/problem-solving skills by responding to various situations you might encounter on the job.

Section III (editing activities) contains reports with embedded errors. Your task will be to proofread the reports, and identify and correct all errors you find. You should consult all types of reference materials while correcting the reports.

Good luck with these challenging activities!

Section I: Transcription Exercises

Directions: Dictation provides opportunities for you to transcribe reports different from those provided in Chapters 2–19. Listen to the audio to complete this section.

Transcription Exercise 1 (TE#1) contains material for a white paper (journal article). In addition to practicing medicine, some physicians write articles for professional journals sharing their expertise with other medical practitioners. Although this article does not contain footnotes or endnotes, on the job you might have to know how to format them. Consult a reference manual for the correct format.

TE#2 presents examples of notes dictated by physicians in the office that would be transcribed and placed in the patients' charts.

Type the information for **TE#3**. Continuation forms are used in various medical offices and/or clinics to enter information on patients each time they visit the doctor. After completing the examination of the patient, the physician dictates information that you would transcribe onto this form.

TE#4 requires you to transcribe sample letters that might be dictated by physicians. You may download a letterhead from the web site and use any letter style unless your teacher specifies a particular one. The block letter style is used most frequently in the business world, however.

Transcribe **TE#5** like you did in the exercises in Chapters 2–19. Just listen to the dictation and transcribe onto plain paper. This information represents dictation you might hear from an emergency room visit.

Section II: Realistic On-the-Job Dilemmas

In your day-to-day activities as a medical transcriptionist, you will encounter problem situations that require you to apply decision-making skills. According to practicing medical transcriptionists, the following scenarios represent typical situations you might face.

Complete the activities as your instructor directs. You may either retrieve the file on the template that corresponds with Chapter 20, Section II, or you may write your responses in the appropriate spaces on the following pages.

Directions: Retrieve the file on the template that corresponds to Chapter 20, Section II, and type your response to the following situations in the space following each question.

Decision-Making Scenarios

For each of the scenarios, what would you do? If you don't know the answer, indicate the steps you would take to solve the problem and/or the references you would consult.

1. The physician dictates: "HEENT: Head normal. Eyes normal. TM apostrophe *s* intact." How would you transcribe?

2. The physician dictates: "Please send a carbon copy to Dr. Joe C. Crumley." What notations would you make on the letter or report?

3. The salutation "Dear Sirs:" is dictated in a letter to the Wilson Medical Group (WMG). (You are aware that there are both female and male physicians in the WMG.) What would be the correct salutation?

4. The physician dictates the physical examination. You have typed the examination of the head, eyes, ears, nose, throat, and lungs, and now are typing the cardiovascular exam. Without any specific instruction, the physician dictates "sinuses show moderate amount of exudate." What would you do?

5. You cannot understand the name of a drug in the dictation. Identify the appropriate steps to solve the problem.

6. The physician dictates the following: "No further bleeding was encountered, and a sterile dry dressing was applied, and the patient returned to the recovery room in a satisfactory condition." What would you do to transcribe the statement accurately?

7. What could you do to improve the connotation of the following? The physician dictates, "The *pussy* contents of the gallbladder were sent to pathology." (The physician means the contents resembled pus.)

8. If the physician said, "This is an operative report on Mr. Andrew Jacobs . . . ," and you recognize that it is actually a history & physical, what would you do?

9. The doctor dictates that the patient is allergic to aspirin in one sentence. Two sentences later, the physician says the current medications include aspirin. What should you do?

10. If the doctor dictates that the patient is white in one place and black in another; or female instead of male; or he instead of she, or right instead of left, etc., what steps should you take to assure that you transcribe the correct words?

11. If the physician dictates punctuation that you feel is wrong (i.e., semicolon, semicolon for everything, and never a period), what should you do?

12. The physician dictates "Destroy the previous report I dictated on Monday, and I will redictate it now." What should you do?

13. If one name is given at the beginning of the report and then another name is used in the middle, which name would you type?

14. If information is dictated under the wrong heading (i.e., social history is included in the family history), what is the correct thing to do?

15. If a physician spells a term incorrectly according to your resource material but the doctor insists that she is right, what should you do?

16. If you consult several different reference books and find different spellings for a term, how would you know which to use?

17. If you are typing a report on someone you know and the physician gives incorrect personal information (i.e., number of children, marital status, etc.), what should you do?

18. If a doctor told you that he is redictating a report because "you lost it," and he used curse words and extremely foul language, what would you do?

19. If verbs, adverbs, nouns, or the like are incorrect in a sentence, what should you do?

20. If a doctor's speech is absolutely unintelligible, what do you do?

Section III: Proofreading Exercises

Directions: The proofreading exercises (PE) included in this section contain numerous errors of all kinds (i.e., punctuation, grammar, format, spelling, etc.). You should follow AAMT guidelines for report formatting.

The following exercises are included:

PE#1	Operative Report
PE#2	Report of Tissue Examination
PE#3	Discharge Summary
PE#4	History & Physical
PE#5	History & Physical
PE#6	White Paper in Dermatology

Examine these reports for inclusion of necessary parts in headings and closing lines. Check for correct punctuation, spelling, number usage, and so. Check for correct AAMT format.

Proofreading Exercise 1

OPERATIVE REPORT

Hill, Suzanne
9022394
Martha Draughn, M,D.
12/19/ - -

SURGEON: Martha Draughn, MD

ASSISTANT: Benjamin West, MD

PREOPERATIVE DIAGNOSIS: Uterine fibroids

POSTOPERATIVE DIAGNOSIS: Uterine fibroids

FINDINGS: Multiple uterine fibroids with the uterus about 10 to 12 week gestational size, 2 cm right ovarian cyst.

PROCEDURE
Laparoscopic assisted vaginal hysterectomy with bilateral salpingo-ophorectomy.

ANESTHESIA: General endotracheal.

ANESTHESIOLOGIST: David Underwood, MD

PROCEDURE IN DETAIL: The patient was taken to the Operating Room and placed in the supin position. After adequate general anesthesia had been obtained, the patient was preped and draped in the usual fashion for laparoscopic assisted vaginal hysterectomy. The bladder was drained with a red rubber catheter. A small infraumbilical skin incision was made with the scalpel and 10-mm laparoscopic sleeve and trocar were introduced without difficulty. The trocar was removed. The laparoscope was placed, and 2 liters of C02 gas was insufflated in the patients abdomen.

A second incision was made suprapubically and a 12-mm laparoscopic sleeve and trocar were introduced under direct visualization. A 5-mm laparoscopic sleeve and trocar were placed in the left lower quadrant under direct visualization. A manipulator was used to examine the patient's pelvic organs. There was a small cyst on the right ovary. Both ovaries were free from adhesions. The ureters were free from the operative field. After measuring the ovarian distal pedicles the endo-GIA staple was placed across each round ligament.

At this time, attention was turned to the vaginal part of the procedure. A waited speculum was placed in the vagina. The anterior lip of the cervix was grasped with a Lahey tenaculum. Posterior colpotomy incision was made and the posterior peritoneum entered in this fashion. The uterosacral ligaments were bilaterally clamped, cut, and Heaney sutured with No. 1 chromic. The cardinal ligaments were bilaterally clamped, cut, and ligated. The anterior vaginal mucosa was then incised with the scalpel and with sharp and blunt dissection, the bladder was freed from the underlying cervix. The bladder pillars were bilaterally clamped, cut, and ligated. The uterine vessels were then bilaterally clamped, cut, and ligated. Visualization was fairly difficult because the patient had a very narrow pelvic outlet. In addition, there were several small fibroids that made placement of clamps somewhat difficult. Using the clamp, cut, and tie method after the anterior peritoneum had been entered with scissors the uterus was then left without vascular supply. The fundus was delivered by flipping the uterus posteriorly and through an a vascular small pedicle, Heaney clamps were placed across and the uterus was then removed enbloc with the tubes and ovaries attached.

(continued)

OPERATIVE REPORT
Patient Name: Suzanne Hill
Hospital No.: 9022394
December 19, 20 - -
Page 2

At this point, the remaining Heaney pedicles were ligated with a free-hand suture of 0 chromic. At this point, sponge and instrument counts were correct. Avascular pedicles were inspected and found to be hemostatic. The posterior vaginal cuff was then closed using running interlocking suture of No. 1 chromic. The anterior peritoneum was then grasped and using pursestring suture of 0 chromic, the peritoneum was closed. The vaginal cuff was then closed reincorporating the previously tagged uterosacral ligaments into the vaginal cuff through the anterior and posterior vaginal cuff. Another figure of eight suture totally closed the cuff. Hemostasis was excellent. A foley was then placed in the patients bladder and clear urine was noted to be draining.

At this point the laparoscope was placed back through the 10-mm sleeve and the vaginal cuff inspected. A small amount of old blood was suctioned away, but all areas were hemostatic.

At this point, the laparoscopic instruments were removed after the excess gas had been allowed to escape. These incisions were closed first with suture of 2.0 Vicryl through the fascia of each incision, and then the skin edges were reapproximated with interrupted sutures of 3.0 plain. Sponge and instrument counts were correct times three. The estimated blood loss for the entire procedure was 450 ccs. The patient was awakened from general anesthesia and taken to the recovery room in stable satisfactory condition with clear urine draining from the Foley catheter.

Marth Draughn, MD

LP:re

D: 12/19/ - - - -
T: 12/20/ - - - -

Proofreading Exercise 2

REPORT OF TISSUE EXAMINATION

PATIENT: Eubanks, Clara SPECIMEN NUMBER: 32402

DOCTOR: Patrick, L. DATE REMOVED: 4/29/ - -

DATE RECEIVED: 4/29/ - -

Lamar Memorial Hospital
Hattiesburg, MS 39401

SPECIMEN: Placenta. DATE REPORTED: 4/30/ - -

CLINICAL HISTORY: Vaginal breach delivery.

GROSS: The specimen consists of one container labeled with the patient's name and identifier and designated "placenta/breach." It contains a placenta with attached umbilical cord and fetal membranes weighing 361 gm. The umbilical cord has a length of 20-cm and has a velamentous insertion into the fetal membranes. Cross section of the umbilical cord reveals three umbilical vessels. The fetal membranes and the fetal side of the placenta demonstrate hemorrhage and attached clot. The placenta is discoid in shape and measures 15-cm in diameter with a depth of 2-cm. The maternal side of the placenta demonstrates maroon colored cotyledons with focal yellowish areas scattered throughout. Serial sectioning of the cotyledons demonstrates unremarkable maroon colored cotyledons. Representatives sections submitted in three cassettes. Cassette 1 - umbilical cord and fetal membranes. Cassettes 2 and 3 - maternal and fetal side of placenta.

MICROSCOPIC DIAGNOSIS
Uterine contents - placenta with three vessel umbilical cord and multifocal areas of calcification within the cotyledons.

Lucinda Patrick, MD
Pathologist

LP:re

D: April 30, - - - -
T: April 30, - - - -

Proofreading Exercise 3

DISCHARGE SUMMARY
Courville, Jannis
5044424
Joseph A. Chevillis, MD

ADMITTED: March 20, - - - -
DISCHARGED: March 27, - - - -

HISTORY OF PRESENT ILLNESS
This 46-year-old right-handed female resident manager for the Ritz Motel presents with a two year history of severe episodic right face pain in a DV2 distribution. She was unable to take Dilantin or Tegretol.

PHYSICAL EXAMINATION
On admission examination, she had mild hyperpathia in right V2 distribution. Her neurological examination was otherwise normal.

HOSPITAL COURSE/TREATMENT
An MRI scan of the head dated 1/16/- -, was unremarkable. She was admitted on 3/20 and on that day underwent a right suboccipital craniectomy with microvascular decompression of the right trigeminal nerve. Immediately postoperatively, she had profound nausea but was awake and alert and exhibited no focal deficits. By 3/22 she was awake, alert, and ambulatory. She complained of headache, nausea, and dizziness when standing but denied any face pain. On 3/25 she continued to have severe headaches and some mild right face pain. Her wound was healing well. By March 26 she was afebrile. Her headaches had decreased. She had only occasional right V2 pain that seemed to be different from her preoperative pain. Her wound was healing well and she showed no focal neurologic deficits. She was discharged on 3/27 on the following medications.

DISCHARGE MEDICATIONS
1. Klonopin 1 mg p.o. q. daily.
2. Prednisone 50 mg po bid
3. Flexeril 10 mg p.o. q.h.s.
4. Bentyl 20 mg po q.h.s.
5. Percocet p.r.n.
6. Ambien prn

DISPOSITION
She was advised to return for follow-up in three weeks.

DISCHARGE DIAGNOSIS
1. Trigeminal neuralgia (right V2).
2. Pulmonary sarcoidosis.

Joseph A. Chevillis, MD

D: 3/20/ - -
T: 3/27/ - -

Proofreading Exercise 4

HISTORY
Long, Daniel
2968287
James Carlton, MD
January 25, - - - -

ADMISSION: 10/25/ - -

INTRODUCTION: This is the first Forrest General admission since birth for this 10 month old child from Hattiesburg. The history is obtained from the patient's parents and seems reliable.

CC: Fever.

REASON FOR HOSPITALIZATION: This is a 10 month old black male who is followed at the Pediatric Clinic with a 4 day history of running nose, which worsened over the next few days to include cough and fever. The day prior to admission, he was treated with Tylenol at home. Fever at home was subjective as the parents had no thermometer. The child reportedly had difficulty breathing secondary to nasal congestion over the past few days. His appetite was noted to be decreased, but he was reportedly taking fluids okay with good urine output. He did have 3 episodes of vomiting the day prior to admission, but on the day of admission was tolerating fluids without difficulty. No diarrhea was reported. He presented to the Forrest General Emergency Room on the day of admission where his temperature was 106, at which time he was given oral Motrin. Numerous attempts at an IV by ER nurses, NICU nurses, the ERP and Respiratory Therapist were unsuccessful, except for a CBC which was obtained by an arterial stick. Chest x-ray was consistent with right middle lobe pneumonia per the ERP. Patient is not clinically dehydrated. A catheterized urine was obtained, which was within normal limits. The patient was treated with IM antibiotics in the Emergency Room and is admitted for further management.

PMH: BIRTH: The patient was a 6 pound produce of a term pregnancy who apparently spent 2 weeks in the NICU for "breathing problems". He was on oxygen in the Emergency Room, but it does not seem that he was mechanically ventilated. He was discharged home on an apnea monitor which he was maintained for 3 to 4 months of life.

HOSPITALIZATIONS: None.
SURGERIES: None.
ILLNESSES: None reported by the parents.
IMMUNIZATIONS: Reportedly up to date.
DIET: Consists of table food and baby food with Infamil with iron.
DEVELOPMENTALLY: The child is appropriate for age.
MEDICATIONS AT HOME: None.
ROS: HEENT: He has had a runny nose and a cough as in the HPI above. No apparent ear pain, no apparent sore throat.
CP: Cough as above. No history of heart murmurs or problems and no congestive symptoms.
GI: No diarrhea, no constipation. He did have vomiting yesterday as above.
GU: No urinary tract infection, no sysuria, no problems voiding.
MS: There have been no injuries or broken bones.

(continued)

HISTORY
Patient Name: Long, Daniel
Hospital No.: 2968287
January 25, - - - -
Page 2

FH: Mother and father are alive and well, except for asthma in the father's side of the family including the father and grandfather. The child has a 4 year old half sister who is reportedly healthy.

SH: The patient lives in Hattiesburg with his mother, grandmother, and half sibling. Mother is unemployed and is the primary care giver. Both mother and father are present with the child and both appear to be appropriately concerned and understand the need for hospitalization.

VS: Temperature 97.8, pulse 168, respirations 56 while crying, blood pressure 88/49 while calm. Weight is 18 pounds.

GENERAL: The child seems to be alert and seems to be a well nourished well developed in no acute distress.

HEENT: Extraocular muscles are intact. Pupils equally round and reactive to light. Tympanic membranes are slightly pink and dull bilaterally. Oropharynx is red appearing and the nose does have a mucoid discharge.

NECK: Supple with a full range of movement.

CV: Reveals regular rate and rhythm without murmurs. Perfusion is good.

LUNGS: Left side is clear, however breath sounds are decreased on the entire right side. The patient is not tachypneic and there are no retractions noted.

GI: Abdominal exam reveals normoactive bowel sounds, is soft and non tender. No masses are noted.

GU: Normal male with testes descended bilaterally.

NEURO: The child is alert and very actively responds to the exam without apparent deficits.

LABORATORY: White blood count 19.6 with 76% segs, 20% lymphocytes. Hematocrit is 25, platelets 349,000. Catheterized urinalysis is within normal limits. Chest x-ray reportedly reveals right middle lobe pneumonia.

IMPRESSION: This is a 10 month old black male with right middle lobe pneumonia and pharyngitis. He was treated with IM antibiotics in the Emergency Room.

PLAN: Will include IV placement which was obtained by ward RN without difficulty. Blood culture was obtained (IM antibiotics were given 2 hours prior to blood culture). CHEM 6, IV fluids and IV antibiotics and will follow up CBC in the morning.

James Carlton, MD

Proofreading Exercise 5

HISTORY AND PHYSICAL
Lang, Charles
5042066
Holly Freman, MD
3/12/ - -

CHIEF COMPLAINT
Gunshot wound.

PRESENT ILLNESS
This 27 year old right handed black male restaurant worker from Dallas presented with the following history. Around 1:45 AM on the day of admission, he was apparently at a bar on Tiffany Street and became involved in an argument. As he was leaving the bar, he was shot allegedly with a shotgun. He apparently fell in the street unconscious. He was brought to the Dallas General Hospital emergency room in a car by his friends. He apparently began to awaken on the way to the hospital. He apparently has not vomited or become agitated since the injury.

PAST HISTORY
He had asthma as a child.

SURGICAL
He has had an appendectomy in the past.

FAMILY HISTORY
His mother has diabetes and hypertension. His grandfather had kidney failure.

SOCIAL HISTORY
He lives with his wife. He was last employed five months ago as a chef in a restaurant. He smokes about one pack of cigarettes per day.

ALLERGIES
None known.

REVIEW OF SYSTEMS
HEENT: Negative.
CARDIORESPIRATORY: He has frequent upper respiratory tract infections, ocassional neck and back pain.
GASTROINTESTINAL: Negative.
GENITOURINARY: Negative.

NEUROLOGIC: Negative.

PHYSICAL EXAMINATION

GENERAL: Blood pressure was 149/84 mmHg, pulse 106/minute. He is a well developed, well nourished black male, moaning and obtunded on a gurney. He has a 3-cm laceration across the mid forehead with small entrance wound in the right parietal area and superficial abrasion on the right cheek.
HEENT: Not examined
NECK: Not examined
CHEST: Not examined
HEART: Not examined

(continued)

HISTORY AND PHYSICAL
Patient Name: Charles Lang
Hospital No.: 5042066
March 12, - - - -
Page 2

NEUROLOGICAL: He was obtunded but arousable. He will answer simple questions appropriately with single word responses. He occasionally follows commands. Motor function in the upper and lower extremities is intact. His deep tendon reflexes are normal. His gaze is conjugate. His pupils are equal and reactive. He fixes on an observer with conjugate gaze.

IMPRESSION
1. Gunshot wound to head
2. Right parietal hematoma
3. Subarachnoid hemorrhage
4. Pneumocephalus
5. Frontal scalp laceration
6. Acute alcohol intoxication

Holly Freman, MD

HF:TR

D: 3/12/ - -
T: 6/13/ - -

Proofreading Exercise 6

INTRODUCTION

The dermatologists differential diagnosis of a purpuric eruption in a patient seen in an office or emergency room is long. This paper will attempt to provide a workable classification of purpuric eruptions.

The term purpura denotes a red to blue-black discoloration of skin or mucous membranes resulting from extravasation of blood located intracutaneously or subcutaneously. Petechia are small purpuric lesions arbitrarily less than one centimeter. Ecchymoses are larger lesions. Purpura do not blanch on diascopic pressure, and this is a helpful aid to distinguish between purpura and erythema.

One important distinction lies in making the diagnosis of an infectious process as the cause of purpura. The physician must suspect an infectious agent (bacterial, viral, or rickettsial) in any acutely-ill patient with systemic toxicity and fever.

I will divide the classification of purpura into two main categories non-inflammatory and inflammatory purpura. Non-inflammatory purpura are usually flat and non-palpable, and inflammatory purpura are usually palpable secondary to accumulation of cells and edema fluid. This is a helpful distinction to make as non-inflammatory or non-palpable purpura are in general associated with platelet abnormalities, coagulation defects, or connective tissue defects, while inflammatory or palpable purpura are often associated with infectious diseases or angitis.

Blood platelets are essential for normal hemostasis. Platelets adhere to areas of subendothelial exposure as well as damaged endothelial cells causing a subsequent aggregation of platelets and formation of a platelet plug. Platelets release factor III which helps activate the clotting cascade (factor 10 and prothromb-thrombin). Platelets also mediate the phenomenon of clot retraction.

Purpura on the basis of platelet abnormalities can have a number of mechanisms. Platelet abnormalities can result from decreased production, increased destruction or decreased qualitative function.

Among the abnormalities that may cause thrombocytopenia secondary to decreased production are marrow infiltration by malignancy (leukemia),granulomas, or lipidoses and marrow depression secondary to drugs - as idiosyncrasy or immunosuppression - or malignancy.

Increased destruction of platelets can come from sequestration secondary to splenomegaly or hemangiomas. Platelet antibodies can be produced in autoimmune disorders like idio-pathic thrombocytopenic purpura or systemic lupus erythematosus or can be secondary to drugs like Quinidine which may combine haptenically with platelets resulting in lysis by antibody and complement. Other drugs that may act similarly include gold, arsenicals, sulfa drugs, Phenacetin, and iodides. Also accelerated intravascular coagulation will consume platelets as well as clotting factors.

The mechanism of qualitative functional defects in platelets secondary to poor adhesion, aggregation or release of granular contents are complex but can be seen with drugs such as acetylsalicylic acid (secondary to inhibition of prostaglandins which decreases levels of thromboxane A2 which is important in aggregation) and penicillin. Diabetes, uremia, liver disease, scurvy and dysproteinemias cause decreased function of platelets as well. Poor platelet function secondary to thrombocythemia as seen in leukemias, primary thrombocythemia and polycythemia vera can also occur. Congenital qualitative disorders such as Glanzmann's disease complete the list.

Platelet abnormalities result in petechiae and ecchymosis commonly but rarely are associated with deep hematomas. Coagulation defects on the other hand commonly show ecchymoses and deep hematomas including hemarthroses.

Defects of factors including factor VIII (classical hemophilia A, von Willebrand's disease) factor IX (hemophilia B or Christmas disease), factors XI, XIII, prothrombin, and fibrinogen can be the cause of purpura. It is important to realize that a significant deficiency of a factor (i.e., 20% of normal) may be present, may produce hemorrhagic symptoms and yet may not prolong the PT or PTT.

Vitamin K deficiency may result from liver disease, malabsorption syndromes and the newborn state. Vitamin K is important in the synthesis of factor VII, IX, X, and prothrombin, therefore, deficiency can result in hemorrhagic manifestations.

Overdosage of Heparin or coumadin will cause bleeding manifestations. It is important to remember an entity called coumadin necrosis which is an idiosyncratic response to coumadin which occurs characteristically approximately seven days after starting the drug and occurs as a vesiculobullous lesion located on the legs. The mechanism of the reaction is unknown and the lesion resolves despite continuation of the drug.

Metabolic causes of purpura such as diabetes and uremia have been discussed. Scurvy results in purpura, classically, perifollicular and gingival bleeding are seen. Ascorbic acid deficiency results in poor platelet aggregation, faulty cement substance; and impaired collagen synthesis. Hyperadreno-corticoidism results in loss of the connective tissue framework around vessels and subsequent purpura. Hereditary disorders of connective tissue frequently present with hemorrhagic manifestations secondary to defects in collagen, elastin or mucopolysaccharides. The seven types of Ehlers-Danlos syndrome are associated with vascular fragility, skin fragility and hyperextensible joints. Osteogenesis imperfecta, Marfan's syndrome and *Pseudoxanthoma elasticum* can also show bleeding and bruisability. These diseases may also show a qualitative platelet defect.

Harrison's *Principles of Internal Medicine* recommends the use of the prothrombin time, partial thromboplastin time, platelet count and bleeding time as screening measures for diagnosing the disorders of hemostasis discussed above. Along with a careful history and physical exam those four tests will provide a valuable presumptive diagnosis.

Mechanical factors are often important in categorizing purpura. The distribution of lesions provide a clue that mechanical factors are working. Such as the purpura seen on exposed and easily traumatized areas of hands and arms in an elderly person. These "Bateman's" purpura are caused by vessel and connective tissue fragility. The purpura associated with stasis dermatitis will be present around the ankles and tibial areas since these are secondary to increased venous pressure. Varicose veins and phlebitis aggregate this condition which can lead to ulceration. Violent muscular contractions as with coughing or vomiting can cause purpura of face and upper chest or purpura may be seen distal to a tourniquet.

Miscellaneous factors such as amyloid can result in purpura and ecchymoses. This is caused by amyloid around vessels leading to fragility. This occurs in primary systemic amyloidosis of unknown etiology or secondary to myeloma. The purpura often involves the periorbital area in plaques or may be seen after scratching or pinching the skin. Amyloidosis can also lead to an acquired factor X deficiency. Paraproteinemias such as cryoglobulinemia or hypergammaglobulinemia may cause purpura by coating platelets causing decreased adhesiveness, by sludging in peripheral vessels or by activating complement leading to a vasculitis. Toxic venoms produced by snakes cause a DIC-like reaction secondary to clot promoting toxins.

Inflammatory purpura as mentioned before are palpable secondary to edema, cellular infiltration and blood components being present in the lesion.

This category includes purpura of an infectious nature secondary to bacteria, viruses, or rickettsia. The appearance of infectious purpura can vary from the slate grey indurated, irregular bordered septic infarcts of acute meningococcemia to the rose spots produced by *Salmonella typhi*. In general, septic lesions begin few in number, are located distally and are distributed asymmetrically. Depending on the illness the patient may have only mild fever and malaise or may show high fever, vomiting, diarrhea, convulsions, meningitis, cyanosis and shock.

Gram positive sepsis possibly with associated endocarditis can be caused by pneumococcus, Staphylococcus, Streptococcus, and Listeria. Gram negative sepsis can be caused by pseudomonas, salmonella, Neisseria meningitis, and neisseria gonorrhae. Leptospirosis, or Weil's disease, causes jaundice, urticaria, and purpura. The meningococcus produces a severe acute infection and less commonly a chronic infection resembling chronic gonococcemia. Chronic gonococcemia characteristically affects women (2/3) and produces a hemorrhagic vesicopustule on the hands and feet and may be associated with a septic arthritis. Blood culture may be positive but no other objective findings of the gonococcus can be found.

Viral diseases can produce petechiae and fever as well. In atypical rubeola syndrome, an acutely-ill young adult with purpura that begins distally is seen. This occurs in partially immunized hosts. Varicella may be hemorrhagic. Echo virus Type IX and Coxsackie Group A type 9 can produce meningitis and petechiae. Mononucleosis produces palatal petechiae and rubella can lead to congenital purpura.

The rickettsia act by invading and damaging endothelium causing infarctive thrombosis and hemorrhage. Epidemic typhus, transmitted by the body louse, causes palatal petechiae and centrally-located erythematous macules. Hemorrhagic changes are a bad prognostic sign. Rocky Mountain spotted fever is transmitted by the tick (Dermacentor endersoni - wood tick, or D. variabilis - dog tick). The onset of disease is abrupt with headaches, shaking rigors, myalgias and fever. On the second to sixth day the rash begins distally and extends centripetally. The rash begins macular and progresses to purpuric.

Infectious agents cause purpura by a mechanism of septic emboli, toxins, damage to endothelium of blood vessels or disseminated intravascular coagulation.

DIC is a consuption coagulopathy secondary to clot promoting material initiating rapid coagulation. Coagulation factors are consumed faster than replaced resulting in bleeding.

DIC can be secondary to any of the above infectious agents either during acute infection or occurring days later, as well as entities such as amniotic fluid embolism, transfusion reaction, hemolytic uremic syndrome, carcinomatosis and leukemia. Purpura fulminans is an entity known to dermatologists. It classically occurs in children is preceded by a relatively benign infection (Strep and varicella most often) has a definite latent period and presents as DIC. The lesions involve skin with large purpura that may lead to bullae, necrosis and ischemic gangrene.

The next group of inflammatory purpuras have inflammation of vessel walls secondary to various mediators rather than acute infection as the cause. I will concentrate on disorders seen by the dermatologist in this part of the discussion.

Large arteries are affected in giant cell or temporal arteritis. Rarely ulcers may be seen overlying the arteritic area.

Medium and small arteries are affected in polyarteritis nodosa. The classic type affects kidneys, peripheral nerves, joints and heart. Tender subcutaneous nodules along the course of vessels may be seen and may result in ulcerated lesions. There seems to be a type of polyarteritis limited to the skin. These patients develop a distinctive blanchible livedo pattern most marked on the legs. Palpable purpura may also be seen.

Medium and small arteries may also be involved in Wegner's granulomatosus, lymphomatoid granulomatosus and allergic granulomatous angiitis of Churg and Strauss. Skin lesions include tender deep cutaneous nodules, infarcts and palpable purpura depending on the size of the vessel involved. A larger deeper vessel that becomes occluded by inflammatory thrombus may lead to an ulcer while a smaller more superficial vessel will cause a palpable purpuric papule.

A very common entity seen by dermatologists is a group characterized by a lymphocytic capillaritis. This group has the broad heading of benign pigmented purpuric eruptions. These are characterized by petechiae, orange to fawn colored macules, and hemosiderin deposits. Occasionally lichenoid papules (Gougerot and Blum) and eczema (Doucas and Kapetanakis) are seen. The most common are referred to as Schamberg's purpura and Majocchi's disease descriptively named purpura annularis telangiectodes. These are idiopathic and chronic persisting for months to years.

The final category of vasculitis is an inflammatory reaction localized to post capillary venules. This group is referred to as leukocytoclastic vasculitis, cutaneous necrotizing angiitis, or hypersensitivity angiitis.

Clinically the type of lesion ranges from urticarial papules to petechia papules, ecchymoses, vesicles and bullae. The skin is most often the only site of involvement which is symmetric and most marked on the lwoer extremities. In severe cases viscera especially the liver and kidneys may be involved. Systemic symptoms except for burning, pruritis, or arthritis are often absent.

Histologically, acumulation of polymorphonuclear leukocytes can be seen about and in vessel walls. Fragmented PMN's (leukocytoclasis), fibrin in vessel walls, and extravasation of red blood cells is also seen.

There is strong evidence for immune complex deposition in the pathogenesis of these conditions. They characteristically occur 7 to 10 days after antigen exposure if the antigen can be identified. Lesions tend to be in the same stage of development as well as occuring in crops indicating episodic exposure. Individual lesions last 1 to 4 weeks with residua being hyperpigmentation, atrophic scar or none. The disease may last weeks, to months, to years.

As mentioned previously there is strong evidence for immune complex deposition in these lesions and indeed immunoglobulins and complement can be detected in early lesions by immunofluorescent techniques. The next slide depicts the pathogenesis showing circulating soluble immune complexes depositing in vessel walls and activating complement with resultant chemotactic attraction of neutrophils. The immune complexes are felt to be soluable by virtue of formation in mild antigen excess. Either prior to this or immediately following, mast cell degranulation adds to the inflammation by releasing histamine, neutrophil and eosinophil chemotactic factor and platelet activating factor. Cell mediated immunity may be activated to participate in chronic lesions and play a role in granulomatous vasculitis.

Though the causative agent of leukocytoclastic vasculitis may not be identified a number of agents have been linked with the phenomenon. Commonly associated are drugs such as Penicillin and sulfa drugs. Infectious agents such as B hemolytic Streptococci, Staphylococcus aureus, hepatitis B virus, mycoplasma, and *mycobacterium leprae* have been associated. Collagen vascular disease as well can be associated with vasculitis, most often rheumatoid arthritis and Lupus erythematosus but occasionally dermatomyositis. Paraproteinemias by virtue of their ability to activate complement can cause vasculitis. In this group are included Waldenstrom's macroglobulinemia and hyperglobulinemia and cryoglobulinemia. Cryoproteins may be essential or associated with malignancy (leukemia, lymphoma), collagen disease, infectious disease (hepatitis, SBE, infectious mononucleosis, syphilis, CMV), cirrhosis, or coronary artery disease. Leukocytoclastic vasculitis can also be directly associated with underlying malignancy. Certain clinical syndromes are distinct enough to be given names such as Henoch-Schoenlein purpura seen as arthritis, gastrointestinal upset and bleeding, palpable purpura and glomerulonephritis; and hypocomplementemic vasculitis seen as urticaria showing vasculitis on biopsy, arthralgias and hypocomplementemia. Treatment of these disorders is treatment of the underlying disease if one is present. Steroids are helpful in managing these disorders.

APPENDIX

Contents

Frequently Used Drugs (partial list)

a
Actifed
Actiq
acyclovir
Adriamycin
Afrin Nasal Spray
aldesleukin
Aldoril
alemtuzumab
Ambien
amifostine
amoxicillin
ampicillin
anastrozole
Apresoline
Ara-C
Aredia
Arimidex
Aromasin
arsenic trioxide
asparaginase
Ativan
Augmentin
Azo Gantrisin
Azulfidine

b
Bactrim
belladonna
Benadryl
Betadine
bexarotene
Bexxar
Bumex
busulfan
Busulfex
Butisol Sodium Elixir

c
C-225
CaldeCORT hydrocortisone cream
Campath
Camptosar
capecitabine
Capoten
carboplatin
Cardizem
Ceclor
Ceftin
Celebrex
celecoxib
Celestone
cephalosporin
Chloromycetin
Choledyl
Cipro
Cleosin
clonidine
codeine
Coly-Mycin
Compazine
Cortef
Coumadin
CPT-11
cyclobenzaprine
cytarabine
Cytoxan

d
Danocrine
Darvocet-N
Darvon
Decadron
denileukin diftitox
DepoCyt
Depo-Provera
Desyrel
dexrazoxane
DiaBeta
Diabinese
Dialose
dicumarol
diethylstilbestrol
diethylstilbestrol diphosphate
Diflucan
digoxin
Dilantin
Dimetane
Dimetapp
dimethyl sulfoxide
docetaxel
Dolobid
dopamine
doxorubicin HCl
Dramamine
Dulcolax
Dyazide

e
Elavil
Ellence
Elspar
Emetrol
epirubicin HCl
Equagesic
erythromycin
Ethyol
etoposide
Evac-Q-Kit
exemestane

f
F-18
Femara
fentanyl citrate
filgrastim
Flagyl
fluconazole
Fludara
fludarabine phosphate
fludeoxyglucose
fluocinonide
Fluorodeoxyuridine
fluorouracil
Furadantin

g
Gantanol
Gantrisin
Garamycin
gemcitabine
gemtuzumab ozogamicin
Gemzar
Genasense
gentamicin
Gleevec
goserelin acetate
granisetron HCl
GVAX

h
Haldol
heparin
hepatitis B immune globulin
Herceptin
Herplex
histamine phosphate
Hycamtin
hydrocodone
hydrocortisone
HydroDIURIL

i
Idamycin
idarubicin

Ilosone
imatinib mesylate
Inderal
Indocin
insulin
iodine I 131 tositumomab
ipecac
irinotecan
Iressa
Isordil
isosorbide
Isuprel

k

K-Dur
K-Lyte
Keflex
Keflin
Kenalog
Kolantyl gel
Kondremul
Konsyl
Kytril

l

L-PAM
Lactinex granules
Lanoxin
Lasix
letrozole
leucovorin
Leukeran
leuprolide acetate
Librax
lidocaine
Lincocin
lithium carbonate
Lopressor
Lortab
Luminal

m

Maalox
magnesium sulfate
Mandol
medroxyprogesterone acetate
Mefoxin
Mellaril
melphalan
mercaptopurine
Metamucil
methadone hydrochloride
methotrexate (MTX)
methoxsalen
Minipress
Minocin
mithramycin
mitotane
Monistat
morphine
Motrin
MTX
Mutalane
Mycostatin
Mycostatin Oral Tablets
Mylicon
Mylotarg

n

Naldecon
nandrolone decanoate
Narcan
Navelbine
Nembutal
NeoDecadron
Neomycin-DEX
Neosporin
Neovastat
Neumega
Neupogen
Nipent
nitroglycerin
Norgesic
Norpace
Novahistine
Novocain
Nupercainal

o

ondansetron HCl
Ontak
Ophthocort
oprelvekin
Oruvail
Orinase
Ornade Spansule
Ortho-Novum
oxytocin

p

Pamelor
pamidronate disodium
Parafon Forte
Paraplatin
Parepectolin
Pathilon
penicillin
pentostatin
Pentothal
Persantine
Phenergan
phenobarbital
Photofrin
Polycillin
porfimer sodium
prednisone
Premarin
Pro-Banthine
procaine
procarbazine
Proleukin
Protamine
Provera
Purinethol
Pyridium

q

Quinidex
quinidine

r

Reglan
reserpine
PhoGAM
Rifamate
Riopan
Ritalin
Rituxan
rituximab
Robaxin
Robitussin
Rubex
Ru-Tuss

s

scopolamine
Seconal
semustine
Serpasil
Similac
Sinequan
Slow-K
sodium bicarbonate
Sodren
Solu-Medrol
sorbide
Sorbitrate

t

TACE
Tagamet
Talwin

tamoxifen
Tarceva
Targretin
Taxotere
Tegopen
Temodar
temozolomide
teniposide
Terramycin
Thick-It
thioguanine
Thioplex
thiotepa
Thorazine
Thyrolar
Tigan
Tofranil
Tolbutamide
topotecan HCl
trastuzumab
Trelstar Depot
triptorelin pamoate
Trisenox
Tuss-Ornade
Tylenol

u
Urised
Urispas
Uvadex

v
Valisone
Valium
valrubicin
Valstar
Viadur
Vibramycin
vincristine
vinorelbine
vinorelbine tartrate
Virulizin
Vitron-C
VP-16
Vumon

w
Wyanoids Relief Factor
Wydase

x
Xanax
Xeloda
Xylocaine

y
Yutopar

z
Zinecard
Zofran
Zoladex
Zovirax

Medical Instruments (partial list)

a
Abadie clamp
ACMI gastroscope
Adair-Allis tissue forceps
Adson forceps
Adson-Brown forceps
Allport-Babcock mastoid retractor
argon laser

b
Babcock forceps
Backhaus dilator
Backhaus towel clamps
Bacon rongeur
Bailey-Gibbon rib contractor
Bainbridge goiter clamp
Bakes common duct dilator
Balfour retractor
Ballenger-Lillie mastoid bur
Ballenger tonsil forceps
Bard-Parker blade
Barraquer iris forceps
Beck-Schenck tonsil snare
Beckman goiter retractor
Bellucci scissors
Benedict gastroscope
Bennett retractor
Berens lens expressor
Berens mastectomy retractor
Bernstein gastroscope
Bethune rib shears
Beyer rongeur forceps
Blanchard hemorrhoid forceps
Blohmka tonsil hemostat
Boettcher antrum trocar
Bonney dissecting forceps
Boucheron ear speculum
Bovie unit
Bozeman forceps
Braasch bulb ureteral catheter
Bronson-Turtz iris retractor
Brown-Buerger cystoscope
Burford rib spreader

c
Cameron flexible gastroscope
Caparosa burs
Carmel clamps
Castroviejo-Arruga forceps
Cavanaugh-Wells tonsil suturing forceps
Chevalier Jackson gastroscope
Church scissors
Cicherelli rongeur/forceps
Clark common duct dilator
Cloward instrument
Collin forceps

Cottle-Neivert retractor
C-P suction (Chaffin-Pratt)
Crile hemostatic forceps
Crutchfield tongs
Cushing retractor
Cushing vein retractor

d

Dandy forceps
Davidson electric bur
Davis-Crowe mouth gag
Deaver retractor
Debakey-Cooley retractor
deCourcy goiter clamp
DeMartel-Wolfson forceps
Depuy-Weiss tonsil needle
Deschamps' ligature needles
Desjardin gallstone forceps
Desmarres lid elevator
Deutschman cataract knife
DeVilbiss cranial rongeur
DeWecker eye scissors
Dormia basket
Doubilet sphincterotome
Doyen intestinal occlusion clamp
Doyen raspatory
Doyen retractor
Duckbill rongeur
Duffield scissors
Dunning periosteal elevator
Duval-Allis forceps

e

Eder gastroscope
Elliott forceps
Ellsner gastroscope
Elschnig cataract knife
Emerson suction

f

Farabeuf periosteal elevator
Faulkner antrum gouge
Fehland clamps
Fein antrum trocar
Fenger forceps
Ferguson needle
Ferris-Robb tonsil knife
Finochietto rib spreader
Foley catheter
Frankfeldt grasping forceps
Frazier retractor
Freer elevator
French catheter
Fritsch's retractor
Furniss-Clute clamp

g

Gavin-Miller forceps
Gelepi retractor
Gerzog mallet
Gifford curette
Gigli saw
Gill scissors
Gomco clamp
Gomco suction tube
Goodell dilator
Goodhill tonsil forceps
Graham scalene elevator
Grover meniscotome
Gruenwald rongeur
Guyton-Park lid speculum

h

Hajek elevator/mallet
Hall air drill
Hank dilator
Harrison-Shea curet
Hartmann forceps
Heaney forceps
Heerman chisel
Hegar dilator
Hemovac drain
Herrick clamp
Heyman-Paparella angular scissors
Hibbs retractor
Hibbs-Spratt curette
Hirschowitz gastroduodenal fiberscope
Holter valve
Hotz ear probe
House-Dieter Malleus nipper
House myringotomy knife
Housset-Debray gastroscope

j

Jaboulay button
Jackson laryngoscope
Janeway gastroscope
Jansen forceps
Jesberg scope
Jewett osteotomy plate
Johns Hopkins forceps
Joker dissector
Judd-DeMartel forceps

k

Kahler forceps
Keeler pantoscope
Kehr's T-tube
Kelly forceps

Kelly-Murphy forceps
Kelman forceps
Kerrison rongeur/forceps
Key periosteal elevator
Kifa skin clip
Kirschner wire
Klebanoff gallstone scoop
Knapp cataract knife
Kocher clamp
Krukenberg pigment spindle
Krwawicz cataract extractor

l

Lahey forceps
Lambotte osteotome
Lane forceps
Langenbeck retractor
LeFort catheter
Lempert knife
Luer bone rongeur
Luer-Korte scoop
Luer-Whiting rongeur forceps

m

MacDonald dissector
Mahoney speculum
Malecot catheter
Mathieu's retractor
Mayo scissors
McCaskey curette
McGuire scissors
McIndoe scissors
McIvor gag
Mentor wet field coagulator
Metzembaum scissors
Meyerding finger retractor
Michel clips
Moersch esophagoscope
Mollison mastoid retractor
Molt mouth gag
Morris retractor
Mosquito forceps
Moynihan artery forceps
Mueller mastoid curette

n

Nesbit resectoscope

o

O'Brien forceps
Ochsner forceps
Olivecrona rongeur/forceps
Ollier rake retractor
O'Sullivan-O'Connor retractor

p

Parker-Heath cautery
Parker ribbon retractor
Payr clamps
Pean forceps
Penrose drain
Pezzer catheter
Potts-Smith forceps

r

Rampley sponge holding forceps
Rapaport common duct dilators
Reich-Nechtow forceps
Reiner rongeur
Rigby self-retaining retractor
Rizzuti iris retractor
Roux retractor
Rubinstein cryoprobe
Ruskin mastoid rongeur

s

Sam Roberts head rest
Sarot needle holder
Satinsky clamp
Sauerbruch box rib rongeur
scalpel
Schiotz tenometer
Schnidt forceps
Schroeder forceps
Schuknecht knife
Sengstaken balloon
Senn retractor
Shallcross forceps
Shambaugh irrigator
Shea curette
Shoemaker thyroid scissors
Siker laryngoscope
Sims probe
Storz-Beck tonsil snare
Sump drain

t

Thorek scissors
Timberlake obturator

v

VanBuren urethral sounds
Varco forceps
Volkmann rake retractor

von Graefe cataract knife
von Petz clamp

w

Wagner antrum punch
Wangensteen clamp
Weiner-Pierce antrum trocar
Weitlaner retractor
Weitlaner self-retaining retractor
Wellaminski antrum perforator
Westcott scissors
Winsbury-White deep retractor
Woodson plastic instrument

y

Yankauer antrum punch
Yankauer suction tube

z

Zeiss operating microscope
Ziegler knife
Zipser clamp

Supportive Web Sites

The following Web sites and books will be helpful in your search for more instruments:

Stedman's Equipment Words, 3rd ed. Baltimore: Lippincott Williams & Wilkins, 2001.

www.sklarcorp.com/
"Search" for "resources"; click on Skylar Surgical Instruments—Surgical Resources or Skylar Surgical Instruments—Site Map and choose links of interest.

www.surgical911.com
Click on any links of interest; this site has an extensive list of instruments.

Laboratory Tests

a

A-1 Antitrypsin
A-1 Fetoprotein (fetoglobulin), quantitative (tumor marker)
A-E-DHA (androsterone, etiocholanoione, dehydroepiandrosterone)
acetaminophen
acetazolamide
acetone
acid phosphatase
aciduria
ACTH
AHT (antihyaluronidase titer augmented histamine test)
albumin, serum
aldolase
aldosterone, serum
alkaline phosphatase
aluminum, serum
amenorrhea profile
amikacin sulfate (Amikin®)
amino acid screen
aminophylline (theophylline)
amitriptyline (Elavil®)
ammonia
amniotic fluid creatinine
amylase, serum or urine
androstenedione
androsterone
angiotensin-converting enzyme
antibody identification panel
anti-DNA antibody
antihyaluronidase
antimitochondrial antibodies
antinuclear antibodies
antiparietal cell antibody assay
anti-smooth muscle antibody
antistreptolysin-O (ASO)
arsenic
ASO (antistreptolysin-O)
AST-aspartate aminotransferase

b

bacteria identification
bacterial meningitis antigens
barbiturates
beta lactamase activity, bacterial isolate
bile acid/cholylglycine
bilirubin, total
bilirubin, total and direct
bleeding time, modified Mielke
blood group-ABO
blood group and type
blood, Rh factor
blood smears, interpretation
bromides, serum
Brucella abortus agglutination
BUN/creatinine ratio

c

C-peptide
C-reactive protein
C-reactive protein, CRP
cadmium, urine
caffeine, serum
calcium-dialysate
calcium, serum, by atomic absorption
calcium, urine
calcium/phosphorus, serum
calcium/phosphorus, urine
calculus, infrared spectroscopy
Campylobacter, stool
cannabinoids, urine
carbamazepine (Tegretol®)
carbon monoxide, blood
carcinoembryonic antigen
carotene
catecholamines, fractionated, plasma
catecholamines, free, urinary
catecholamines, total, urine
CBC (hemoglobin, hematocrit, RBC, WBC, MCH, MCV, MCHC, platelet count)
CBC with differential
cell count
Celontin® (methsuximide)
ceruloplasmin
chloral hydrate/trichloroethanol
chloramphenicol
chlordiazepoxide
chloride, serum
chloride, urine
chlorides, iontophoresis
chlorinated pesticides
chlorpromazine
cholesterol, total
cholinesterase, dibucaine number
cholinesterase (pseudo), serum
clonazepam (Clonopin®)
clorazepate (Tranxene®)
cold agglutinins
complement, (beta 1a) c-3
complement, c-3 and c-4
complement, c-4
compound 5 (deoxycortisol)
Coombs' test direct
Coombs' test, indirect
copper, serum
copper, urine
copro-protoporphyrins, feces
cortisol, plasma
cortisol, urinary free
cosyntropin test (cortisol x3)
CO_2/carbon dioxide, content
CPK isoenzymes
CPK isoenzymes and LDH isoenzymes (D-9)
creatine phosphokinase (cpk)
creatine, serum
creatine, urine
creatinine clearance
creatinine, serum
creatinine, urine
cryofibrinogen
cryoglobulins
Cryptococcus antigen
crystals, fluid
culture, acid-fast bacilli
culture, blood
culture for Neisseria
culture, spinal fluid
culture, sputum
culture, stool
culture, throat
culture, urine
cyclic amp, plasma
cyclic amp, urine
cystine
cytochemistries for leukemia classification, with interpretation
cytologic exam for presence of sperm
cytology breast, fluid aspirate
cytology, bronchial washings or brushings
cytology, cerebrospinal fluid
cytology, cervical
cytology, esophageal brushings
cytology, fluid, not specified
cytology, gastric
cytology, sputum
cytology, urine
cytomegalovirus, CMV-G
cytomegalovirus, CMV-M

d

D-xylose, blood
D-xylose, urine
dehydroepiandrosterone
deoxycorticosterone
deoxycortisol (compound s)
Depakene® (valproic acid)
desipramine
DHEA
DHEA, sulfate
digitoxin
digoxin
Dilantin® (phenytoin)
diphenylhydantoin (phenytoin)
diphenylhydantoin, free
Disophyramide (Norpace®)
Doriden® (glutethimide)
doxepin
drug screen, blood, GLC
drug screen, gastric, GLC
drug screen, gastric, TLC
drug screen, miscellaneous, GLC
drug screen, miscellaneous, TLC
drug screen, serum, TLC
drug screen, urine, GLC
dyphylline

e

Elavil® (amitriptyline)
electrolytes, urine
electrophoresis, CSF (oligoclonal bands)
electrophoresis, serum
electrophoresis, urine
eosinophils, total
estradiol (E2)
estriol, serum
estriol, urine
estrogens, total urine
estrone (E1)
estrone and estradiol
etiocholanolene

f

factor V assay
factor VII assay
factor VIII assay
factor IX assay
factor X
factor XIII
fat globules, serum
fat globules, urine
fat stain, stool
febrile agglutination series
febrile agglutination, tube titer
ferritin
fibrinogen
fluoride, serum
folates (folic acid)
folates, red cell
follicle stimulating hormone
free T4 (thyroxine), includes total T4
fructose, semen
FSH/LH
FSH/LH/porolactin
fungal antibodies, R.I.D.
fungus identification

g

galactose
gamma glutamyl transpeptidase
gastrin
glucagon
glucose
glucose, fasting and 2-hour postprandial
glucose, fractionated, 24-hour urine
glucose, postprandial
glucose, 6-phosphate dehydrogenase
glucose, spinal fluid
glucose, 24-hour urine
glucose tolerance
glutamic oxalacetic transaminase-GOT
glutamic pyruvic transaminase-GPT
glutethimide (Doriden®), GLC
gold, serum
gold, urine
gram stain
growth hormone (HGH)

h

H-1 profile
H-2 profile
H-3 profile
H-4 profile
H-5 profile
H-6 profile
H-7 profile
H-8 profile
haloperidol
Ham's acid serum test
haptoglobin
HCG-beta subunit
HDL-cholesterol
HDL/LDL-cholesterol
heavy metal screen, urine
hemoglobin
hemoglobin A-2
hemoglobin A-2 and F
hemoglobin and hematocrit

hemoglobin electrophoresis
hemoglobin F
hemoglobin, glycosylated
hemoglobin, plasma or serum
hemophilus influenzae antigen
hemosiderin
hepatitis A antibody
hepatitis B core antibody
hepatitis B "E" antigen and B antibody
hepatitis B surface antibody
hepatitis B surface antigen
herpes simplex virus culture
herpes smear
heterophile antibodies, absorption
histochemistry enzyme battery, muscle biopsy
histochemistry stains, Class I, miscellaneous
histochemistry stains, Class II, miscellaneous
histoplasmosis, titer
HLA phenotype
HLA-B27
homocystine, urine
homogentisic acid, urine
homovanillic acid, urine
human placental lactogen, serum
5-hydroxyindoleacetic acid, urine
17-hydroxycorticosterone, urine
17-hydroxyprogesterone, serum
hydroxyproline, free and total, urine
hydroxyproline, total, urine

i

immunoelectrophoresis, serum, K&L chains
immunoelectrophoresis, urine, K&L chains
immunoglobulin A (IgA)
immunoglobulin E
immunoglobulin G (IgG)
immunoglobulin G in CSF
immunoglobulins (IgA, IgG, IgM)
immunoperoxidase, special stains
India ink preparation
indican, as potassium indoxyl sulfate
insulin by RIA
iron and iron binding capacity
iron binding capacity
iron in miscellaneous solutions
iron, serum
iron stain
iron, urinary, excretion
isohemagglutinin titer

k

17-ketogenic steroids
17-ketosteroids, full fractionation
17-ketosteroids, 17 hydroxycorticoids
17-ketosteroids, 17 ketogenic
17-ketosteroids, total neutral
Kleihauer-Betke, stain

l

lactic acid (lactate)
lactic dehydrogenase isoenzymes
lactose in urine
LDG isoenzymes CSF
LE latex
lead, blood
lead, urine
lecithin-sphingomyelin ratio, includes phosphatidylglycerol
leucine aminopeptidase
leukemia, cytochemistry classification, with interpretation
leukocyte alkaline phosphatase
lipase
lipids, total, feces
lipids, total, serum
lipoproteins
lithium in erythrocytes
lithium, serum
luteinizing hormone

m

magnesium (water soluble), feces
magnesium, serum
magnesium, urine
malaria, blood smears
manganese, serum
melanin, random urine
mercury, urine
metanephrines, fractionated
metanephrines, total
metanephrines, 12 hours
methemalbumin
methemoglobin
MHPG (methoxyhydroxyphenylglycol)
micro assay, water/dialysate
minimal inhibitory concentration (MIC)
mono test
mucopolysaccharide screen, urine
muscle fibers, stool
mycobacterium identification
myoglobin, serum
myoglobin, urine

n

NA+, K+, water soluble, stool
5-nucleotidase

o

oligoclonal bands, CSF (electrophoresis)
osmolality, serum or urine

osmolality, stool
ova, parasites, occult blood
oxalate as oxalic acid

p

paramethadione
parathyroid hormone C-terminal
parathyroid hormone mid-molecule
partial thromboplastin
PAS for fungus
pesticides screening, miscellaneous
PH, NA+, K+, osmolality, stool
PH, stool, meter
PH, urine, meter
phenol, total, urine
phenothiazines, serum
phenylalanine, quantitative
phosphorus, inorganic, serum
phosphorus, inorganic, urine
pinworm preparation
PKU-Guthrie
platelet count
PN-1 profile
PN-2 profile
PN-3 profile
PN-4 profile
PN-5 profile
PN-6 profile
pneumococcal bacterial antigen
porphobilinogen
porphyrins, fecal
potassium in water
potassium, serum
potassium (water soluble), stool
potassium, urine
pregnancy screen, serum
pregnancy test, urine
pregnanediol, urine
pregnanetriol, urine
progesterone
prolactin
prostatic acid phosphatase RIA
protein, CSF
protein, miscellaneous substances
protein, serum
protein, total urine
proteus agglutinins
prothrombin time
protoporphyrin, zinc
protoporphyrins, fecal
protriptyline

r

renin activity
reticulocytes
RH titre/antibody identification
rheumatoid factor
rotavirus antigen
RPR (serological test syphilis)
rubella antibodies

s

S. pneumoniae bacterial antigen
salicylates, serum
sedimentation rate modified, Westergren
sensitivity
serum inhibitory level
sex chromatin (Barr bodies)
sialic acid, serum
sickle-cell preparation
SGOT-serum glutamate oxalacetate transaminase
SGPT-serum glutamate pyruvate transaminase
smear, acid-fast bacilli
sodium and potassium, serum
sodium and potassium, urine
sodium, serum
sodium, urine
stains, cytochemistries
stains, histochemistry
stercobilinogen-urobilinogen, stool
streptococcus group B latex
Streptonase-B
streptozyme
strychnine, qual, identification
sugars, fractionated in urine
sulfa
sulfhemoglobin

t

T3 total circulating
T3 uptake
T3 uptake and T4 (D-18)
T4 (thyroxine) by RIA
T4, free
T4, neonatal
testosterone
testosterone/luteinizing hormone
thallium
thrombin time
thyroglobulin antibody
thyroid antibody group (D-20)
thyroid microsomal antibodies
thyroid stimulating hormone (TSH)
thyroxine binding globulin
thyroxine (T4) by RIA
thyroxine, free
tissue exam, gross
tissue exam, gross and micro
tissue, stains
total protein and A/G ratio, serum

total protein, fluid
toxicology study, miscellaneous
Toxoplasma antibodies, IgG specific
Toxoplasma antibodies, IgM specific
transferrin
treponemal antibodies-FTA/ABS
TRH stimulation (cortisol X3)
triglycerides
trimethadione
trypsin, stool
TSH, neonatal
tubular reabsorption phosphorus
tularemia agglutination
tyrosine

u

urea nitrogen, serum
urea nitrogen, urine
uric acid, serum
uric acid, urine
urinalysis
urine isolate
urobilinogen, fecal
urobilinogen, urine
uroporphyrinogen-1 synthetase
uroporphyrins, fecal
uroporphyrins, urine

v

valproic acid (Depakene®)
vanillylmandelic acid
vanillylmandelic acid, 12 hours
VDRL, CSF
VDRL, quantitative
VDRL, serum
vibrio, stool
viscosity
vitamin B-12
volatiles

w

water quality analysis, aluminum
water quality analysis, calcium
water quality analysis, iron
water quality analysis, sodium
white blood cells and differential

y

Yersinia, stool

z

zinc, serum or urine

Types of Sutures and Suture Materials (partial list)

Acier stainless steel
Acufex bioabsorbable Suretac
Acumed suture anchor
Ailee
Anspach suture anchor
ArthroSew suturing system
Atralease
atraumatic
bioabsorbable
BioSorb
Biosyn
Bondek absorbable
Bralon braided nylon
bridle
buried
buried-knot
chromic catgut
coaptation
colposuspension
Connell
continuous
Cushing
Cutalon
cutaneous
Dacron
Dafilon
Dagrofil
Deklene II
Deknatel
Dermalene
Dermalon
Dexon
Ethibond
Ethicon
Ethiflex
Ethilon
Ethistrip skin closures
everting
figure-of-eight
Flexon
Giampapa
Grams nonabsorbable
Halsted
hemostatic
Investa
Kelly plication
Lembert
limbal
Linatrix
Littre
lock-stitch vertical mattress
Lukens PGA
mattress
Maunsell
Maxon
Mersilene
Mersilk black silk
Micrins microsurgical
MicroMite anchor
Miralene
Mitek
Mitek Mini GII
Monocryl
monofilament
Monosyn
multifilament
Novafil
Nurolon
Palfyn

Panacryl
PDS
PeBA
Petit
PGA
plication
Polydek
polyethylene
Polysorb
Prolene
Pronova
pursestring
Ramdohr
Rapide
Reddick-Saye
retention
right-angle
Ritisch
running lock
Safil
Serralene
Serralnyl
Serralsilk
Silkam
silk-braided
Sofsilk
Softcat
stainless steel
Statak
Steelex
steel mesh
stick tie
subcuticular
superior rectus
Supramid
Suretac
Surgilon
Sutralon
SutraSilk
Suture Clinch
Suture Lok
Sutured-Clip
Sutureloop
Synthofil
Tevdek
through-and-through
tongue-in-groove
traction
Tycron or Ti-Cron
Ultrasorb
undyed
Vascufil
Vicryl
Vicryl Rapide
visceroparietal
Y-sutures
Zimmer Statak

Anesthetic Agents (partial list)

Anestacon
Brevital
Carbocaine
cocaine
Demerol
Ethrane
fentanyl
Fluothane
Forane
halothane
ketamine hydrochloride
lidocaine
Marcaine hydrochloride
morphine
Nembutal
Nescacaine
Nisentil
nitrous oxide
Novocain
Nupercaine hydrochloride
Pontocaine
procaine hydrochloride
sodium pentothal
sufentanil
tetracaine hydrochloride
thiopental sodium
topical cocaine
Valium
Xylocaine

Supportive Web Sites

The following Web sites provide an extensive list of anesthetic agents:

www.anesthesia-nursing.com/
On the Site Menu, click on "Web Links"; click on "The Worldwide Anaesthetist," then on "Anaesthesia," then on "Drugs, volatiles & anaesthesia" for other helpful links.

www.nlm.nih.gov/medlineplus/
Click on "Health Topics"; search for "anesthesia" and select links of interest.

Types of Dressings (partial list)

ABD pad
Adaptic
Aeroplast
Desault bandage, ligature
Esmarch bandage, tourniquet
Kerlix gauze
Kling bandage, dressing
Kos-House
Owen cloth
Robert-Jones compression bandage
Sayre bandage
scultetus binder
Semken dressing
spica cast
stent surgical dressing
Steri-Drape (3-M drape)
Steri-Strip skin closure
Steri-tape
Telfa
Unna paste boot
Vaseline wick dressing
Velpeau bandage
Xeroform gauze dressing

Supportive Web Sites

The following Web site will be helpful in locating other dressings:

www.mtdesk.com/
For an extensive list of dressings, search on "dressings"; click on "Medical Dictionary—Surgical Glossary—D."

Types of Incisions (partial list)

ab-externo
Auvray
buttonhole
Cherney
circumferential
collar
coronal
crosshatch
cruciate
cuvilinear
Deaver
Dührssen
elliptical
endaural
Fowler
gridiron
hockey-stick
infraumbilical
intracapsular
Kehr
Kocher
Küstner
Langenbeck
lateral flank
lateral rectus
Mackenrodt
McBurney
median
midline
muscle splitting
paramedian
Parker
Pfannenstiel
racquet or racket
rectus muscle splitting
Rockey-Davis
Schuchardt
suprapubic
transverse
Vischer lumboiliac
Z-flap
Z-shaped

Operative Positions (partial list)

decubitus
dorsal recumbent or dorsorecumbent
jackknife
knee-chest
Kraske
lateral
lithotomy
Proetz
prone
Sims
supine
Trendelenburg

Medical Prefixes and Meanings (partial list)

Prefixes are always located at the beginning of a word and are generally one or two syllables. A prefix can never stand alone; it is always used in conjunction with a medical combining form or with a combining form and suffix.

Prefix	Meaning
a-	without
ab-	from, away
ad-	to, toward
ambi-	both
ante-	forward, before
antero-	in front of
apo-	away, from
arter-, arteri-	artery
arthr-	joint
auto-	self
bi-, bis-	twice, double
bio-	pertaining to life
carcin-	cancer
cardi-	heart
cata-	down, lower
cervic-	neck
circum-	around, about
contra-	against, counter
crani-	skull
cyst-	bladder
de-	down from
derm-	skin
di-	double
dia-	through
dis-	apart from
dys-	bad, painful
e-, ec-, ex-	out of
ecto-	outside
endo-	within
entero-	intestine
epi-	upon
gastr-	stomach
gyn-	woman
hemi-	half
hemo-, hema-	blood
hyper-	increased, over, excessive
hypo-	decreased, below
hyster-	womb, uterus
infra-	below, beneath
inter-	between, among
intra-	within, into
intro-	into
iso-	equal
laryng-	windpipe
leuk-	white
lig-	tie
macro-, mega, megalo-	large, great
mast-	breast
meso-, media-	in middle of, center
meta-	from one place to another
micro-	small
myo-	muscle
neur-	pertaining to nerves
ortho-	normal, straight
oss-, oste-, osteo-	bone
ot-, oto-	ear
ov-	egg
patho-	disease
peri-	around
phleb-	vein
pneumo-	lung
postero-	in back, behind
psyche-	the mind
pulmo-	lung
retro-	backward
supra-, super-	upon, above
thorac-	chest
thromb-	lump, clot
tox-	poison
ultra-	excess

Medical Suffixes and Meanings (partial list)

A suffix is always located at the end of a word. It may be found in combination with a prefix and combining form(s) or with only a combining form. A suffix should never be used alone.

Suffix	Meaning
-able, -ible	denoting an ability or tendency toward
-ac	pertaining to
-aemia	condition of blood
-algia, -dynia	painful
-asis, -iasis	state resulting from
-cele	pouching, hernia
-centesis	puncture for aspiration

Suffix	Meaning
-cle	expresses diminution
-cyte	cell
-ectomy	excision; surgical removal of
-edema	swelling
-emia	blood
-genic	producing
-ia	denoting state or condition
-ic	pertaining to, resembling
-id	state or condition
-ist	one who practices a skill
-itis	inflammation
-logy, -ology	science of
-mania	madness or insane desire
-megaly	enlargement
-ness	state of being
-oma	a swelling, usually a tumor, either benign or malignant
-opia	sight
-oscopy	observation by means of an instrument
-osis	condition, state, process
-otomy, -ostomy	opening, incision
-pexy	fixation
-phagia, -phagy	eating, swallowing
-phasia	speaking
-phobia	fear, dread of
-plasty	plastic surgery
-plegia	paralysis
-ptosis	falling, downward displacement
-rhagia	hemorrhage
-rhea	discharge, flow
-rrhaphy	suture
-scope	instrument for inspection or examination
-scopy	examination
-sis	denoting condition; act of
-trophy	nutrition or growth

Medical Combining Forms and Meanings (partial list)

The combining form is the main stem of each medical term. Combining forms are always found in conjunction with a prefix, suffix, another combining form, or any combination of these.

Combining Form	Meaning
abdomino	abdomen
acro	extremity
adeno, aden	gland
adreno	adrenal gland
aero, aer	air, gas
angio, angi	vessel
arterio	artery
arthro, arthr	joint
atrio	atrium of the heart
brady	slow
broncho	bronchus, bronchi
carcino	carcinoma
cardio, card	heart
celio	abdomen
cephalo, cephal	head
cheilo, cheil	lip
chole, chol, cholo	bile
chondro, chondr	cartilage
chordo	cord
colpo, colp	vagina
costo	rib
cranio	cranium, skull
cyano, cyan	blue
cysto, cyst, cysti, cystido	sac, bladder
cyto, cyt	cell
dermato, dermat, derma, dermo	skin
duodeno	duodenum
encephalo	brain
entero, enter	intestines
episio	vulva
erythro	red
eu	normal
fibro	fibers
ganglio, gangli	ganglion
gastro, gastr	stomach
glosso, gloss	tongue
gluco	glucose
glyco	sugar
gyneco, gyn, gyne, gyno	woman
hem, hema, hemo, hemat, hemato	blood
hepato, hepat	liver
hydro, hydr	water
hystero	uterus, hysteria
ileo	ileum
ilio	ilium, flank
jejuno	jejunum

Combining Form	Meaning
kerato	cornea, horny tissue
laparo	flank, abdomen
laryngo	larynx
leuco, leuko	white
lipo	fat
litho, lith	stone, calculus
lyso	breaking down, dissolution
macro	large, long
malaco	softening
mammo, masto, mast	breast
melano	black
meningo	meninges
meno	menses
micro, micr	small
myelo, myel	bone marrow, spinal cord
myo, my	muscle
myringo	eardrum
naso	nose
necro	death
neo	new
nephro, nephr	kidney
neuro, neur	nerve
oculo	eye
oligo	few, deficient
oophoro, oophor	ovary
ophthalmo, ophthalm	eye
orchio, orchi, orchido	testis, testes
oro	mouth
ortho	straight, normal, correct
osteo, oste	bone
oto, ot	ear
patho	disease
pedo	child, foot
phago	eating, engulfing

Combining Form	Meaning
pharyngo	pharynx
phlebo, phleb	vein
phono, phon	sound
pleuro, pleur	pleura
pneo	breathing
pneumo	lung
poly	many, excessive
procto, proct	rectum
psycho	mind
pulmo, pulmono	lung
py, pyo	pus
pyelo, pyel	pelvis of the kidney
recto	rectum
rhino, rhin	nose
salpingo, salping	tube, uterine or eustachian
sclero, scler	hard, sclera
splanchno	viscera
spleno, splen	spleen
steno	narrowed
sterno	sternum
tachy	fast
thoraco	chest
thrombo	clot
thyro	thyroid
toxico, toxo	poison
tracheo	trachea
tropho	nourishment
uretero	ureter
urethro	urethra
uro, ur	urine
utero	uterus
vaso	vessel
veno	vein
ventriculo	ventricle of the heart or brain

Suggested Readings

GENERAL

Chabner DE. *The Language of Medicine.* 6th ed. Philadelphia: W. B. Saunders Company; 2001.

Davies J. *Essentials of Medical Terminology.* 2nd ed. Clifton Park, NY: Delmar Learning; 2002.

Dorland's Illustrated Medical Dictionary. 29th ed. Philadelphia: W. B. Saunders Company; 2000.

Drake E. *Sloane's Medical Word Book.* 4th ed. Philadelphia: W. B. Saunders Company; 2001.

Drake E, Drake RF. *Saunders Pharmaceutical Word Book.* Philadelphia: W. B. Saunders Company; 2002.

Medical Phrase Index. 4th ed. Los Angeles: Practice Management Information Corporation; 2002.

Physicians' Desk Reference (most current edition). Los Angeles: Practice Management Information Corporation.

Pyle V. *Current Medical Terminology.* 8th ed. Modesto, CA: Health Professional Institute, 2000.

Quick Look Drug Book 2002. Baltimore: Lippincott Williams & Wilkins; 2002.

Sloane, SB. *Medical Abbreviations and Eponyms.* 2nd ed. Philadelphia: W. B. Saunders Company; 1997.

Stedman's Concise Medical Dictionary for the Health Professions. 4th ed. Baltimore: Lippincott Williams & Wilkins; 2001.

Stedman's Equipment Words. 3rd ed. Baltimore: Lippincott Williams & Wilkins; 2001.

Stedman's Medical Speller. 3rd ed. Baltimore: Lippincott Williams & Wilkins; 2001.

Taber's Medical Dictionary. 19th ed. Los Angeles: Practice Management Information Corporation; 2002.

Tessier C. *The AAMT Book of Style for Medical Transcription*. Philadelphia: W. B. Saunders Company; 2003.

Tessier C. *The Surgical Word Book*. 3rd ed. Philadelphia: W. B. Saunders Company; 2003.

CARDIOLOGY

Cardiology Words and Phrases. 2nd ed. Modesto, CA: Health Professions Institute; 1995.

Stedman's Cardiovascular & Pulmonary Words. 3rd ed. Baltimore: Lippincott Williams & Wilkins; 2001.

DENTISTRY/ORAL SURGERY

Dorland's Dentistry Speller. Philadelphia: W. B. Saunders Company; 1993.

Stedman's Plastic Surgery/ENT/Dentistry Words. Baltimore: Lippincott Williams & Wilkins; 1998.

DIAGNOSTIC IMAGING/ INTERVENTIONAL RADIOLOGY

Carlton, R, Adler, A. *Principles of Radiographic Imaging*. 3rd ed. Clifton Park, NY: Delmar Learning; 2001.

Dorland's Radiology/Oncology Word Book for Medical Transcriptionists. Philadelphia: W. B. Saunders Company; 2001.

Radiology Imaging Words and Phrases. Modesto, CA: Health Professions Institute; 1997.

Stedman's Radiology Words. 3rd ed. Baltimore: Lippincott Williams & Wilkins; 2000.

GASTROENTEROLOGY

Dorland's Gastroenterology Speller. Modesto, CA: Health Professions Institute; 1993.

Stedman's GI & GU Words. 3rd ed. Baltimore: Lippincott Williams & Wilkins; 2002.

HEMATOLOGY/INFECTIOUS DISEASES

Calisher CH, Fauquet CM. *Stedman's ICTV Virus Words*. Baltimore: Lippincott Williams & Wilkins; 1992.

Human Diseases. Modesto, CA: Health Professions Institute; 1997.

Laboratory/Pathology Words and Phrases. Modesto, CA: Health Professions Institute; 1996.

Sloane SB, Dusseau JL. *A Word Book in Pathology & Lab Medicine*. 2nd ed. Philadelphia: W. B. Saunders Company; 1995.

Stedman's Organisms & Infectious Disease Words. Baltimore: Lippincott Williams & Wilkins; 2002.

NEUROLOGY/NEUROSURGERY

Orthopedic/Neurology Words and Phrases. 2nd ed. Modesto, CA: Health Professions Institute; 2000.

Stedman's Psychiatry/Neurology/Neurosurgery Words. 2nd ed. Baltimore: Lippincott Williams & Wilkins; 1999.

OBSTETRICS/GYNECOLOGY

OB-GYN and Genitourinary Words and Phrases. Modesto, CA: Health Professions Institute; 2002.

Stedman's OB-GYN & Genetics Words. 3rd ed. Baltimore: Lippincott Williams & Wilkins; 2000.

ONCOLOGY

Dorland's Radiology/Oncology Word Book for Medical Transcriptionists. Philadelphia: W. B. Saunders Company; 2001.

Stedman's Oncology Words. 3rd ed. Baltimore: Lippincott Williams & Wilkins; 2000.

OPHTHALMOLOGY

Adams J. *Saunder's Ophthalmology Word Book*. Philadelphia: W. B. Saunders Company; 1991.

Stedman's Ophthalmology Words. 2nd ed. Baltimore: Lippincott Williams & Wilkins; 1999.

ORTHOPEDICS

Orthopedic/Neurology Words and Phrases. 2nd ed. Modesto, CA: Health Professions Institute; 2000.

Stedman's Orthopaedic & Rehab Words. 3rd ed. Baltimore: Lippincott Williams & Wilkins; 1999.

OTORHINOLARYNGOLOGY

Stedman's Plastic Surgery/ENT/Dentistry Words. Baltimore: Lippincott Williams & Wilkins; 1998.

PATHOLOGY

Medical Phrase Index. 4th ed. Los Angeles: Practice Management Information Corporation; 2002.

Sloane SB, Dusseau J. *A Word Book in Pathology & Lab Medicine*. 2nd ed. Philadelphia: W. B. Saunders Company, 1995.

PEDIATRICS/NEONATOLOGY

Klaus MH, Fanaroff AA. *Care of the High-Risk Neonate*. 2nd ed. Philadelphia: W. B. Saunders Company; 2001.

Stedman's Pediatric Words. Baltimore: Lippincott Williams & Wilkins; 2001.

PLASTIC SURGERY

Stedman's Plastic Surgery/ENT/Dentistry Words. Baltimore: Lippincott Williams & Wilkins; 1998.

PSYCHIATRY

Psychiatric Words & Phrases. 2nd ed. Modesto, CA: Health Professions Institute; 1998.

Stedman's Psychiatry/Neurology/Neurosurgery Words. 2nd ed. Baltimore: Lippincott Williams & Wilkins; 1999.

SURGERY

General Surgery/GI. Modesto, CA: Health Professions Institute; 2001.

Stedman's Equipment Words. 3rd ed. Baltimore: Lippincott Williams & Wilkins; 2001.

Tessier C. *The Surgical Word Book*. 3rd ed. Philadelphia: W. B. Saunders Company; 2003.

INDEX

f

g